The

WHOLE FOOD
BIBLE

The
WHOLE FOOD
BIBLE

How to Select & Prepare
Safe, Healthful Foods

CHRIS KILHAM

Recipes compiled and edited by Catherine Conniff
Recipe development by Catherine Conniff, Rachel Reid, and Johna Albi

Healing Arts Press
Rochester, Vermont

Healing Arts Press
One Park Street
Rochester, Vermont 05767
Web Site: http://www.gotoit.com

*Note to the reader: This book is intended as an informational guide. The remedies, approaches,
and techniques described herein are meant to supplement, and not to be a substitute for,
professional medical care or treatment. They should not be used to treat a serious ailment without
prior consultation with a qualified health care professional.*

LIBRARY OF CONGRESS CATALOGING-IN-PUBLICATION DATA

Kilham, Christopher S.
The whole food bible : how to select and prepare safe, healthful foods / Christopher Kilham.
p. cm.
Rev. ed. of: The Bread & Circus whole food bible. Reading, Mass.: Addison-Wesley, c1991.
Includes bibliographical references and index.
ISBN 0-89281-626-0
1. Natural foods. 2. Cookery (Natural foods). 3. Food contamination.
I. Kilham, Christopher. Bread & Circus whole food bible. II. Title.
TX369.K53 1997
641.5'63–dc20   96–38263
CIP

Printed and bound in Canada

10 9 8 7 6 5 4 3 2 1

Text design by Peri Champine
Layout by Virginia L. Scott
This book was typeset in Minion with Mesozoic Gothic and
Galahad as the display typefaces

Healing Arts Press is a division of Inner Traditions International

Distributed to the book trade in Canada by Publishers Group West (PGW), Toronto, Ontario

Distributed to the health food trade in Canada by Alive Books, Toronto and Vancouver

Distributed to the book trade in the United Kingdom by Deep Books, London

Distributed to the book trade in Australia by Millennium Books, Newtown, N. S. W.

Distributed to the book trade in New Zealand by Tandem Press, Auckland

Distributed to the book trade in South Africa by Alternative Books, Randburg

To Wolf Dog Medicine Woman,
my native queen

CONTENTS

Part Two
RECIPES

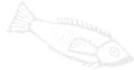

ACKNOWLEDGMENTS

This work has required an enormous commitment of time, energy, and concentration, and would not have been possible without the generous support of many individuals. Special thanks go to my mother, Elizabeth Kilham, for unflagging support and encouragement; to Martha Moutray, editor extraordinaire; to Anna Chapman, Mary Elder Jacobsen, and Rowan Jacobsen for their valuable contributions; to Cate Conniff for her culinary flair; and to Craig Weatherby, who is just plain gold. Thank you all.

Part 1

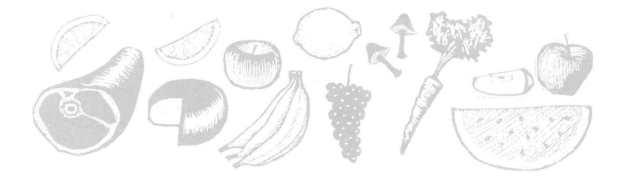

WHOLE FOOD BIBLE

1

WHAT'S HAPPENED TO FOOD?

*I*t used to be that all food was whole food, retaining its natural nutritional value without chemical additives of any kind. For millions of years, food was natural and nutritious; however, in the last century food has changed so radically that much of it is almost unrecognizable as food at all. Today our food is grown with the use of carcinogenic agricultural chemicals. Much of the nutritional value of food is processed out of it by high-tech methods. Chemical additives, including artificial colors, flavors, and preservatives, adulterate most of the foods on grocery store shelves. Many of these chemical agents are known or suspected carcinogens. As a result, unhealthy dietary intake is pandemic, causing dozens of serious health disorders, from cardiovascular disease to colon cancer. *What's happened to food?*

The answer to this question has to do with the growth and development of modern culture. As humans have evolved, we have developed a great capacity to invent. Through invention we have changed our relationship to food and the way in which it is obtained. Hunter-gatherers in the Paleolithic period ate roots, berries, and shrubs; they trapped fish and game for food. In this earliest and longest period of human development, there was no other way to survive. Humans spent much of their lives searching for edible plants and hunting game.

In the Mesolithic and Neolithic periods, humans made a gradual transition from food gathering to food production. Early cultures learned to cultivate land and livestock, causing them to produce more abundantly. They learned to plant seeds and to raise large groups of animals. Agriculture developed and flourished, and the course of human history was altered forever. For the first time, people could produce a steady supply of food. Agricultural inventions, including the hoe, scythe, and plow, opened the door to serious, large-scale food production, enabling farmers to grow a surplus of food to trade as a commodity. Food commerce sprang up in all developing cultures as people began to trade surpluses of food crops for other valuable items, including clothing, tools, household comforts, and eventually money. Ingenious methods of transportation, storage, and product manufacturing arose as larger quantities of food entered the marketplace.

Caravans of camels crossed great plains bearing loads of grains, beans, and spices. Vessels of all kinds, from crockery pots to wooden barrels, were produced to store food crops. Breads were baked, seeds were crushed for oil, and other food products were made. The primitive beginnings of food retail developed, enabling people to purchase food without turning the soil or raising animals.

The advancement of food production methods is the seed from which modern society has grown. Freedom from the labor of food production has afforded thousands of other lifestyle opportunities and has enabled people to pursue previously unexplored arts and sciences. Culture has flourished as our methods of food production have advanced. Advances in technology through continuous invention have changed society and changed our relationship to the environment. From shovels to tractors, from wood-burning hearths to gas-fired furnaces, we have created tools and processes that make our lives easier in a multitude of ways, but at the same time these devices distance us from an intimate relationship with the natural environment.

A Tainted Food Supply

Our many inventions and cultural developments have altered the face of the planet on which we live, and not always for the better. Refrigeration and improved methods of sanitation and hygiene have aided us greatly in keeping food fresh and wholesome. Meanwhile, advances in other areas of food technology have had devastating effects. In our pursuit of more, bigger, better, and faster food, we have ruined our environment and seriously jeopardized our food supply. Chemical-based, energy-intensive, high-tech food production methods have polluted our soil, water, and air; have lowered the quality of the food we eat; and have imperiled our health. The four primary factors that have contributed to the deterioration of our food and the environment in which it is produced are chemical agriculture, drugs in livestock, food processing, and chemical food additives.

Chemical agriculture became more widely practiced after World War II, when the post-war chemical industry decided that food production was an excellent field in which to earn peace-time dollars. Agricultural chemicals, including fertilizers and pesticides, were created to increase the fertility of the soil and reduce destruction of crops by insects, rodents, fungi, and other pests. Today, farmers in the United States spend more than $8 billion annually on fertilizers and apply some 2.6 billion pounds of pesticides to crops. The heavy use of toxic agrichemicals has destroyed the critically important microbial life in the soil. As a result, much of the topsoil in the United States now under cultivation is brittle and dusty and is blowing away at an alarming rate. Many agronomists say that we are headed for another dust bowl in several of the major agricultural states. The soil, water, and air in agricultural areas are heavily polluted with chemical residues that kill wildlife. Cancer rates among farm workers are inordinately high because of exposure to carcinogenic agricultural chemicals. Meanwhile, pesticide residues in food crops increase the probable risk of cancer and other serious degenerative disorders among the general public.

Ironically, our chemical-saturated farmland is no more productive than if it were cultivated organically, without the use of agrichemicals. In 1989 the National Academy of Sciences released a report on a five-year study that analyzed farming methods. The report, entitled *Alternative Agriculture,* stated that farmers who apply little or no chemicals to their crops achieve as high a production level as those who use synthetic fertilizers and pesticides. Pest damage is not controlled any better with pesticides than by natural, sustainable methods. The academy recommended that government farm programs turn their attention from chemical-dependent production toward promotion of natural farming techniques. Clearly, chemical agriculture is a failed system of production.

Drug-dependent animal production is a major part of the chemical farming industry. Most livestock today are raised according to factory farming methods in crowded living conditions. Animals are subjected to a heavy dietary intake of antibiotics and implants of anabolic steroids, or growth hormones, residues of which can remain in meats. The annual use of more than 18 million pounds of antibiotics in livestock feed breeds antibiotic-resistant strains of bacteria. These bacteria are a major cause of food poisoning in humans, resulting in serious illness or death. Food and Drug Administration microbiologists estimate that food-borne bacteria account for

Twenty-Eight Carcinogenic Agrichemicals

According to the National Academy of Sciences' report *Regulating Pesticides in Food,* 90 percent of the total pesticide-related risk of cancer comes from twenty-eight commonly used agrichemicals. For chemicals with single manufacturers, trade names are given.

Fungicides Zineb, Captafol, Captan, Maneb, Mancozeb, Folpet, Chlorothanlonil (Bravo), Metiram, Benomyl (Benylate), Ophenyphenol, Fosetylal (Aliette).

Insecticides Permethrin (Ambush, Pounce), Chlordimeform (Fundal, Galecron), Acephate (Orthene), Parathion, Cypermethrin (Ammo, Cymbush), Cyromazine (Larvadex), Azinphosmethyl (Guthion).

Herbicides Linuron (Lorox), Alachlor (Lasso), Metolachlor (Dual), Oxadiazon (Ronstar), Oryzalin (Surflan), Pronamide (Kerb), Ethylfluralin (Sonalan), Diclofop methyl (Hoelon), Terbutryn, Glyphosate (Roundup).

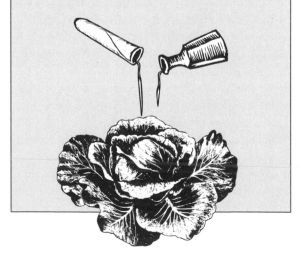

approximately 75 million cases of illness in the United States each year. Meat from animals raised with growth hormones is banned for import by the European Economic Community and many other nations. Factory farming of livestock delivers millions of pounds of animal-based foods to market every day and is an extremely energy-intensive industry. The production of animal foods consumes a disproportionately high amount of plant energy. Sixteen pounds of grain are required to produce one pound of beef. One pound of beef can feed three people for one meal. Sixteen pounds of grain can feed twenty people for three meals. The National Academy of Sciences found that drug-dependent animal farming methods are no more productive than natural ones.

Modern food processing methods are a far cry from the simple grinding of grains and pressing of oils that occurred when food commerce first started. Today these methods are the primary cause of the nutrient devaluation of foods in developed nations. From oil-refining methods that involve the use of toxic solvents and extremely hot temperatures, to high-volume grain-refining techniques, modern food processing strips away precious vitamins, minerals, fibers, and flavor from our food.

With the aid of advanced, high-tech laboratories, food manufacturers have also developed **chemical food additives** such as preservatives, artificial colors and flavors, emulsifiers, lubricants, bleaching agents, flavor enhancers, and synthetic sweeteners. By the time an American child is five years old, he or she will have consumed more than 7.5 pounds of food additives. None of these additives is necessary to keep food wholesome and nutritious, nor do they contribute to our health. Many of these additives are synthetic and thus exist outside of the natural food chain. They are foreign to the body and can produce undesirable effects. Since 1959 more than twenty-five chemical food additives have been banned because they cause cancer or other serious diseases in laboratory animals, and dozens of other additives are currently under review by the FDA.

Our farmland is choked with toxic agricultural

chemicals, and our foods are tainted with chemical residues and drugs. Our food supply is systematically stripped of many essential nutrients during processing and is pumped full of chemical food additives. Under these conditions, *how do we eat healthily in a poisoned world?*

Diet and Nutrition

The primary cornerstone of good health is a nutritious diet. The body is sustained by water, food, and air; it requires a steady dietary intake of nutritional substances for fuel, growth, and repair. Every function of the body, from muscle contraction to thought, requires healthy dietary intake. To understand what constitutes a healthy eating program, it is essential to know something about nutrition.

Carbohydrates

The primary fuels of the body, carbohydrates are a group of simple and complex hydrated carbon chains containing carbon, hydrogen, and oxygen and known as sugars and starches. Carbohydrates are found primarily in plant foods, including grains, beans, fruits, and vegetables, and ideally compose the greater part of the human diet. Carbohydrates are our primary dietary energy source and are absolutely essential to metabolism, the process by which the body breaks down and utilizes nutrients.

In our world today, carbohydrate consumption is directly related to economics. The lower the per capita income in a culture, the higher the percentage of carbohydrate intake overall. In less developed cultures, more than 70 percent of the diet is composed of carbohydrates. For these populations, the primary sources of carbohydrates are whole grains and beans. In the United States and other developed nations, less than 50 percent of the total dietary intake is carbohydrates, and most of that 50 percent comes from refined grains and sugars. The average American consumes in excess of 150 pounds of refined sugars per year and eats grains primarily in the form of highly refined, fiber-deficient white flour.

The more we learn about carbohydrates, the more we discover how important they are to health. Unrefined plant foods not only provide energy but also contain soluble and insoluble fibers. The soluble fibers, including pectins, gums, and mucilages, are known to reduce serum cholesterol and help regulate the use of sugars in the body. Insoluble fibers, including cellulose, lignin, and hemicelluloses, aid intestinal elimination and help to prevent diverticulosis, various gastrointestinal cancers, arthritis, and peptic ulcers. A more detailed discussion of the role fiber plays in the diet can be found in the "Grains" chapter.

Protein

Protein is the primary structural material of the body and is found in our bones, muscles, connective tissue, hair, and brains. Protein molecules are composed of chains of amino acids from food that enables our bodies to create the various protein-based tissues.

Our bodies can synthesize the amino acids they need, converting them from other amino acids available in the diet. But there are nine essential amino acids that are critical to life. These amino acids, which cannot be produced by the body and must be obtained from the diet, are phenylalanine, valine, tryptophan, threonine, isoleucine, leucine, histidine, methionine, and lysine. They are obtained from grains, beans, vegetables, meats, fish, dairy products, and eggs. The object of eating protein foods is to obtain all the essential amino acids in a balance, forming what is known as a complete protein. It is the ratio of the essential amino acids to one another that determines the extent to which a dietary protein is usable by the body.

The most widely consumed sources of dietary protein worldwide are from the plant kingdom. Grains and beans (and to a lesser extent, vegetables) in combination supply a proper ratio of all nine essential amino acids, forming a complete protein. Animal source foods and flesh foods are already complete proteins and are important dietary protein sources. They also provide vitamin B_{12}, which cannot be obtained from any known vegetarian dietary source.

In technologically developed cultures, the ratio of animal-based to plant-based proteins is the reverse of the ratio in undeveloped cultures. We derive approximately 70 percent of our protein from animal foods. This reversal has a far-reaching impact on human health. While animal-based foods are excellent sources of complete protein, they also contain saturated fats as well as residues of drugs and agrichemicals. By weight, meats contain as much as thirteen times the amount of pesticide residues found in plant foods, and dairy products contain six times as much. At the same time, animal foods contain no fiber, which is critical to proper digestion and the prevention of disease. In the ideal diet, animal foods make up no more than one third or less of total dietary protein.

Fats

Fats are lipids, which, along with carbohydrates and protein, constitute the principal components of all living cells. Fats can be manufactured by the body or obtained from plant and animal sources. Dietary fats are composed of fatty acids, which are important for metabolic functions including digestion, maintenance of cellular integrity, energy, hormone production, and lubrication of tissues and membranes.

Fats contain a combination of saturated, monosaturated, and polyunsaturated fatty acids. The extent to which a fat is saturated, or bound to hydrogen, determines the extent to which it will increase cholesterol production in the body. Dietary fats are best obtained from unrefined grains, nuts, seeds, and fish. These sources contain lower amounts of saturated fats than meats or dairy products.

By weight fats contain twice the calories of protein or carbohydrates. While fats should ideally constitute only 15 to 20 percent of our caloric intake, they currently account for a full 40 percent or more of the total calories in the standard American diet (SAD). Today foods are filled with saturated fats from both plant and animal sources. Lard is used for frying in commercial food production, while shorten-

ing and hydrogenated oils appear in thousands of popular packaged foods. This tremendously high intake of saturated and processed fats has led to epidemic obesity, cancer, and coronary disease. A more thorough consideration of the role fats play in the healthy diet can be found in the "Oils" chapter.

Vitamins

Essential to human survival, vitamins must be obtained from the diet because they are produced by the body in insufficient quantities or not at all. Vitamins act as precursors or coenzymes to millions of metabolic functions, but they do not provide caloric energy or building blocks. Vitamins can be water-soluble or oil-soluble and are obtained from all natural foods. The fat-soluble vitamins are A, D, E, and K, while the water-soluble vitamins are C and the B complex. An inadequate dietary intake of vitamins can lead to poor eyesight, impaired bone growth, muscle spasms, reproductive failure, liver degeneration, beriberi, muscular weakness, skin eruptions, pellagra, dizziness, nausea, pernicious anemia, scurvy, and hundreds of other metabolic problems.

Ideally, all vitamins should be obtained from a healthy diet, but because so much of our food is grown in nutrient-deficient soil, its actual vitamin value is greatly reduced. Transportation and storage time also reduce the vitamins in food, as does processing. Many foods wind up on the dinner table with only a fraction of their original vitamin value. One answer to this has been fortification, by which pharmaceutically engineered vitamins are added to cereals, breads, and other packaged foods to bolster low vitamin levels. This, however, is a palliative measure. What is needed instead is nutrient-rich soil in agricultural areas, along with food processing methods that do not remove vitamins. Food processors cannot accurately add vitamins to foods in the proportions best utilized by our bodies, because such proportions are not fully understood. In addition, they cannot fortify foods with all the other nutritive factors that are removed from foods by processing.

Minerals

Minerals are of neither plant nor animal origin but are compounds resulting from the inorganic processes of nature. They occur in the environment in soil, sand, and stone, and are absorbed up the food chain into plants and animals. The principal minerals in the human body are calcium, potassium, phosphorus, magnesium, and sodium. Many other minerals, however, including sulfur, manganese, chloride, copper, iodine, zinc, fluorine, chromium, selenium, and molybdenum, are also essential to our health. They cannot be manufactured by the body and must therefore be obtained from dietary sources. Other trace minerals, including boron and germanium, are currently being studied by nutritional biochemists and are believed to play important roles in health.

Minerals are active in digestion, reproduction, brain activity, and all aspects of metabolism. They help to build and repair tissue, and act as catalysts in millions of biochemical functions in the body. A deficiency of dietary minerals can lead to stunted bone growth; weakness; loss of appetite; heart irregularities; cramping and spasms in muscles; kidney disease; swelling and edema; anemia; fatigue; weakness; loss of hair, nails, and teeth; sexual dysfunction; abnormal sugar metabolism; and death.

Most foods today contain appreciably fewer minerals than they would had they been grown by sustainable organic methods. Processing further devalues the mineral value of foods. Thus, it is no longer easy to obtain all the minerals we need from the foods we eat. Some minerals, like selenium and chromium, are extremely difficult to obtain from today's processed food supply. Partial mineral fortification is employed by food processors, along with vitamin fortification. But as with vitamins, fortification does not restore the original mineral value of foods.

Other Nutritive Factors

A diet composed of whole foods from all major groups (grains, beans, nuts, seeds, fruits, vegetables, meats, fish, eggs, and dairy products) will provide other nutritional factors besides vitamins and minerals. There are additional substances in food that contribute to health and well-being, though they are not essential nutrients. These include octacosanol, a stamina factor from wheat (see "Grains" chapter), chlorophyll from plants, bioflavonoids from citrus, and thousands of compounds from herbs. The plant kingdom in particular is a source of potent nutritive and medicinal factors that not only meet our nutritional needs but provide us with an extensive pharmaceutical repertoire.

The current food pyramid developed by the U. S. Department of Agriculture places a welcome emphasis on grains, fruits, and vegetables and encourages limited consumption of meats and fish; dairy products; and fats, oils, and sweets.

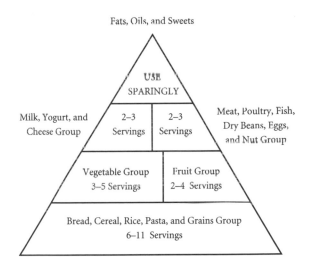

From the production of crops in nutrient-deficient soil to food processing methods, the more we tinker with the food system the more we reduce, eliminate, or somehow alter these other nutritive factors in food. Our modern food system does not preserve these valuable substances.

Our Nutritional Report Card

In July 1988 the Surgeon General's *Report on Diet and Health* delivered a scathing nutritional report card to the United States. The report blamed the poor diet of the nation for increased incidence of coronary heart disease, high blood pressure, cancer, diabetes, obesity, skeletal diseases, dental diseases, kidney diseases, gastrointestinal diseases, infections and lowered immunity, anemia, and neurological disorders. According to the Surgeon General's report, Americans can reduce the likelihood of developing any of the above diseases by dietary modification alone. The key recommendations in the Surgeon General's report are these:

- **Eat a variety of foods.** A healthy, nutritious diet consists of fruits, vegetables, whole grains, beans, nuts, seeds, lean meats, poultry, fish, and low-fat dairy products.
- **Maintain desirable weight.** To control weight, reduce intake of high-calorie foods, including fats, sugars, and alcoholic beverages. At the same time, increase your energy expenditure with regular physical exercise.
- **Avoid too much fat, saturated fat, and cholesterol.** Reduce consumption of fat, saturated fat, and cholesterol. Eat a diet high in fruits, vegetables, whole grains, fish, poultry, lean meats, and low-fat dairy products. Use little or no fat in food preparation.
- **Eat foods with adequate starch and fiber.** Increase your consumption of whole grains, beans, fruits, and vegetables.
- **Avoid too much sugar.** Restrict consumption of foods high in sugars, especially candies, soft drinks, and desserts.
- **Avoid too much sodium.** Reduce your sodium intake by eating low-sodium foods and using little or no sodium in food preparation.
- **If you drink alcoholic beverages, do so in moderation.** Consume no more than two alcoholic drinks daily.

According to the Surgeon General's report, diet was the primary cause of 2.1 million deaths in the United States in 1987. While our diet-related health problems are serious, the corrective recommendations made in the Surgeon General's report are nothing more than commonsense whole-food dietary guidelines. The message is clear: we are overdue for a diet change.

Emerging Food Awareness

According to a study of nutrition conducted by the Food Marketing Institute and *Better Homes and Gardens,* Americans are increasingly interested in the freshness and nutritional value of foods, including increased fiber, low cholesterol, reduced fat, reduced sodium, reduced sugar, and increased calcium. This new food awareness is a hopeful sign for a culture that is eating itself to death.

A Food Marketing Institute report entitled *Consumer Attitudes & the Supermarket* describes the responses of consumers surveyed in regard to the food they buy. Nearly 95 percent of those surveyed say that nutrition is an important factor in making food purchasing choices. Food safety is also a concern to 74 percent. A survey conducted for *Prevention* magazine by Louis Harris & Associates also encountered an increased food awareness among the general public. Americans are beginning to restrict alcohol consumption: an estimated 50 percent consume fewer than three drinks daily, while another 39 percent abstain from alcohol altogether. While a whopping 64 percent of adult Americans are overweight according to height-and-build weight tables, 48 percent of adults are trying to be more aware of the amount of fat and cholesterol they consume. Almost half of those surveyed say they are trying to reduce their intake of sodium and sugar.

While this emerging awareness is a healthy sign, people are confused about what to do. Fifty percent of Americans surveyed are so confused about the food information they hear that they don't know which foods to eat and which to avoid. The same percentage admits that they would like to live by a healthier regimen of diet and exercise but can't get themselves together to actually do so.

Whole Foods: Eating Healthily in a Poisoned World

A whole-foods diet is the answer to today's dietary health crisis and an important key to a cleaner environment. Whole foods are minimally refined, thus retaining their maximum nutritional value. They contain no chemical additives such as preservatives and artificial colors or flavors. Whenever possible, whole foods are grown by sustainable methods that regenerate and nourish the soil while imparting no toxic chemical residues to crops. The primary whole-food groups include grains, beans, nuts, seeds, fruits, vegetables, meats, poultry, fish, dairy products, and herbs. From these groups, all prepared and packaged whole foods are made.

In the following chapters, the world of whole foods is explored in detail. Every category of whole foods is considered, along with issues of food production, processing, contamination, handling, safety, nutrition, and labeling. Recipes and guidelines for selecting and preparing whole foods are also included, making a flavorful, wholesome,

Harris Poll on Organically Grown Food

A Harris poll of 1,250 adults throughout the United States shows that a large majority of Americans would choose organically grown food over chemically grown food if the price were the same. The survey, conducted for *Organic Gardening* magazine, found that 84 percent of those surveyed would choose organically grown food if they had that option, 12 percent would not, and 4 percent were unsure. Forty-nine percent said they would pay more for organically grown food.

nutritious diet immediately accessible to the reader. By becoming familiar with whole foods, along with the broader issues of food production, you will have all the basic information you need to eat heathily in a poisoned world.

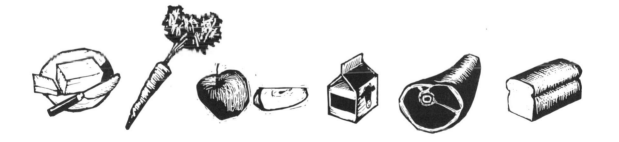

2

SUSTAINABLE AGRICULTURE

$\mathcal{S}$oil is the surface layer of the earth that contains organic matter. It is capable of supporting vegetation and is cultivated and planted by farmers for food production purposes. Topsoil may be less than a single inch deep or as deep as several yards. The specific composition of soil varies from one location to another, but it consists of disintegrated rock material, the organic remains of decomposed vegetation and animal material, air, and water. Inorganic rocks and minerals of various kinds are found in soil as sand, clay, gravel, and stone. In addition, soil contains aerobic bacteria (bacteria that need air to live), earthworms, and insects.

The fertility of soil depends upon its organic matter content, moisture, air, temperature, pH, and other soil composition factors. Methods of fertilization and cultivation also affect soil fertility. Fertile soil is a complex living material capable of supporting and promoting life. Since the advent of chemical and industrial methods of agriculture, however, the soil in our major growing areas has been treated like dirt.

Non-ecological Methods of Food Production

Current methods of agriculture include monoculture (the growing of just one crop on the same piece of land over and over again), chemical fertilization, and the heavy application of insecticides, fungicides, herbicides, and rodenticides. The result of these practices is nutrient depletion of the soil. This has disastrous effects, both on the health of the soil itself and on the nutritional value of foods grown in that soil. Since the 1940s, the nutritional value of crops grown in major farming areas of the United States has deteriorated at an alarming rate. Many fruits, vegetables, grains, and beans no longer contain sufficient amounts of their important nutrients because of soil depletion. Additionally, abused soil dies. The aerobic bacteria, earthworms, insects, and other essential life within soil are destroyed by the application of poisonous agrichemicals. Soil that was previously soft, fertile, and alive becomes hard, brittle, and dead. This soil must be pumped full of chemical fertilizers in an increasingly aggressive, chemical-based effort to keep land productive.

Health and Environmental Hazards of Current Farming Methods

Farmers are the first victims of chemical agriculture. The toxic agrichemicals used in modern farming expose farm workers to respiratory and neurological disorders, bizarre skin diseases, and allergies. The cancer and leukemia rates in major agricultural areas are as much as five times the national average because of the intensive use of carcinogenic pesticide sprays. Cases of acute toxicity due to exposure to pesticides are common among farm workers. Children in agricultural areas suffer the most. They are particularly sensitive to pesticides in the air and in drinking water. The leukemia rate among children in some agricultural areas is extraordinarily high. Yet, the spraying of toxic chemicals goes on. Of course, the food chain is affected as well. Pesticides find their way to the dinner table of every American family. The National Academy of Sciences estimates that approximately 1.4 million cancer deaths are due to the consumption of pesticide residues in foods.

Meanwhile, our farmland is literally disappearing because of abusive nonsustainable farming methods. Dead, overworked, nutrient-deficient soil leads to the erosion of land, an ecological disaster of immense proportions. Topsoil in all the major farming areas of the United States is blowing away and washing away, and a dust bowl phenomenon similar to that of the 1930s is developing. If erosion and land development continue at present rates, only 4 percent of the earth's surface will be fertile farmland by the year 2000. Every day in America twelve square miles of farmland are developed. Approximately 35 percent of the world's farmland is currently undergoing serious erosion. Desertification is a problem on all six continents because of poor land management. Where forests and grasslands have been destroyed for agricultural purposes, floods and droughts have resulted. Considering that the world's current population of 4.6 billion people will double in thirty years, it is reasonable to predict that we are heading toward a time of inadequate food production, irreversible environmental pollution, and widespread starvation. We have precious little time to stop treating our soil like dirt.

Farmers Wake Up

Wendell Berry, in *The Unsettling of America,* says ". . . the care of the earth is our most ancient and most worthy and, after all, our most pleasing responsibility. To cherish what remains of it, and to foster its renewal, is our only legitimate hope." An increased number of food growers have begun to recognize that current methods of food production are nonsustainable and therefore irresponsible. It is because of this recognition that some farmers have begun to produce food by sustainable organic methods.

I know several farmers who were literally forced into organic food production. One western Massachusetts vegetable grower discovered, after fifteen years of chemical farming, that his land was dead. He searched for earthworms in the soil but could find none. The soil on his farm looked nothing like it had when he had started farming. It was hard, like packed graphite. It felt like linoleum when he walked on it. He realized that if there was any hope of reviving the land he farmed, he would have to institute organic farming practices. Today, the farm that was once dead is fertile and productive, and the former chemical-dependent farmer is now a successful organic food producer.

Another grower I know in South Dakota was riding on a tractor spraying insecticides on one of his fields. He was behind his father, who was also spraying on a tractor. Suddenly his father's tractor stopped, and his father tumbled to the ground, gasping for breath, in convulsions from exposure to the chemicals they were spraying. The use of agrichemicals of all kinds ended on that farm that day. Today the family successfully farms organically. Their crops are healthy, their yields are high, and their soil is alive.

These stories are not unusual. They are typical of what is taking place in agriculture today. Some farmers are forced out of chemical farming because the cost of chemicals is simply too high. Though supplementary nitrogen, for example, costs only about twenty-five cents per pound, a farmer may be advised to apply as much as two hundred pounds of nitrogen per acre. The per-acre cost of potassium, phosphorus, and pesticides can be astronomical. A farmer can spend hundreds of dollars per acre on chemicals alone. This reduces profitability for food producers and is one of the main reasons that family farming is disappearing in the United States. Toxic chemicals, besides being dangerous to human health and the environment, are expensive.

There is nothing scientific about the use of chemicals on farmland. In fact, no two soil-testing companies can agree on what to apply to the same piece of land. Rodale Press of Emmaus, Pennsylvania, conducted a test in which they sent soil samples from the same piece of land to sixty-nine major soil-testing laboratories for recommendations of fertilization. No two tests were the same, and recommendations for the amount of nitrogen to be applied ranged from absolutely none at all to as high as 230 pounds per acre. There is no such thing as a reliable soil test for nitrogen. Nonetheless, farmers annually are duped into spending millions of dollars on supplementary nitrogen for their farms, based on recommendations made by soil-testing laboratories.

Organic Farming

Before chemical agriculture, there was organic farming. Today, in the face of aggressive promotional campaigns by Monsanto, Cargill, Dow, Union Carbide, Mobil, Du Pont, and other purveyors of toxic agrichemicals, organic farming is on the increase. More than twenty states have adopted specific standards for organic agriculture, and several organizations are working together to standardize organic production nationwide.

Organic farming involves maintaining the health and fertility of soil by natural methods, and growing crops without the use of chemical fertilizers, insecticides, fungicides, herbicides, or rodenticides. The following organic production standards are those of Farm Verified Organic. FVO is a Connecticut-based farm certification program for organic growers worldwide. Their standards are typical of those being adopted by independent certification programs.

1. **The soils upon which production is grown** shall have been treated in accordance with the following standards for a continuous period of at least thirty-six months from the time of production harvest. Adherence to the standards must be attested to by the affidavit of the producer.
2. **Soil enrichment.** Products acceptable for use on land shall be only (a) organic matter products that have not been chemically fortified, (b) natural rock products that have not been mined or processed with the addition of synthetic chemicals, (c) beneficial bacteria and algae cultures that are not chemically fortified, and (d) earthworms.
3. **Rotation.** The fields from which a product is harvested shall be part of a rotation program that precludes repetition of the same crop during the previous year. This does not apply to such perennial crops as alfalfa, orchard trees, maple trees, or crops that require more than one year to mature.
4. **Insect control.** Products acceptable for use on land shall be only (a) predatory insects, (b) insect disease cultures, (c) attractants, and only in case of emergency (d) rotenone, pyrethrum, ryania, or sabadilia.
5. **Weed control.** Weed control on land shall be done only by crop rotation, hand or mechanical cultivation techniques, or cutting of weed patches.
6. **Rodent control.** Rodent control on land shall be done by the introduction of the rodent's natural enemy, natural repellent techniques, or traps.

7. **Fungal or bacterial diseases** can be controlled only by the use of any products acceptable under item 2 (soil enrichment products).

8. **Drying of a product** shall be done by natural field drying bin aeration or by artificial drying at temperatures not to exceed 160°F.

9. **In storage,** if fumigation is needed, only diatomaceous earth shall be used.

10. **All production must meet standards** set by the U.S. Food and Drug Administration and must comply with state organic standards if applicable.

A National Organic Standard

In 1991, Congress passed the Organic Foods Production Act as part of the national farm bill. Critics said the bill would never fly. But it did, in a meteoric fashion. The Organic Foods Production Act of 1991 recognizes organically produced foods as a separate and distinct category of foods, deserving of a special seal of identity. The bill sets specific uniform standards for organic food production, and assigns implementation of the organic law to the USDA. That's the good news. The bad news is that the USDA, which should be renamed the United States Department of Foot-dragging and Obfuscation, has thus far failed to provide adequate funding for the implementation of the bill.

When USDA officials finally get off their butts and do the right thing, the bill will require organic verification that includes questionnaires, affidavits, on-site inspeciton by third parties, laboratory analyses, and audits. Organic foods will be readily identified by a single, easily recognizable seal, and both organic producers and the general public will benefit.

The Organic Future

Organic food production is on the increase because it makes ecological sense. Farmers want to keep the

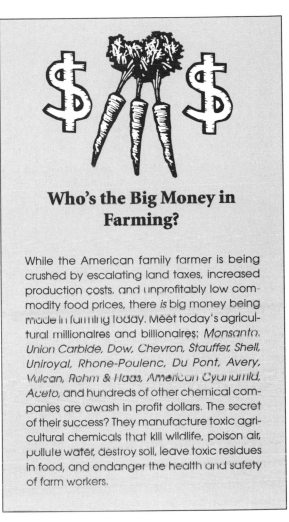

Who's the Big Money in Farming?

While the American family farmer is being crushed by escalating land taxes, increased production costs, and unprofitably low commodity food prices, there *is* big money being made in farming today. Meet today's agricultural millionaires and billionaires: Monsanto, Union Carbide, Dow, Chevron, Stauffer, Shell, Uniroyal, Rhone-Poulenc, Du Pont, Avery, Vulcan, Rohm & Haas, American Cyanamid, Aceto, and hundreds of other chemical companies are awash in profit dollars. The secret of their success? They manufacture toxic agricultural chemicals that kill wildlife, poison air, pollute water, destroy soil, leave toxic residues in food, and endanger the health and safety of farm workers.

soil alive and productive, and there is a growing demand for foods grown without toxic chemicals. Consumers, increasingly aware of the alarming problem of pesticide residues in foods, are seeking organically produced foods at an unprecedented rate. Yet, current organic production represents only a tiny fraction of agriculture in the United States. How quickly this fraction will increase is unknown. What is known is that farmers, farmland, and consumers are all at risk from the hazards of chemical agriculture. Organic production is a viable and sustainable solution to this crisis. Organically produced foods are the key to our future survival, and we need them now.

3

ECO REPORT: PESTICIDES

esticides are poisons composed of a broad category of chemical agents that include insecticides, fungicides, herbicides, and rodenticides. Their function is to kill pests of all kinds that interfere with the growth cycle of agricultural crops. They are used to increase crop yields and improve the appearance of fruits, vegetables, herbs, nuts, seeds, grains, and beans by controlling insects, fungi, weeds, rodents, and other pests. Only a fraction of the pesticides used actually reach the target pests they are supposed to control. The rest simply pollute the environment; contaminate our soil, air, water, and food; kill wildlife; and endanger human health.

The use of agrichemicals is on the rise and is escalating rapidly as the effectiveness of pesticides continues to decline. Pesticides are used today far more liberally than in 1945. Yet, pests of all kinds are destroying more crops and, since World War II, crop losses from insects have increased. Some previously insignificant pests have become major crop destroyers now that their predators have been killed by chemicals. The tobacco budworm is an example. The number of insecticide-resistant insects and mites has increased over 4,000 percent. Pesticide-resistant species of weeds, fungi, rodents, and other pests have also increased greatly.

The production of this volume of pesticides deposits millions of tons of toxic waste into the air as well as into surface water and ground water. Exposure to pesticides is a particularly serious threat to agricultural workers. Pesticide exposure can cause cancer, birth defects, nervous disorders, and other serious diseases.

Pesticides are frequently used illegally. Seed treated with pesticides has repeatedly been fed to livestock, even though doing so violates federal law. In 1986, meat and milk in Arkansas were contaminated after animals ate feed treated with heptachlor, a deadly pesticide. Since 1983 the use of heptachlor has been legally restricted to the eradication of termites. Nonetheless, a 1986 investigation showed that the treatment and sale of heptachlor-contaminated livestock feed was widespread.

The Delaney Amendment

The Delaney Amendment, which is found in Section 409 of the Food, Drug and Cosmetic Act, states

Acceptable Risk?

Tolerances for the use of pesticides on food crops are based on estimates of the amount of pesticide that may actually be ingested by consumers and the resulting toxic effects. "Acceptable risk," as defined by the Environmental Protection Agency, is one case of cancer out of one million people exposed to any chemical. According to the National Academy of Sciences (NAS), the actual risk of developing cancer due to exposure to toxic pesticide residues is much higher than EPA stan-

dards ostensibly permit or than federal health and safety officials admit.

The following table illustrates the NAS estimates of actual cancer risk from consuming eight different toxic pesticide residues. The estimates assume that exposure occurs over a seventy-year life span, that residues are at tolerance levels, and that 100 percent of acres with appropriate crops are treated.

Pesticide	Risk per Million	Pounds Used Annually	Major Crop Uses
Acephate	37	1,900,000	Citrus
Benomyl	113	2,000,000	Citrus, stone fruits, rice
Captafol	594	6,000,000	Apples, cherries, tomatoes
Captan	474	10,000,000	Apples, almonds, peaches, seeds
Chrorothalonil	237	6,000,000	Fruits, vegetables, peanuts
Mancozeb	338	16,000,000	Fruits, vegetables, grains
Maneb	442	10,000,000	Fruits, vegetables, grains
Pronamide	8	100,000	Lettuce

"No additive shall be deemed safe if it is found to induce cancer when ingested by man or animal." If an additive is deemed unsafe, it cannot legally be used. However, the Delaney Amendment has been seriously abused and largely ignored. According to a 1984 National Academy of Sciences report entitled *Toxicity Testing: Strategies to Determine Needs and Priorities,* 71 to 80 percent of all pesticides sold in the United States have not been sufficiently tested to determine whether or not they are cancer-causing agents. Furthermore, pesticides and other agrichemicals that are known carcinogens remain in use because they were approved prior to the passing of the Delaney Amendment. This use of carcinogenic chemicals in food production poses a serious threat to the public. An Environmental Protection Agency report entitled *Unfinished Busi-*

ness: A Comparative Assessment of Environmental Problems ranked pesticide residues in food as the number three cancer risk in the environment today, after radon in the home and toxins in the workplace.

Pesticide-Residue Testing

According to the General Accounting Office (GAO), the investigative arm of Congress, the Food and Drug Administration samples only 0.8 percent of imported fruits and vegetables for pesticide residues. The FDA reported that, among the 14,923 samples analyzed in 1992 and 1993, 4.0 percent of these samples were found to be pesticide-contaminated, but a separate analysis of the data done by an independent group found a 7.4 percent rate of pesticide contamination.

Similarly, the FDA reported an illegal contamination rate of 1.5 percent for domestic produce, but the numbers indicate that 3.1 percent contained illegal pesticides.

In thirty-eight cases during those two years, residues of chemicals banned in this country appeared on imported foods. This is because many chemicals banned for use in the United States are still produced here, and are sold for export to foreign nations. Those countries use the chemicals, then ship foods grown with them back to the United States for sale. Since the FDA sampled only 0.8 percent of imported shipments during this time, we can estimate that approximately 4,750 shipments of food containing banned pesticides entered the U.S. food supply.

Inadequate Testing Methods

Standard Food and Drug Administration residue tests are not capable of detecting many pesticides currently in use. Furthermore, 310 pesticides currently monitored by the FDA have not even been classified with regard to the threat that they may

Putting Produce to the Test

Recent issues about the hazards of pesticide residues in food have raised public concern about food safety and the effectiveness of government testing programs. To ensure an extra margin of safety, many food retailers are employing independent testing companies to analyze fruits and vegetables for traces of pesticides. Supporters of independent testing programs claim that these efforts substantially improve the safety of produce, while detractors say that these programs conduct tests that are inferior to those performed by federal officials.

The most highly visible testing company is NutriClean of Oakland, California, founded by chemist Stan Rhodes. NutriClean's seventeen full-time employees conduct inspections for approximately four hundred growers, primarily in California. The inspectors monitor pesticide use throughout the full production cycle of various fruit and vegetable crops and work with growers to greatly reduce or eliminate applications of pesticides. In addition, the company provides weekly pesticide residue testing of produce for approximately one thousand grocery stores nationwide. NutriClean has taken the position of being an independent auditor, much like a Good Housekeeping Seal of Approval for safe food.

Detractors view the company's efforts as opportunistic and inferior to government programs. They cite NutriClean's "multi-residue screen" test, which looks for only 108 pesticides out of the more than three hundred currently in use. The Food and Drug Administration, when it does test, uses a multi-residue screen plus analyses for other specific pesticides. Supporters of the NutriClean program argue that some testing is far better than no testing at all, and that the multi-residue screen tests detect those pesticides that are most commonly applied. NutriClean also tests for specific chemicals not covered by the multi-residue screen. Their tests are conducted in the state-of-the-art facilities owned and leased by the National Food Processors Association.

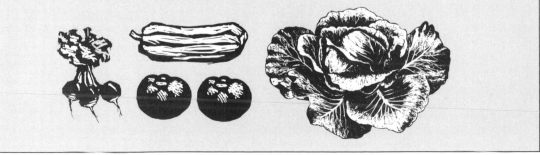

pose to human health. Most of these 310 chemicals (according to the General Accounting Office) cannot be detected by standard FDA residue tests.

Sale of Contaminated Foods

Though the Food and Drug Administration tests very little produce for chemical residues, even tested items with illegal quantities of toxins, as well as residues of banned chemicals, still wind up on the consumer's dinner table. A General Accounting Office publication on FDA food testing procedures reported that "in a current review of pesticide residues in foods, we found that the FDA was not able to prevent any violative foods from reaching the consumer because of untimely laboratory processing. By the time the FDA identified the products as violative, they were often no longer available, because most agricultural products are perishable and therefore move rapidly from farms to consumers."

Between October 1983 and July 1985 the FDA had jurisdiction over 179 cases involving the interstate marketing of food found to contain illegal pesticide residues. In 107 cases, the FDA took no action whatsoever to prevent the food from being sold to the public. The average time for lab analysis of these products, according to the GAO, was twenty-seven days.

Bad Imports

General Accounting Office investigators report that the sale of contaminated imported food is even worse. Technically, Food and Drug Administration policy demands that imported foods should be kept from the marketplace until they have been tested and deemed safe. In actuality, these foods are sold immediately to prevent spoilage. Even when a shipment of food is suspected to contain dangerous chemical contaminants, the FDA orders to hold the shipments are summarily ignored, according to GAO officials. An increasing amount of fruit consumed in the United States is produced by foreign countries, and the incidence of crops contaminated with illegal chemical residues is on the rise. None-

theless, the FDA has been unable to prevent contaminated foreign fruit from reaching consumer dinner tables.

Bogus Safety Tests

The General Accounting Office reports that the safety of many pesticides has been established on the basis of false information. Food and Drug Administration tolerance standards (safe levels) are arrived at by toxicity tests conducted in analytical laboratories. The FDA discovered, however, that ninety pesticides still in use today were approved with information submitted by Bio-Test Laboratories in Illinois, which was found to have provided fraudulent test data for several years. Bio-Test was convicted in 1983 of falsifying or inventing the bulk of its data.

Illegal residues and poor testing methods are not the only problems. There are four other problems with *legal* residues:

1. Legal pesticide tolerances most likely put consumers at risk of developing cancer. According to the National Academy of Sciences, current tolerance levels of pesticides in foods can be assumed to cause cancer and other diseases. This is because many agrichemicals known to cause cancer are used widely and are consumed in unpredictable quantities by the general population.

2. Current tolerance levels are based largely on consumption. If a person eats more than the FDA-assumed amount for a food, he or she may consume more than the presumed "safe" limit for certain chemicals. The FDA's "average diet" assumes 7.5 ounces of cantaloupe, 1 avocado, $1^1/_2$ cups cooked summer squash, $2^1/_2$ tangerines, 1 mango, and similarly tiny amounts of other fruits and vegetables per person per year. These estimates are obviously ridiculously low.

3. Some pesticides and other agricultural chemicals that may or may not be carcinogenic by themselves may become harmful

Food Consumption Estimates

The Environmental Protection Agency determines "negligible risk" of pesticide residues in foods based on food consumption data. Pesticides that are known or suspected carcinogens are registered for use on specific food crops according to estimates of how much of these foods we eat in a year. The EPA estimates are widely criticized, for good reason.

The EPA assumes that the average American eats less than $\frac{1}{2}$ pound of the following foods per year: almonds, avocados, blackberries, boysenberries, eggplant, figs, honeydew melons, leeks, mushrooms, summer squash, Swiss chard, tangelos, tangerines, walnuts, winter squash. How much of these items do you actually eat?

According to the Natural Resources Defense Council, children are appreciably more sensitive to pesticide residues than adults. Children's immune systems are more delicate, their organs are still in the process of developing, and their nervous systems are more sensitive. Children consume significantly more fruit and fruit juices than adults.

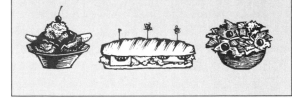

when combined with other chemicals. Cooking and digestion can also turn relatively harmless substances into carcinogens. Alar, a growth regulator once used on apples, forms the more potent carcinogen UDMH (unsymmetrical dimethylhydrazine) when cooked. UDMH was suspected to be particularly harmful to children, who consume large quantities of cooked apple products.

4. Certain populations may be at higher risk than FDA tolerances address. Children, the elderly, and pregnant women are often more highly sensitive to chemical toxicity and are thus at greater risk of developing disease conditions due to chemical consumption.

PESTICIDES:
THREE CASE STORIES

Alar: An Apple a Day

In 1986 the manure hit the fan for Uniroyal, manufacturer of daminozide, a plant-growth regulator marketed under the name Alar. Alar, which has been in widespread use since 1963, inhibits the growth of molds and fungus. Alar allows apples and other fruits to ripen more uniformly, keeping the fruit colorful and firm and making harvest easier. It is also a suspected carcinogen—a charge that Uniroyal vigorously denies.

The flap surrounding Alar drew unprecedented public reaction and was widely publicized. As a result of strong consumer concern over the suspected carcinogen, many food processors publicly declared that they would no longer accept Alar-treated apples for use in their products. Heinz, Beech Nut, and Gerber rejected Alar-grown apples, as did the makers of Mott's apple products, Red Cheek apple juice, and Veryfine apple juice. The Washington State Apple Commission urged growers to voluntarily suspend use of the chemical, and many supermarkets throughout the United States announced that they would no longer permit the sale of Alar-treated apples or apple products in their stores. The Environmental Protection Agency attempted to ban the use of Alar nationwide but was thwarted by a substantial Uniroyal lobbying effort.

In May 1986 Uniroyal sold its farm chemical division to Avery International, a New York–based holding company. Uniroyal officials deny that the controversy over Alar played any role in their decision to unload the beleaguered division. The sale of the farm chemical division came after an aggressive but unsuccessful campaign to bolster rapidly declining Alar revenues. Uniroyal mounted a major public relations effort to restore food industry and consumer confidence in the growth regulator, but the effort could not combat the widespread distrust of Alar. Next, Uniroyal urgently directed its efforts toward rapidly expanding foreign sales of the product in an attempt to unload surpluses on the international market. Other countries, however, had already begun to consider bans on both Alar use and the import of foods grown with the chemical.

Contrary to Uniroyal's claims, the undoing of Alar was not based on frivolous hysteria. In 1978 a report published by the Eppley Institute of the University of Nebraska's Medical School indicated a direct link between the ingestion of Alar and cancerous tumors in laboratory animals. Dr. Bela Toth, who published the paper in the medical journal *Cancer Research,* also discovered that Alar in the body breaks down into UDMH, or unsymmetrical dimethylhydrazine, a recognized carcinogen. Alar also breaks down into UDMH upon cooking.

Subsequent studies conducted by both the National Cancer Institute and the United States Air Force confirmed Dr. Toth's report, establishing a link between Alar and cancer. Not until 1984, however, under pressure from environmental activists, did the EPA began its special review of Alar. In 1985, the EPA announced its intent to cancel Uniroyal's license to sell Alar for use on food crops. This would have effectively banned the chemical. Uniroyal, facing an estimated annual revenue loss of $20 million, fought back vehemently. When the dust cleared, additional studies of Alar were ordered, and the EPA cut the permissible amount of Alar in apples by a third. In 1989 the Apple Grower's Association volunteered to stop the use of Alar industry-wide, and this carcinogen was finally phased out of the food system.

The Alar case is typical of what happens when a profitable chemical is discovered to be hazardous. Chemical industry pressure has kept literally hundreds of toxic compounds in widespread use throughout the United States and the world. Legal wrangling, governmental foot-dragging, and clever but deceptive media campaigns can keep a danger-

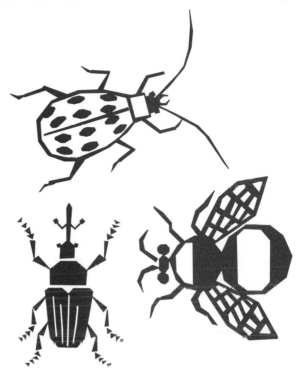

ous chemical in use long after it has been shown to pose a significant threat to human health and the environment.

Malathion vs. the Mediterranean Fruit Fly, Mosquitos, and You

Malathion, an organophosphate pesticide, is widely used in California against the Mediterranean fruit fly, which endangers fruit crops. It is also commonly sprayed by municipal mosquito-control projects throughout neighborhoods all over the United States. Touted by chemical industry experts as one of the least toxic pesticides in use today, malathion is at the center of a storm of controversy over its short- and long-term health effects.

The EPA reported in February 1988 that 15 to 20 million pounds of malathion were used in the United states between 1985 and 1986. The EPA's Pesticide Incident Monitoring System reported 962 malathion-related incidents from 1960 to 1980. From 1981 to 1985 malathion was the third most common cause of pesticide-related illness in California.

Furthermore, the EPA has noted that available toxicology data indicate that food residue tolerances for malathion should be reassessed, and probably need to be lowered. In the 315-page EPA publication entitled *Guidance for the Reregistration of Pesticide Products Containing Malathion as the Active Ingredient,* the EPA states that "pesticide incident data show that spray drift is a principal source of poisoning risk from this chemical." Spray drift occurs with aerial crop spraying, as well as when local mosquito control projects fog neighborhoods with malathion to kill mosquitos. The EPA says that "Malathion is a cholinesterase inhibitor, reducing plasma and red blood cell cholinesterase." Cholinesterase is an important human enzyme that is crucial to healthy brain function. Inhibition of this enzyme can lead to brain disorders.

Nor does the EPA mince words regarding the threat that malathion poses to wildlife. "There is sufficient information to indicate that current registered uses of malathion may adversely affect endangered species." The EPA goes on to clarify the point: "The Agency is concerned about the potential hazards to nontarget organisms (fish and wildlife, domestic animals and humans) caused by the drift from aerial and ground applications of malathion." While national environmental groups such as Pesticide Watch are working to reduce or eliminate the use of malathion on agricultural crops, there is no coordinated effort to eliminate the direct spraying of neighborhoods by this toxic chemical. If mosquito-control trucks are spraying your neighborhood, they are most likely spraying your home and yard with malathion. If this is the case, get active. Start by phoning the mosquito-control project in your local area and request that it stop spraying your street. Contact your town council members and apprise them of the hazards of malathion. In addition, contact your local newspapers and provide them with information on the hazards of malathion spraying. While chemical warfare is banned according to the Geneva Convention, malathion spray trucks may be rumbling through your neighborhood, endangering the health of your family.

How Many Chemicals?

As chemical-based agriculture becomes increasingly sophisticated, the number of toxic agrichemicals in use increases. As a result, the number of chemicals used on individual crops has soared. Moreover, many pesticides that are banned or restricted because of the risks they pose to health are still found on foods, because the Food and Drug Administration lacks effective procedures and authority to enforce the regulations. Among these restricted or banned pesticides are captan, which is classified as a probable human carcinogen; chlorpyrifos (Durshan), which is a potent neurotoxin; and endosulfan, which is related to DDT and has an action in the human body very much like that of estrogen.

Pesticides are often found in great amounts on produce imported from other countries: Guatemala, Mexico, Korea, Argentina, Colombia, and others. Because many such pesticides are not registered for use in this country, we have little or no knowledge of their effects on health or the environment. The FDA and the U.S. Customs Service monitor imported produce on a spot-check basis, but like the FDA with domestic produce, their efforts are not comprehensive or reliably effective.

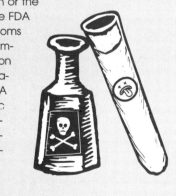

Monsanto Dumps Parathion

Monsanto, manufacturer of ethyl parathion, an acutely toxic organophosphate insecticide, announced in November 1985 that it would phase out production of the chemical. Parathion is one of the twelve pesticides targeted by the Pesticide Action

Network (PAN) in their international "Dirty Dozen" campaign. The campaign drew attention to twelve acutely toxic pesticides currently used extensively worldwide. Parathion is believed to be responsible for as many as half of all the pesticide-related deaths in Central America.

Despite Monsanto's statements to the contrary, it appears that the company did in fact drop the beleaguered parathion because of mounting pressure from the PAN campaign. This demonstrates that persistent aggressive public action can be valuable in curbing or eliminating the use of harmful chemicals in the environment. Despite the power and wealth of large chemical manufacturers, it is possible for environmental organizations to combat the production of toxic products and succeed in getting them removed from the marketplace.

The Pesticide Dilemma

Despite the fact that pesticides are toxic and are known to contribute significantly to the number of cases of cancer in the United States today, they cannot be summarily dropped overnight. United States agriculture is currently primarily chemical based. The soil in major agricultural areas is as dependent on the continued use of pesticides as a heroin addict is on a regular daily supply of that potent opium-derived drug. To go "cold turkey" from the use of pesticides in the United States would create a monumental agricultural disaster that would result in serious food shortages and possible widespread starvation.

Sustainable agricultural practices, including biodynamic and organic farming methods, can be adopted on a widespread scale. These methods, however, require an entirely different approach to farming than current chemical-based methods. Natural methods of soil regeneration, integrated pest management, crop rotation, and other sustainable practices must be cultivated for several years to successfully resurrect deficient, depleted, overworked farmland. During this transition, farmers often experience lower crop yields and increasingly

difficult pest problems. To initiate these practices, either one must innately understand the ultimate value of sustainable agriculture, or one must be delivered to these methods via a chemical disaster. Many organic farmers in production today were virtually forced into organic farming because of serious health problems or the deterioration of the soil due to chemical use. As a nationwide movement, organic agricultural practices will become widespread only when we as a society face repeated,

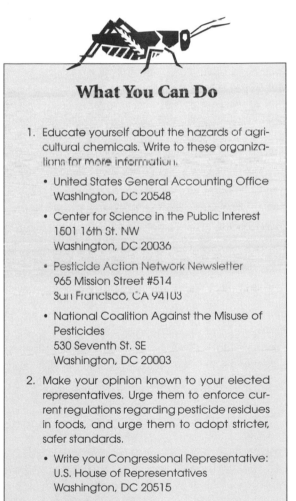

What You Can Do

1. Educate yourself about the hazards of agricultural chemicals. Write to these organizations for more information.

   - United States General Accounting Office
     Washington, DC 20548

   - Center for Science in the Public Interest
     1501 16th St. NW
     Washington, DC 20036

   - Pesticide Action Network Newsletter
     965 Mission Street #514
     San Francisco, CA 94103

   - National Coalition Against the Misuse of Pesticides
     530 Seventh St. SE
     Washington, DC 20003

2. Make your opinion known to your elected representatives. Urge them to enforce current regulations regarding pesticide residues in foods, and urge them to adopt stricter, safer standards.

   - Write your Congressional Representative:
     U.S. House of Representatives
     Washington, DC 20515

   - Write your Senators:
     U.S. Senate
     Washington, DC 20510

highly publicized, chemically generated disasters that severely affect the public health. Otherwise, many farmers will continue to be unaware of the grave hazards of pesticides and other agricultural chemicals and will not be inclined to adopt the more labor-intensive methods of organic farming. In addition, the multibillion-dollar agrichemical industry is not likely to lie down, roll over, and play dead, voluntarily making way for organic farming.

We can be assured that chemical-based agricultural practices will remain firmly in place into the foreseeable future. Pesticides will continue to be widely and heavily used, and they will continue to cause cancer and other diseases. Food retailers who wish to sell only or primarily organically produced foods will be thwarted in their efforts by inconsistent supplies of these products, despite the ever-expanding organic farming industry and the increased consumer demand for these goods.

Pesticides are one group of hazardous chemicals that compromise public health and safety. The extent of the danger they pose may never by fully understood. You can help in the fight against pesticides by making sure your voice is heard.

4

GRAINS

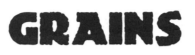

The most widely consumed staple foods in the world are whole cereal grains such as wheat, oats, rice, buckwheat, and corn. Grains are the seeds and fruits of cereal grasses; they grow in a wide variety of climates and conditions, from hot, wet, tropical paddies to cold, barren, rocky mountains. The cultivation of grains goes back as far as ten thousand years. They are central to the lore of virtually all ancient civilizations and are still highly revered by the people of nonindustrialized cultures.

From a nutritional standpoint, grains are the most valuable of all foods. They contain protein, fats, carbohydrates, fiber, vitamins, and minerals. These nutrients are found in the various layers of whole grains. Although the actual number of layers found in the kernels of grains varies from one grain to another, there are four types of layers common to whole grains:

The **hull** of a grain is its protective outer coating. In general, this outer shell is hard, tough, and inedible. This does not mean, however, that grain hulls have no value. In India grain hulls are used as fuel for cooking fires. They are often included in

animal feed or in bedding. In addition, some grain hulls are a source of furfural, which is used commercially in the manufacture of lacquers and dyes. The Japanese stuff pillows with the inedible hulls of buckwheat groats.

The **bran** layers of a grain contain fiber and B vitamins. Much attention has been paid to fiber in the last several years. The dietary fiber in grains adds bulk to the digestive system, speeding up the transit time of food from consumption to elimination, and increasing the ease and size of bowel movements. Fiber is a key to the relief of constipation, a condition caused by the consumption of a diet composed of processed, refined foods. Eating fiber reduces the risk of intestinal diseases, including colon and rectal cancers, and hemorrhoids. Because fiber adds bulk to the digestive system, it enhances the feeling of fullness during eating, thus curbing the tendency to overeat. The fiber in the bran layers of grains also helps to stabilize blood sugar by regulating the absorption of nutrients and sugars in the digestive tract. Lastly, the water-soluble dietary fiber found in the bran layers of some grains has been shown to reduce blood cholesterol as effectively as any known cholesterol-lowering drugs.

The **germ** layers of whole grains contain vitamins, minerals, protein, and oils. Germ oils are an important source of vitamin E, an antioxidant nutrient that prevents the destruction of cells by compounds known as free radicals. Vitamin E is critical to reproductive function, circulation, and healthy skin. The protein found in the germ layers of grains needs to be complemented by other protein foods like beans, dairy products, or meats. This is because the protein in grains is usually low in one or more of the essential amino acids, the building blocks of protein. Beans and other protein foods contain the amino acids that are typically deficient in whole grains. This is why grains and beans are eaten together in the diets of virtually all traditional cultures.

The **endosperm** of whole grains is the interior, starchy kernel. This is the source of complex carbohydrates, which break down in the digestive process into sugars that are eventually converted into blood glucose to fuel the body. Although some people believe that starch is a fattening food, it has no more calories than protein and only half as many as fat. Starch consumed in the form of whole grains is entirely healthful and difficult to overeat because of the filling effects of the accompanying bulk-enhancing dietary fiber.

When buying whole grains, look for whole, intact kernels that are not scratched, dented, or gnarled. When storing grains at home, keep them cool, dry, and shaded in a closed container. Remember that the enemies of food are air, light, moisture, and time. Stored properly, grains will last for several months.

Organically produced grains are readily available in most natural food stores because of the increased demand for whole foods grown without toxic agrichemicals. Organic grains usually have more flavor than their conventionally grown counterparts.

Amaranth is not a true cereal grain. It comes not from a grass but from a broad-leafed plant with multiple seed heads. The heads of the amaranth plant are packed with thousands of seeds. The seeds are tiny, about the size of millet, and their color ranges from purple to yellow. An unusually hardy plant, amaranth grows well under harsh conditions and in hostile terrain and is resistant to pests and drought. The harvesting of the seed is labor intensive; thus, amaranth is expensive.

No one knows how long amaranth has been cultivated, although there is evidence that it has been grown for as long as eight thousand years in Central and South America. For several hundred years amaranth has been cultivated in the high-altitude terrain of the Himalayas and the hill regions of India, Nepal, Pakistan, China, and the Tibetan plateau. A staple food of the Aztecs, amaranth was highly revered as a life-giving, strength-endowing food. In Aztec sacrificial rituals amaranth was mixed with human blood and fashioned into cakes in the shape of Aztec gods. An end to the Aztec cultivation of amaranth was decreed by Cortez as part of his campaign to systematically destroy the Aztec culture.

After the campaign led by Cortez, amaranth production declined until the middle of this century, and was limited to just a few small regions in Mexico and Central and South America. Since 1967, however, amaranth production has been vigorously promoted by the United States Food and Agriculture Organization. The seed is now cultivated in North America, and worldwide production is on the increase.

Amaranth is now making regular appearances in cereals, crackers, cookies, and baking mixes. Higher in fiber than wheat or rice, it is also fairly high in protein (around 16 percent). This is a very favorable protein value for a seed or grain, although there are some strains of wheat that achieve an 18 to 19 percent protein value. To compare, wheat usually comes in at about 12 percent.

The protein quality of amaranth is superior to that of most grains. Much of amaranth's protein is concentrated in the germ. It is rich in lysine and methionine, two essential amino acids. Amaranth combines extremely well with beans to make a high-quality, complete-protein food.

To cook, place 1 cup amaranth and 3 cups cold

water in a pan, and bring to a boil. Simmer, covered, for 25 minutes. Cooked plain, amaranth is a relatively unappetizing food with a gooey, mucilaginous consistency that does not improve its appeal. It truly needs to be flavored. Add herbs and spices, vegetables, or other grains to it. Or cook it in broth instead of plain water.

Amaranth can also be popped like corn. Heat a dry wok, skillet, or large pan and place a tablespoon of amaranth in the dry pan. Stir the seeds until they have popped.

Barley was one of the first cultivated grains. It is known to have been planted in Asia about 7000 B.C. Used as currency by the Sumerians about 4000 B.C., barley has been a primary grain in the Middle East for centuries. It is a staple food of the Tibetans and hill people of the Himalayas, where it is made into tsampa, a ground mixture cooked into a gruel and pounded in a churn with yak butter and brick tea. Prior to the partial genocide of the Tibetan people by the invading Chinese in the 1960s, tsampa was the primary food throughout the extensive Tibetan Buddhist monastic community. In Europe barley was the principal grain for several centuries until it was displaced by wheat. The grain was brought by British and Dutch colonists to America for beer brewing, which is its primary use to this day.

Barley has two inedible outer hulls. The outer hulls are typically removed by machine. The remaining hulled whole barley is nutritionally intact. The next layer after the inedible hulls is the **aleurone,** which is rich in protein, B vitamins, and fiber. Most barley, however, is subjected to further abrasion to remove more of the outer layers of the grain. This abrasive process, known as pearling, removes the nutrient-rich aleurone. Thus, pearled barley is nutritionally inferior to hulled whole barley.

According to researchers at the University of Wisconsin, barley contains a substance that inhibits cholesterol production. Pigs and chickens fed barley show reduced cholesterol values in their meat and eggs.

Besides being used in beer brewing, barley is commonly cooked in soups and stews. It is relatively easy to digest and is recommended for individuals with sensitive stomachs.

Barley comes in several forms. Pearled barley is commonly available but offers poor nutrition. Hulled whole barley is less commonly available but is the preferred form. Barley grits are the toasted, cracked whole grain and are used in salads and casseroles. Barley flour is excellent for baking but is low in gluten and so must be used in combination with wheat. Sprouted barley is an excellent salad garnish and is also found in sprouted multigrain breads. The Japanese make a health drink from barley grass. The grass is juiced, and the juice is then dehydrated and granulated. The granules are prized for their rich chlorophyll value.

To cook whole barley, add 1 cup barley to 3 cups water. Simmer, covered, for about 1 hour. *cooking*

Bulgur is wheat that has been steamed, dried, and cracked into pieces. It is commonly used in Middle Eastern foods, including tabouli. Bulgur is not always made from whole wheat. It is important to check the label on the bulgur you purchase to make sure that it is made from unprocessed whole wheat.

Because it is precooked, bulgur cooks quickly. Add 1 part bulgur to 2 parts water, and cook for 15 minutes. Or bring 2 cups of water to a boil, pour the boiling water over 1 cup bulgur, cover, and let stand off heat for 20 minutes. *cooking*

Buckwheat is technically not a cereal grain, but an edible fruit seed. It comes from a plant that resembles a bush rather than a grass. Buckwheat is closely related to rhubarb, has more than eight hundred species in its botanical family, and grows easily in varied climates. The three-cornered seed has an inedible black outer hull that must be removed, yielding a tan-colored interior kernel that is used for poultry and stock feed, cereal, and flour. Buckwheat originated in Asia and has been cultivated since the Middle Ages. It was brought to America by Dutch colonists who first planted it along the banks of the Hudson River. Toasted buckwheat is known as kasha.

Buckwheat is fairly high in protein, with about half as much per gram as beef. It is a good source of B vitamins, potassium, calcium, iron, and dietary fiber. The primary outstanding characteristic of buckwheat as a protein food is that it is high in the essential amino acid lysine—more than any other known cereal grain. The protein profile of buckwheat compares favorably with those of nonfat milk solids (92 percent) and whole egg solids (81 percent), according to the Agricultural Research Service in Madison, Wisconsin. Buckwheat can be cooked as a whole-grain cereal or used in baking. Because it is low in gluten, buckwheat must be mixed with wheat flour to make bread. Some people recommend combining uncooked buckwheat with egg before cooking it in water. This is because when boiled, the groats swell and rupture, losing their shape. Egg albumin seals the uncooked buckwheat with a binding that keeps the shape of the groats intact and separate during cooking. This does not prevent the groats from absorbing water in the cooking process, but it does add to the protein value of this food.

To cook, add 1 cup buckwheat to 2 cups boiling water, cover, and simmer for 15 to 20 minutes.

Corn (maize), the only cereal grain native to the American continents, is a tall, thick grass that was cultivated in America long before the arrival of Europeans to the New World. Native American peoples developed a highly refined system of corn agriculture. They grew corn for meal; sweet corn; popcorn; and yellow, red, blue, and white corns. Corn is the basic starch food of Central and South America and is typically ground into tortillas, tamales, and other unleavened breads. In the United States corn is traditionally eaten as grits, hominy, and mush.

The types of corn used for grain purposes are flint, dent, and flour corn. The variety of edible corn eaten as a vegetable is sweet corn, which is softer, moister, and sweeter than the grain varieties. Popcorn, yet another strain, is a well-known snack food.

Despite its great food value for humans, corn is primarily used as livestock feed. It is a major source of oil, sugars, and starches for literally thousands of different uses. Cornstarch, which is devoid of nutritional value, appears as a filler and thickener in packaged and processed foods, adding only calories to those items.

Corn is a highly exploited plant. It is used in the manufacture of paints, lacquers, textiles, paper, and plastics. Corn agriculture is extremely energy intensive, and the plant itself removes a tremendous amount of nutrients from the soil in which it is grown. The corn belt in the United States runs through Ohio, Illinois, Indiana, Iowa, Kansas, Missouri, and Nebraska. Most of the corn grown today is in the form of highly refined hybrid strains, developed for their high yields and resistance to pests. Very few original native strains are currently being grown; however, heirloom seeds are available through a few specialized seed companies that recognize the value of preserving and promoting original botanical genetic species.

Corn is low in the essential amino acids lysine and tryptophan. Traditionally corn is combined with beans, which have adequate amounts of these nutrients, thereby making a complete protein food of good quality.

Popcorn is a particular strain of corn in which each kernel is sealed in its own tiny husk, locking in moisture. When heated, the moisture in the kernel expands, and the kernel explodes or pops. Popcorn is high in fiber, low in calories, and very healthy. Keep it in a sealed container so that it retains its moisture, or it won't pop. You can snack regularly, shamelessly, and healthfully on popcorn. Be aware, though, that flavoring popcorn with salt and butter turns this healthful snack into a high-calorie cardiovascular antagonist. Keep it simple.

Blue corn, traditionally grown by native peoples of the southwestern United States for centuries, is making a comeback because of its novel color and its nutritional value. Found in chips, tortillas, pancake and baking mixes, and as popcorn, blue corn is higher in protein, potassium, and manganese than yellow corn.

Couscous, a traditional food of North Africa, where it is most often cooked with meats, is a product made from semolina, the refined endosperm (inside starch) of durum wheat, without the germ or bran. The semolina is ground and mixed with water into thin strands, which are broken into tiny pieces, steamed, and dried. The result is little round yellow granules that cook quickly and have a delicate flavor.

Because couscous is a refined grain product, it is not recommended as a nutritionally useful food. A few companies, however, are now offering a nonrefined couscous with the bran and germ intact. This alternative is a truly nutritious food. Durum wheat, from which couscous originates, is high in protein.

To cook, add 1½ cups boiling water to 1 cup couscous, and let stand off heat for 15 minutes.

Cooking

Quinoa (pronounced *keenwah*) is a small, flat, disk-shaped seed, ranging in color from yellow to orange, red, pink, purple, and black. Not actually a cereal grain, quinoa is the fruit of an annual herb of the Chenopodiaceae family, the seed fruit of which grows in clusters at the end of the stalk. There are literally hundreds of different strains of quinoa, all differing somewhat from each other in color, shape, and flavor.

Quinoa is naturally covered with inedible saponin, a resinous substance that can be used as soap. It is believed that saponin, which has a bitter taste, protects the tiny quinoa seeds from invasion by insects and consumption by birds. This saponin must be removed by a labor-intensive washing process before quinoa is ready for human consumption.

Referred to as the "Lost Grain of the Incas," quinoa has been farmed in the mountain regions of Peru and Bolivia for three thousand years. In the Inca Empire, only potatoes were more widely cultivated. Quinoa was regarded as a sacred plant, and its annual cultivation was conducted with ceremony. After Pizarro's conquest of the Incas in the 1500s,

quinoa production declined until the twentieth century. Today, quinoa is being recultivated in South America and to a lesser extent in the United States, where it is grown in the Rocky Mountains of Colorado. Previous attempts to grow it outside its natural habitat have been unsuccessful.

Quinoa has traditionally been used in several ways by the indigenous peoples of the Andes. It is boiled like rice, cooked in soups and stews, and ground into flour for tortillas, breads, and biscuits. The stalks of the quinoa plant are burned for fuel, the saponin is used for soap and shampoo, and the leaves of the herb are fed to livestock.

Quinoa has about twice the protein of barley, corn, and rice and is a good source of calcium, iron, vitamin E, phosphorus, and some B vitamins. It cooks quickly, has a delicious flavor, and goes well with virtually all vegetables, beans, and meats. The only drawback to quinoa is its price.

To cook, rinse the quinoa in a strainer. Combine 2 cups water with 1 cup quinoa in a saucepan. Bring to a boil, then reduce the heat, cover the pan, and simmer for about 15 minutes or until all the water is absorbed.

Cooking

Millet is a name for several cereal grasses grown for both human consumption and livestock feed throughout the world. Millet has a long history of cultivation. It is known to have been grown by lake dwellers in Switzerland during the Stone Age, and it has been part of Chinese agriculture for almost three thousand years.

Pearl millet is the variety available in natural food stores. Grown in the north central United States and Canada, pearl millet is always hulled. Millet, one of the grains highest in protein, grows well under adverse climatic conditions. It is gluten free, is the only alkaline grain, and is very easy to digest. Despite its excellent nutritional profile, millet is generally ignored as a food in the United States.

To cook, combine 2 ½ cups water with 1 cup millet. Simmer, covered, for approximately 30 minutes.

Cooking

Oats are among the most recently cultivated cereal grasses and are not known to have been domesticated prior to 2500 B.C. A major grain crop in the United States, oats rival wheat and corn in production volume. Only 5 percent of the oats grown commercially are for human consumption. The greatest percentage of oats are used in animal feed. The hulls yield furfural, a widely used industrial solvent. Oat straw is a common animal bedding, and oat flour is used in ice creams and dairy products.

Oats have received attention because of the cholesterol-lowering effects of oat bran, which is a source of soluble fibers. As little as half a cup of oat bran daily can lower serum cholesterol by as much as 20 percent. This means that oat bran rivals the finest and most expensive cholesterol-lowering drugs ever devised, most of which were developed with millions of dollars of research. That's not a bad performance for the outer layer of an inexpensive grain! Actually, nobody should be surprised. Foods are consistently the best products available for reversing or correcting health problems, especially metabolic disorders.

Oats have a hard, inedible hull that must be removed before they can be eaten. The remaining grain, with its bran and germ layers intact, is known as the groat. Rolled oats are made by slicing and steaming the groats, which are then crushed between rollers and dried. The amount of pressure used in the rolling process determines how much the groats are flattened. Flatter, more finely rolled oat groats (so-called quick oats) cook faster than the thicker, less finely rolled groats. Regular rolled oats are used to make oatmeal. They usually take only about 15 minutes to cook, and the consistency of the resulting cereal is more pleasing than that of the quick oat products. However, the nutritional values of the regular and quick varieties are the same.

Steel-cut oats are hulled groats that are sliced but not rolled. Steel-cut oats should be soaked prior to cooking. To cook rolled oats, boil 2 ½ cups water, add 1 cup oats, stir for 2 minutes, cover, and cook over low heat for approximately 15 minutes.

Rice is the most widely consumed staple food in the world. Half of the world's population subsists primarily on rice. Cultivated in China for more than four thousand years, rice was introduced to India prior to the time of the Greeks. Rice was already the staple crop in China at the time that Chinese language was taking form, as indicated by the fact that the words for *rice* and *agriculture* are the same in some Chinese dialects. The original form of rice is not known, but thousands of strains currently exist throughout the world. Numerous ceremonies celebrating or worshipping the grain exist worldwide, and rice appears frequently in Asian art as a symbol of life and abundance.

Rice grows most easily in subtropical regions, rather than in hot or cold areas. It requires moisture for successful cultivation, and irrigation and flooding are commonly used to grow rice crops. Ninety percent of all the rice in the world is grown in India, China, and Japan. In densely populated areas of the East, entire forests have been cleared to accommodate rice cultivation. This deforestation has had devastating effects and is the cause of disastrous flooding, particularly in India.

Rice cultivation in the East is accomplished by ancient methods. The plows are pulled by water buffalo, fertilizing is done with manure, the smoothing of the land is accomplished by dragging logs over the soil, and planting is done by hand. In the United States rice is grown in Arkansas, Louisiana, Texas, and California entirely by modern agricultural methods. Rice with the hull intact is known as *paddy,* which is also the name of rice fields. In the West, rice is usually hulled, then stripped of the outer brown layers, which include the bran and germ. This removes most of the vitamins, minerals, and protein from the grain, leaving only the carbohydrate endosperm. In many parts of Asia, rice is left intact except for the removal of the outer inedible hull. Because rice is an incomplete protein, it must be combined with either beans or meat to supplement its nutritional profile.

Rice bran, straw, and meal are fed to livestock, and the hulls are a source of furfural, a commercial

Cooking

solvent. In Japan, rice is brewed to make sake, the traditional liquor of that country. In the United States, rice is used by some breweries in beer making, although barley is the preferred grain for that purpose.

White rice is not a whole food. The removal of the bran and germ layers of the grain render a nutritionally inferior food that is almost exclusively starch. The nutritionally intact brown rice varieties are legion, but the most popular ones are described here. Brown rice is an excellent source of the B vitamins and contains calcium, phosphorus, vitamin E, iron, and much-needed dietary fiber as well. Brown rice comes in short-, medium-, and long-grain varieties. There is no significant difference in nutritional value between these sizes of rice.

Short-grain rice tends to be the chewiest of all brown rices. Some people claim that short-grain varieties are sweeter than longer-grain varieties, although this is debatable. Cooked medium-grain brown rice is fluffier than short-grain brown rice. Long-grain brown rice most closely approximates the texture of white rice when cooked. Long-grain rice is generally the preferred rice for salads.

Basmati rice originated in India, where the many varieties of this rice are typically polished white. Brown basmati rice is available, however. It yields a nutty flavor and a delicate aroma. It is excellent for Indian cuisine and for all other rice uses.

Texmati rice, a sweet, nutty-tasting basmati variety, is grown mostly in Texas.

Sweet brown rice is a sticky short-grain variety that is used in Asian desserts and is mixed with regular brown rice to make sushi. The consistency of sweet brown rice makes it ideal for rice balls and croquettes.

Instant brown rice has been cooked and then dried. This makes for a very fast-cooking brown rice, with most of the nutrients intact.

To cook brown rice, combine 2 cups water and 1 cup rice. Bring to a boil, lower heat, and simmer, covered, for approximately 45 minutes. *Cooking*

Wild rice is not a rice at all but the fruit seed of a tall aquatic grass, *Zinzania aquatica,* which is na-

tive to the northern United States and southern Canada. It grows in shallow ponds and lakes and is believed to have been eaten by Native Americans as much as ten thousand years ago. *Zinzania aquatica* is a habitat for waterfowl and fish and is sown for this purpose.

Indians traditionally harvested wild rice by canoeing into wetlands and bending the grass into the canoe. The seeds were then flailed off the grass with paddles. The seeds were sun-dried or parched to crack the hulls, then trampled and winnowed. Today some wild rice is still grown in natural wetlands without chemical fertilizers or other agricultural chemicals and harvested in a traditional manner.

Most "wild" rice sold in grocery stores is not wild at all and is therefore mislabeled. It is grown in commercial diked paddies from hybrid seeds, with the use of toxic agrichemicals, and is mechanically harvested by caterpillar-tracked combines. This farmed wild rice is sown and harvested for commercial purposes. To be sure that the wild rice you are buying is actually wild and harvested by hand, look for that specific information on the package. Some states require paddy-cultivated, pseudo-wild rice to be labeled as such. For further information on traditionally grown and harvested wild rice, you can write to Northern Lakes Wild Rice Company, P.O. Box 392, Teton Village, Wyoming 83025.

Wild rice offers protein, iron, and B vitamins. It has a nutlike taste and is often mixed with other rices. To cook wild rice, combine 4 cups of water and 1 cup wild rice. Simmer, covered, 45 to 60 minutes. *Cooking*

Rye, domesticated later than wheat and other staple grains, is a principal ingredient in breads and baked goods. Easily grown under conditions that are unsuitable for producing a satisfactory wheat crop, rye is used as a cover crop, as livestock feed, and as a distiller's grain in the manufacture of gin and whiskey.

Rye is high in the amino acid lysine and contains B vitamins, iron, vitamin E, and protein. It is not usually cooked by itself as a cereal. Rye has been bred with wheat to produce the hybrid grain triticale.

Triticale. Wheat and rye often grow together in the same fields, where they produce hybrid offspring. These offspring do not naturally produce seeds, however. In the late 1800s, scientists experimented with natural rye/wheat hybrids until they developed a seed-bearing strain known as triticale. (Wheat is *Triticum.* Rye is *Secale.* Thus, *triticale.*) Today triticale is grown primarily in the midwestern United States.

Triticale is higher in lysine and lower in gluten than wheat, and higher in protein than either wheat or rye. It has a nutty flavor and is used in breads and baking mixes.

Wheat is a primary staple food worldwide and a huge commodity on the international market. Modern wheat varieties are classified as winter wheat and spring wheat. Winter wheat is planted in the fall, lies dormant in winter, and is harvested in early summer. Spring wheat is planted in early spring and is harvested in the late fall. There are three basic strains of wheat: hard, soft, and durum. Hard wheat is higher in gluten than soft wheat and thus has a

higher protein value. Hard wheat is preferred for bread baking. Soft wheat is lighter in color than hard varieties and, while not ideal for making bread, is used widely in pastries. Soft-wheat flour is known as pastry flour. Durum wheat is used for making pasta because it holds its shape without dissolving in water while cooking.

In the United States, wheat is widely consumed in its least nutritional form. It is typically stripped of its nutritionally rich bran and germ layers and is pulverized into a fine starchy powder for the manufacture of white bread. It is bleached, manipulated with "dough conditioner," adulterated with carcinogenic preservatives, and must have synthetic vitamins added to it in order to make bread that has any nutritional value at all. The very notion that such a useless product builds strong bodies is an insult to the health and intelligence of every person. It's a wonder that such products can legally be sold as food.

Although whole-wheat berries are not typically cooked as cereal, they can be. Combine 2 cups water and 1 cup wheat berries. Simmer, covered, for about 45 minutes.

Wheat is also available as cracked wheat. As the name implies, this is wheat that has been cracked into small pieces. Cracked wheat is used in cereals and breads, and cooks somewhat more quickly than whole-wheat berries.

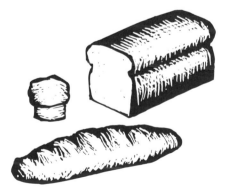

5

BEANS AND SPROUTS, NUTS AND SEEDS

BEANS

Along with cereal grains, legumes—or beans—are among the most widely consumed foods in the world. Beans contain more protein than any other foods in the vegetable kingdom; yet, they have none of the cholesterol found in animal-source protein foods. They complement whole grains well, making high-quality protein that rivals protein from meats and other animal foods. Beans have abundant complex carbohydrates, which we need for energy, and they are an excellent source of cholesterol-lowering soluble fibers. Unlike grains, beans do not go through processing methods by which they are stripped of their nutrition. Thus, you do not need to look for "whole" beans versus "refined" beans; all beans are whole foods.

Beans are available in three forms: dried, canned, and retort-cooked. Whole dried beans of all varieties can typically be found in supermarkets and natural food stores. When buying whole beans, look for intact whole beans that are not scratched, dented, or gnarled. To test a dried bean for quality, bite into it. The bean should crack and shatter. If you only dent the bean, that is an indication that the bean has not been adequately dried.

Canned beans may contain sugar or artificial additives. Check the label of canned beans to make sure that the product you are buying does not contain them. Canned beans should be rinsed prior to cooking.

Retort-cooked beans are a great breakthrough in nutrition for precooked beans. Retort-cooked beans are cooked thoroughly inside the sealed glass bottles in which they are sold; thus, all the nutritional value of the beans remains inside the bottle. Retort-cooked beans are definitely preferred if you are going to buy precooked beans. Nonetheless, check the labels to make sure that the product you are buying does not contain chemical additives.

Cleaning beans is simple. Put dried beans into a pot filled with water and pour off any debris, such as dust, dirt, and camel hair, that may float to the surface of the water. Also sift through dried beans to remove any tiny stones that may be present.

Almost all dried beans should be soaked prior to cooking. Presoak beans in water 3 to 4 times their volume, either by letting them sit overnight or for a

Buying

preparing

minimum of 8 hours, or by bringing them to a boil for 3 minutes and letting them sit for 2 hours off the heat. Strain the beans after soaking, and use fresh water for cooking. If you do not soak beans prior to cooking them, it will take many hours for them to cook thoroughly.

Cooking

Beans and Gas

Beans have long been known to produce flatulence (intestinal gas) when eaten by humans. This is due to the presence of certain carbohydrates in beans that humans cannot digest. These carbohydrates include raffinose, stachyose, and verbascose, sugars that pass undigested into the lower intestine and are fermented by bacteria, thus producing gas. That's the bad news. The good news is that you may be able to reduce the gas-producing effects of beans by the above-mentioned method: soaking them, pouring off the soaking water, and cooking the beans thoroughly in fresh water.

Organically Grown Beans

The following organically grown beans are increasingly available in natural food stores. In preparing them, be sure to presoak them, as discussed above, before cooking as detailed here.

Aduki These small, dark red beans are prized by Asian doctors for their alleged medicinal value. They are said to be useful in treating kidney ailments. An excellent protein food, aduki beans are a good source of calcium, phosphorus, potassium, iron, and vitamin A. To cook, add 1 cup beans to 4 cups water. Cover and simmer for 60 minutes or until tender.

Black Turtle This black bean, served in Mexican restaurants from El Paso to Boston, is delicious with melted cheese. Add some hot chilies if you like, and you'll have a meal that tastes as if it came from south of the border. To cook, add 1 cup beans to 4 cups water. Cover and simmer for 60 minutes or until tender.

Black-eyed Peas Also known as cow-peas, black-eyed peas are popular throughout the southern United States, and are the staple bean of "soul food." To cook, add 1 cup beans to 4 cups water. Cover and simmer for 60 minutes, or until tender.

Garbanzo Also known as chick-peas, garbanzo beans are a staple food in the Middle East and are used to make hummus, a spread that also contains sesame tahini. Garbanzos are an interesting-looking bean and are high in potassium, calcium, iron, and vitamin A. To cook, add 1 cup beans to 4 cups water. Cover and simmer for 80 minutes or until tender.

Great Northern One of several types of white beans, Great Northern beans are used in New York baked beans and in cassoulets. To cook, add 1 cup beans to 4 cups water. Cover and simmer for 40 minutes or until tender.

Kidney Beans In the famous Boston baked beans, these deep red beans are simmered slowly with molasses. To cook, add 1 cup beans to 4 cups water. Cover and simmer for 40 minutes or until tender.

Lentils A member of the pea family, these small, lens-shaped seeds have been found in excavations dating from the Bronze Age. You'll find green, red, and brown lentils, each somewhat different in flavor. In the Bible, Esau sold his birthright for a bowl of Egyptian red lentils. High in calcium, magnesium, potassium, phosphorus, chlorine, sulfur, and vitamin A, lentils are a nutritional super food. Unlike other beans, lentils do not need to be presoaked. To cook, add 1 cup beans to 4 cups water. Cover and simmer for 20 minutes or until tender. For a delicious variation, add garlic and oil as the lentils cook. *Do not need to be presoaked*

Lima Beans Unjustly accused of having a bad flavor, lima beans are delicious when cooked properly. They have a distinctive flavor and are loaded with potassium, phosphorus, and vitamin A. To cook, add 1 cup beans to 4 cups water. Cover and simmer for 60 minutes or until tender.

Mung Beans These tiny green beans are grown in India, where they are widely used. Delicious with rice and vegetables, mung beans are one of those foods you can eat repeatedly without growing tired of the taste. Sprouted, they are the mainstay of Chinese vegetable dishes and wok cooking. To cook, add 1 cup beans to 4 cups water. Cover and simmer for 60 minutes or until tender.

Navy Beans These big white beans are delicious in soups and stews. To cook, add 1/2 pound beans to 2 1/2 quarts water. Cover and simmer for 40 minutes or until tender.

Pinto Beans Rich in calcium, potassium, and phosphorus, pinto beans are a favorite from the Southwest, where they are used liberally in chili. They are great with grains, in soups and stews, with vegetables, or by themselves. To cook, add 1 cup beans to 4 cups water. Cover and simmer for 60 minutes or until tender.

Split Peas, Green and Yellow Splits, as they are called, are typically used to make split pea soup. This hearty food is especially welcome on cold days when your body needs something hot and substantial. Split peas do not have to be soaked. To cook, add 1 cup beans to 4 cups water and cook, covered, for 60 minutes or until they are completely soft.

Do not need to presoak

Soybeans Of Chinese origin, the soybean has been a major source of food and oil in China and Japan for thousands of years but was unknown in Europe and America until 1900. The only bean that is a complete protein by itself, soy is the most versatile bean known. With 40 percent protein, soybeans are 20 percent lecithin, which is essential to every cell in the body. Soybeans are used to make tofu, miso, tempeh, and tamari. To cook, add 1 cup beans to 4 cups water. Cover and simmer for 3 hours or until tender.

SPROUTS

Almost everyone is familiar with sprouts, the initial germinated form of all seeds. Mung bean sprouts are common in Chinese and Thai food, and alfalfa sprouts are popular in salads and sandwiches. Fresh sprouts are excellent foods, high in vitamins and live enzymes. Sprouting greatly increases the nutrient value of seeds. Whole soybeans, for example, contain only a trace of vitamin C compared with 13 milligrams of vitamin C per 100 grams of beans when sprouted. This is equivalent to the vitamin C content of tomatoes or lettuce. The thiamine value increases over 300 percent, and the riboflavin content increases over 900 percent.

While any seed that is alive can be sprouted, some sprouts are more commonly available than others. Alfalfa, red clover, mung beans, and radish sprouts are most widely available in natural food stores.

In the market, look for bright, healthy, firm sprouts. Sprouts that are withered, dry, brown, yellow, or slimy should be avoided. It is preferable to buy sprouts in bulk rather than in packages because then you can see what you are buying. Some stores sell sprouts in trays and allow you to pick your own with tongs. If you can find only pre-packaged sprouts, look them over carefully. If you see any slime or yellowing, avoid them. There are few tastes worse than that of a slimy sprout. Store sprouts in an airtight plastic container.

While you can buy a variety of sprouts at the produce counter, you can also grow them at home. The following chart is for growing sprouts by the jar method. Just follow these easy steps:

1. Using either a quart- or gallon-sized jar, soak your sprout seeds for 6 hours.
2. Drain the water. Rinse the seeds in fresh cool water and drain them again.
3. Cover the top of your jar with cheesecloth, secured with an elastic band, and store the jar upside down at a 70-degree angle to allow for continuous drainage and circulation of air.

4. Rinse the sprouts with fresh water at least 2 times daily. If the weather is hot or humid, rinse them 3 times daily.
5. On the last day of growth, expose the sprouts to plenty of light, so they will become green with natural chlorophyll.
6. Drain the sprouts completely before harvesting them, and keep them refrigerated in an airtight container.

NUTS AND SEEDS

Nuts and seeds are concentrated foods that can make a valuable contribution to a healthy diet. Brimming with vitamins, minerals, protein, and polyunsaturated fats, nuts and seeds are among the most nutritious foods in the world. They are the very core of plant life, containing most of the essential ingredients needed to produce a mature plant. To quote J. I. Rodale, the well-known nutritional authority, "The seed is the crucible wherein the alchemy of life works its magic."

Seeds and nuts are available raw, roasted, unsalted, salted, chopped, or still in the shell. Their flavors vary greatly, but in general nuts and seeds are somewhat sweet, heavy, and satisfying. Because they are high in oil, they can be ground into "butters" such as peanut butter, almond butter, pistachio butter, and sesame tahini. The high oil content of nuts and seeds also means that they are high in calories and are thus fattening. Some dietary enthusiasts advocate the heavy use of nuts and seeds in the diet, particularly as a replacement for meats and dairy products. Such replacement should be approached judiciously, because nuts and seeds are very high in fat. Lean meats and low-fat or nonfat dairy products should not be completely replaced by high-fat nuts and seeds.

What to Look For

When shopping for nuts and seeds, buy only whole nuts. This does not mean that nuts should be purchased in the shell but that the actual "meat" of the nut should be whole and intact rather than sliced,

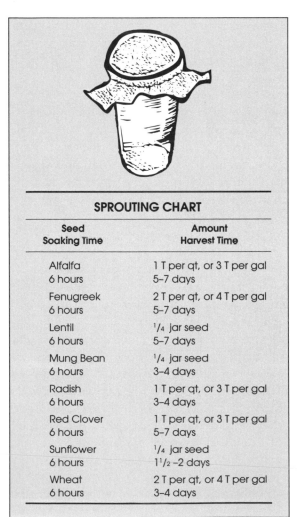

SPROUTING CHART

Seed Soaking Time	Amount Harvest Time
Alfalfa 6 hours	1 T per qt, or 3 T per gal 5–7 days
Fenugreek 6 hours	2 T per qt, or 4 T per gal 5–7 days
Lentil 6 hours	¼ jar seed 5–7 days
Mung Bean 6 hours	¼ jar seed 3–4 days
Radish 6 hours	1 T per qt, or 3 T per gal 3–4 days
Red Clover 6 hours	1 T per qt, or 3 T per gal 5–7 days
Sunflower 6 hours	¼ jar seed 1½ –2 days
Wheat 6 hours	2 T per qt, or 4 T per gal 3–4 days

chopped, or in pieces. Nuts and seeds store well and will keep for several months under refrigeration in a sealed container. When they are sliced or broken in any way, however, their oily flesh is exposed to air, and oxidation occurs. In a relatively short period of time, sometimes as quickly as a couple of days, this produces rancidity. Any rancid food is a toxic food and can cause liver damage.

Most of the time you will not encounter rancid nuts and seeds, but you should know that a rancid nut or seed will have a sharp or bitter taste. Sunflower seeds and cashew nuts are particularly susceptible to rancidity and are often stored poorly. Discard any dark or discolored sunflower seeds. Rancidity is common in cashew pieces, which will have dark edges or spots. If any nut is dark or contains dark gray or black areas, it is most likely rancid and should be avoided. The same is true for any rubbery or moldy nuts.

Purchase unsalted nuts and seeds. You don't need the extra sodium, and you will discover that these foods have enjoyable, varied flavors that do not require salting. Also check the label of any dry-roasted nut or seed product for added salt, sugar, starches, MSG, and preservatives. Avoid these whenever possible; you don't need the additives.

Although some advocates of the macrobiotic diet claim that nuts and seeds are most digestible when toasted, this claim seems to be unsubstantiated. Toasting appears to have no beneficial effect upon the "digestibility" of nuts and seeds, but it will reduce their vitamin content. High heat always reduces the vitamin value of a food.

Here is a list of some of the nuts and seeds you will find in a natural food store:

Alfalfa Seed Rich in vitamins A, E, D, and K, alfalfa seeds are used primarily for sprouting. The sprouts are delicious in sandwiches, in salads, or as garnishes for soups and entrees.

Almond Often referred to as the "king of nuts," almonds are grown primarily in California and Spain.

The almond is high in potassium, magnesium, and phosphorus, and one-fifth of its weight consists of protein. Almond oil is among the finest and most nutritious of all nut oils, and almond butter is one of the sweetest nut butters (protein 18.6 percent, carbohydrate 19.5 percent, fat 54.2 percent).

Brazil Nut High in potassium, phosphorus, and sulfur, in the shell this is the hardest of all nuts to crack. Brazil nuts are grown in soil that has a high level of naturally occurring radionuclides; thus, the nuts themselves are among the most naturally radioactive of foods. In 1988 National Public Radio reported that 1 dozen Brazil nuts exceeds the safety limit for radiation exposure set by the Occupational Safety and Hazard Administration (protein 14.3 percent, carbohydrate 10.9 percent, fat 66.9 percent).

Cashew The evergreen cashew tree is related to both poison ivy and poison sumac. Indigenous to Central and South America, the cashew is now grown primarily in India. In preparation, the seed of the cashew apple is heated until the outer shell bursts, dispelling the poisonous properties of the seed. The inner shell is then broken, and the kernels are ready to be eaten raw or roasted. The cashew is high in potassium, phosphorus, magnesium, and vitamin A (protein 15 percent, carbohydrate 33 percent, fat 46 percent).

Chestnut (marron) Chestnuts may be eaten raw, boiled, or roasted. Dried chestnuts are often milled into flour and used in making soups, breads, and confections. The dried nuts can be soaked in water and cooked with grains. Chestnuts are low in fat (protein 2.9 percent, carbohydrate 42.1 percent, fat 1.5 percent).

Coconut Fresh or dried coconut has a unique flavor that enhances the taste of salads, curries, desserts, and fruit salads. Recently coconut has acquired a bad reputation for its high saturated fat content. Coconut oil contains more saturated fat than beef lard. Saturated fats are associated with overly high blood cholesterol production (protein 3.5 percent, carbohydrate 23 percent, fat 64.9 percent).

Filbert Also known as hazelnuts, these pea-shaped nuts have a lovely mild flavor and are often cooked with vegetables and grains. They are high in potassium, phosphorus, sulfur, and calcium (protein 12.6 percent, carbohydrate 16.7percent, fat 62.4 percent).

Flaxseed A mucilaginous (sticky, slippery) food, flaxseeds are laxative in their action. They are rich in nutrients and aid the digestion of heavy fiber foods such as whole grains. Flaxseed meal is often used in baking. Flaxseeds are a source of soluble fibers, which have been shown to lower serum cholesterol levels (protein 22 percent, carbohydrate 16 percent, fat 45 percent).

Hickory Nut An important part of the diet of many Native Americans, hickory nuts are used as a meat substitute because of their high protein value (protein 13.2 percent, carbohydrate 12.8 percent, fat 68.7 percent).

Macadamia Nut The macadamia nut is indigenous to Australia but is now grown commercially in Hawaii. Its subtle, sweet flavor makes it one of the most delicious of all nuts (protein 7.8 percent, carbohydrate 15.9 percent, fat 71.6 percent).

Peanut Despite its name, the peanut is a legume, not a nut. Pound for pound, peanuts have more protein, vitamins, and minerals than beef liver; more fat than heavy cream; and more food energy (calories) than sugar. The protein of the peanut has tissue-building properties equal to those of eggs and milk (protein 26.3 percent, carbohydrate 17.6 percent, fat 48.4 percent).

Pecan The pecan is a member of the hickory family, and its meat looks like that of a walnut. The pecan's taste, however, is unique. Cultivated mostly in the southeastern United States, pecans are high in phosphorus, potassium, and vitamin A (protein 9.2 percent, carbohydrate 14.6 percent, fat 71.6 percent).

Pine Nut *(pignolia)* Harvested from the European stone pine, the pine nut is used in Middle Eastern and Italian cooking in particular. Soft, chewy, and sweet, these nuts are delicious in salads or with dried fruits (protein 9.2 percent, carbohydrate 14.6 percent, fat 47.4 percent).

Pistachio Nut A native of the Mediterranean region, the pistachio differs from other nuts in the characteristic green color of its kernel. It has a sweet, mild flavor. Grated pistachios make a lovely garnish for desserts. Oil of pistachio is used in traditional Ayurvedic medicine, the original Hindu system of health practiced widely in India (protein 19.3 percent, carbohydrate 19 percent, fat 63.7 percent).

Pumpkin Seed *(pepita)* Besides being a tasty snack, pumpkin seeds are an excellent vermifuge: if eaten regularly, they help to dispel intestinal pinworms and other parasites. They are high in phosphorus and vitamin A and are beneficial to the prostate gland (protein 29 percent, carbohydrate 15 percent, fat 46.7 percent).

Sesame Seed High in calcium, potassium, phosphorus, magnesium, and vitamin A, sesame seeds are certainly a super food, reputed to increase endurance and stamina. They are eaten in some cultures in place of milk or cheese because of their exceptionally high calcium content. Per 100 grams, sesame seeds contain 1,125 milligrams (mg.) of calcium, compared with 1,086 mg. in 100 grams of Swiss cheese or 590 mg. per pint of milk. Sesame seed has been highly prized throughout the Middle East for thousands of years and is believed by some to possess magical properties (protein 18.6 percent, carbohydrate 21.6 percent, fat 49.1 percent).

Sunflower Seed A staple food in some regions of Russia, sunflower seeds are high in potassium, phosphorus, silicon, calcium, and vitamin A (protein 24 percent, carbohydrate 19.9 percent, fat 47.3 percent).

Walnut The common walnut has been eaten as a food since early times, and its oil is used in cooking. The English walnut differs slightly from the black walnut in that it contains more fat and less protein. Walnuts are high in potassium, phosphorus, magnesium, and vitamin A (protein 14.8 percent, carbohydrate 15.8 percent, fat 64 percent).

6

ECO REPORT: FOOD IRRADIATION

Sci-Fi Food Processing

Food irradiation is a technology designed to extend the shelf life of foods by exposing them to radioactivity from nuclear waste. The food irradiation process, which is currently approved for meats, grains, some produce, herbs, and spices, involves sending food on a conveyor belt into a concrete chamber, where it is exposed to radiation for 1 to 2 minutes. The levels of radiation involved are between five thousand and 4 million rads (radiation absorbed dose, a standard unit of measure for radiation). By comparison, a chest X ray gives off less than 1 rad. Irradiated foods must be labeled as such, but products containing irradiated ingredients need not be labeled. It is estimated that there will be approximately one thousand irradiation plants operating in the United States by the end of the 1990s unless the food irradiation industry is stopped.

Making the World a Better Place

According to proponents of food irradiation, including the FDA, this technology is a major blessing to humankind and can replace pesticides and eradicate hunger at the same time. Furthermore, proponents claim that food irradiation is being used successfully worldwide, and that thirty years of careful study and evaluation have proved that food irradiation is safe. None of these claims is true.

And Now a Few Facts

Virtually all of the agricultural pesticides are used in the food-growing stage of the agricultural process. Since food irradiation has nothing whatsoever to do with agriculture, it would not have any impact on the amount of pesticides used to produce food. Most post-harvest pesticides are fungicides like those used in waxes that are applied to produce. Irradiated fruits and vegetables are more susceptible to infection by molds and fungus. Thus, the use of post-harvest fungicides will increase because of food irradiation.

The claim that food irradiation can play a major role in eradicating hunger is patently untrue. A March 1986 report published by the World Bank entitled *Poverty and World Hunger* concluded that there is *no* shortage of food and that hunger is a problem of distribution, economics, and politics.

The U.S. federal government stores more than 2 million tons of surplus food in limestone caves outside Kansas City. Silos throughout the United States are filled with surplus grains, and farmers are paid by federal price support programs not to grow food. The European Community currently has more surplus food than it can store. Despite more than adequate food production, people are starving to death all over the world. Food irradiation has nothing to do with this atrocity and offers no relief.

Despite claims that food irradiation is being used successfully worldwide, there is no evidence that this technology is actually in use anywhere in the world on anything other than a small-scale experimental basis. Some pork, herbs, and spices are being irradiated, a few small batches of tropical fruits have been irradiated, and the Japanese are irradiating small quantities of potatoes. That's it. This does not constitute successful worldwide use.

Last, it is claimed that food irradiation has been studied carefully for thirty years and has been proved safe. In fact, the FDA approved food irradiation technology after it had rejected virtually all of the animal-food-consumption studies that have been conducted to determine the safety of eating irradiated foods. Studies from around the world have shown adverse effects when animals have been fed irradiated food. These effects include tumors, kidney damage, chromosome damage, lower birth rates, and higher infant mortality. According to a 1978 General Accounting Office report entitled *The Army's Food Irradiation Program: Is It Worth Continuing?*, the FDA's approval of food irradiation has been based on mistaken interpretations of safety reports, poorly devised studies, and fraudulent data. The FDA contracted with Bio-Test Laboratories to study food irradiation, but Bio-Test was subsequently convicted of generating fraudulent food-safety study results. Virtually all of the food-safety data generated by the Bio-Test was found to be fictitious.

No Nutrition, Either

Proponents of food irradiation say that this technology keeps food in a wholesome, unspoiled, nu-

tritious condition. Wrong again. Vitamins A, C, E, K, B_1, B_2, B_3, B_6, and folic acid are depleted or destroyed by this process. Several amino acids, which are the basic building blocks of protein, are broken down. Other nutrients are damaged or destroyed. On top of this, food irradiation produces free radicals, which accelerate the aging process in our bodies by chewing up cells. Considering the fact that the primary purpose of eating food is to nourish the body, it seems imprudent to subject food to a process that reduces or destroys its nutritional value.

Unknown Chemical Compounds

Food irradiation not only damages the nutritional value of foods but also produces previously unknown chemical compounds in foods known as URPs, or unique radiolytic particles. Created by radiation, these strange compounds exist only in irradiated foods. Researchers at both the FDA and the U.S. National Bureau of Standards say that URPs have never undergone toxicological testing. In irradiated foods URPs occur at 3 parts per million. This doesn't sound like a lot, but when compared with the pesticide EDB, which causes cancer at the parts per billion level, or the herbicide 245T, which causes cancer at the parts per trillion level, URPs may represent a significant health risk.

We know that many animal-feeding studies report cancer, tumors, kidney damage, and genetic damage when animals are fed foods containing low concentrations of URPs. Toxicology tests, however, need to be conducted with high concentrations of these compounds. According to Dr. John Gofman, former director of research at the Lawrence Livermore National Laboratory and founder of its Biomedical Division, "stable products could be extracted

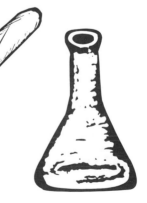

from irradiated foods by various solvents which could then be concentrated and subsequently tested. Until such fundamental studies are undertaken, there is little scientific basis for accepting industry's assurances of safety."

At Least the Plants Are Safe

Proponents of food irradiation technology claim that food irradiation facilities are safe to operate and pose no hazard to the environment. Nothing could be further from the truth. One worker has already died because of radiation exposure, and numerous "accidents" at food irradiation facilities have resulted in the release of radioactive waste into the environment in populated areas. An irradiation facility in Dover, New Jersey, was discovered to have dumped five thousand gallons of radioactive water into a public sewer one block away from an elementary school.

Workers in irradiation facilities are not required to receive special training. Nonetheless, they are expected to handle radioactive materials safely and carefully. Furthermore, facilities can be built anywhere—even next to schools and playgrounds. They are subject only to standard business zoning regulations. Irradiation plants are not required to maintain strict security standards, and they are permitted higher emissions than are nuclear power plants. So much for safety.

What You Can Do

A strong public reaction against food irradiation has already made an impact on the proliferation of this technology. Some states have banned the sale of irradiated foods, and other states are considering similar legislation. Some supermarket chains have promised not to sell irradiated foods, but the Food Marketing Institute in Washington, D.C., is still promoting this dangerous process.

To step up the battle against food irradiation, tell your grocer that you don't want irradiated foods and that you want the store to promise not to sell them. Try to get your friends to do the same. This can really have an impact. Then write to the Food Marketing Institute in Washington and urge it to oppose food irradiation. Last, write or call your state senator and representative and urge them to support legislation that forbids the operation of food irradiation facilities in your state and prohibits the sale of irradiated foods.

7

VEGETABLES AND FRUITS

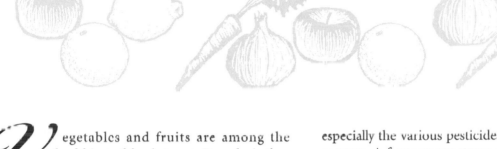

egetables and fruits are among the healthiest of foods to eat. Per calorie they contain more vitamins and minerals than any other food group, with very little fat (olives, coconuts, and avocados excepted) and no cholesterol. Fruits and vegetables are excellent sources of carbohydrates, which are needed for energy. They contain a high amount of indigestible cellulose, a dietary fiber that improves digestion and enhances intestinal regularity. In addition, fruits and vegetables are loaded with live enzymes, which are catalysts involved in virtually every bodily function. The enzymes from fresh produce enhance digestion and the absorption of nutrients, thus enhancing the body's own natural activities.

Conventional, Transitional, and Organic Produce

Today there are three types of produce available in grocery stores, differentiated by whether or not they were grown with agricultural chemicals. Because fruits and vegetables are among the most heavily sprayed of all food crops, the use of agrichemicals,

especially the various pesticides, is a major health concern. A few grocery stores are now starting to label produce according to growing methods, thus enabling consumers to make informed, healthy food choices.

Conventionally grown produce is grown with chemical fertilizers and pesticides. At present, most of the produce sold in the United States is conventionally grown.

Transitionally grown produce is grown without the use of chemical fertilizers and pesticides but comes from land that has not yet been certified for organic production. Most third-party verification programs require that the land has not received chemical applications for three years in order to qualify for organic certification. Transitional crops are grown by farmers who are switching from chemical-based agriculture to organic farming. This is usually a tough period for farmers, who must learn an entirely new way of managing soil, crops, and pests. When you buy transitionally grown produce you support those farmers who are making a change to sustainable agriculture.

Organically grown produce is certified to have

been grown without chemical fertilizers or pesticides. Certification is done by either independent organizations or state governments. While standards vary, the general rule for certification of crops as organically grown is that chemicals have not been applied to the field for three years. Because some agricultural chemicals linger in the soil, even certified organically grown crops can contain traces of some pesticides. In addition, some organic farms are situated near conventional farms and may receive "chemical drift" from aerial spraying or contaminated groundwater. Thus, organically grown fruits and vegetables cannot be considered "chemical free."

Organic farmers use soil-enriching techniques such as crop rotation and the application of composted organic matter such as waste crops, manure, leaves, and mulch. Pest management is accomplished by planting crops in alternating rows and by the use of natural predators such as ladybugs, wasps, and microbes.

Freshness: What to Look For

When you walk into the produce section of a grocery store, look for loose produce. You should be able to pick up individual fruits and vegetables rather than having to examine them through a cellophane wrapper. Prewrapping produce makes it difficult to inspect and increases the cost of goods.

Fresh fruits and vegetables are crisp, firm, and fully hydrated. They should not appear bruised, wilted, rotten, shriveled, molded, sprouting, mushy, blackened, cracked, split, flabby, or yellowing. Any produce with these features should be avoided.

How to Select Ripe Avocados, Mangoes, Melons, Pineapples

Although most people can select a fresh green pepper or a ripe peach, they find it more difficult to pick ripe avocados, mangoes, melons, and pineapples. How do you know when they are ready for the table?

The Myth of the Farm Stand

In the summer months, people go out of their way to get to a local farm stand where fresh fruits and vegetables are displayed in wooden baskets and crates. They go there because the produce seems fresher, crisper, maybe even grown on the spot. Or so they think. While there are still some farm stands that sell produce actually grown by their owner/operators, the truth is that many farm stands sell fruits and vegetables obtained from exactly the same wholesalers who service supermarkets.

The farm stand is an American tradition. A farmer's family grows produce for market and erects a simple wooden stand to sell a small portion of the crops directly to individuals. The farmer makes a little extra money and feels a greater sense of pride than when he sells to a large packing house. But today many farm stands are owned by business people, not farmers. There's nothing wrong with this, except that the implication is that what the farm stand sells is fresher or tastier than what is available in sterile supermarkets. Even farm stands that offer some crops grown by the owner may supplement their selection with other fruits and vegetables purchased from the local wholesaler. If you occasionally shop at a local farm stand, ask the owners whether they grow any of the food they sell. If they do, find out which items they grow and which they buy through a food wholesaler. You may choose to buy all your produce there, but at least you will know exactly what you are getting.

What You Can Do to Reduce Your Pesticide Risk

Although produce is the most heavily pesticide treated of the major food groups, there are some things you can do to reduce your risk of exposure to pesticide residues on fresh fruits and vegetables.

Buy Organically Grown Produce Whenever Possible Make sure that your grocer knows where the produce comes from and that it is certified by a reputable organic-certification program.

Wash All Produce Although many pesticides enter fruits and vegetables and cannot be washed away, others remain on the surface and can be washed off. No matter where it comes from or how it's grown, produce should be washed with water. Environmental groups and the Food and Drug Administration disagree on whether to use soapy water. My recommendation is that you not use soap on produce. You may wish to use a soft brush to scrub the outside of tough or fibrous fruits and vegetables.

Peel Produce By peeling fruits and vegetables you can eliminate surface residues of pesticides. The downside to this is that you also remove many of the valuable nutrients that are found in or under the peel.

Get Active! Don't wait for someone else to clean up the food system. Buy organic when you can. Talk with your neighbors, friends, and grocer. Help to make more people aware of the risks of exposure to toxic pesticide residues in produce. Additionally, write your senators and congresspersons to tell them you want a safer food system with decreased use of agricultural chemicals.

Avocados should be firm but somewhat soft when you apply gentle pressure. Very soft avocados are either overripe or rotten. A strong, musty smell indicates an avocado too far gone.

Mangoes will be firm, but soft to pressure all around. Some not-yet-ripe mangoes smell sweet; however, a mango with a slightly fermented smell is overripe.

Melons

Canary melons should be deep yellow. Light or very bright yellow means that the melon is unripe. When a ripe canary melon is shaken, the seeds will rattle.

Cantaloupe skins should be more beige than green. The stem end should yield slightly to gentle pressure and should smell sweet.

Cranshaws have a flat end that should yield to gentle pressure. The skin should be yellow, and the melon should smell sweet. A green skin indicates unripe fruit.

Honeydews should smell sweet. Sometimes, however, you cannot smell a sweet honeydew. Unripe honeydews have a greenish-white smooth skin. As the melons ripen, the skin tends to yellow and gets stickier or tackier. If you shake a ripe honeydew, you can hear the seeds rattle.

Watermelon can be tested for ripeness in this way: Hold a watermelon in your arm like a baby. With one hand, tap the bottom of the melon. You will feel the melon vibrate or ring. A dull thud usually indicates an overripe melon. A deep, full ring indicates a watermelon at its peak.

Pineapple stems should be more pink than green and should smell sweet. The leaves of a ripe pineapple will pull out easily.

A Calendar of Seasonal Produce

In-season fruits and vegetables should be your first choice whenever they are available. Out-of-season produce either has spent time in storage or is imported. In either case, the item will be less flavorful and/or more costly than when in season. Produce that can be found fresh all year long includes bananas, carrots, celery, coconuts, eggplants, garlic, ginger, kiwi, lemons, limes, cultivated mushrooms,

The Bionic Tomato

Has the Flavr-Savr tomato hit your supermarket yet? This product of biotechnology, which has genes that have been modified to retard spoilage and produce a supposedly superior flavor, was approved for distribution in the U.S. by the FDA in 1994 and in 1996 was approved for distribution in the U.K. as well.

Biotechnology is being used to "immunize" potatoes and other crops against disease and to improve the yields of third-world cash crops such as bananas, papayas, melons, and sweet potatoes. It's even been suggested that coffee plants can be genetically engineered to produce naturally decaffeinated beans.

Genetic engineering is not without its problems, however. Recently a tomato that had been combined with a fish gene to prevent spoilage was found to cause allergies in people allergic to fish. Vegetarians also objected. And the Flavr-Savr itself has been a mixed blessing for its manufacturer, Calgene. The tomato has suffered from thin skin that easily bruised on the way to market and that contributed to fast decay. Consumers have been unimpressed by the 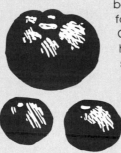 average price of $2.00 per pound. Explaining a net loss of $16,104,000 in the second half of 1995, Calgene stated that "Most of the early Flavr-Savr tomato varieties that Calgene had available for production did not have acceptable yield and disease resistance performance. Consequently, Calgene plans to temporarily limit its tomato growing operations beginning in the Spring of 1996 until it is able to complete its development of Flavr-Savr varieties that have enhanced commercial agronomic qualities."

Reading between the lines, one bioengineering analyst gives a more succinct summary of Calgene's situation: "This tomato has brought them to their knees."

onions, parsley, snow peas, pineapples, potatoes, radishes, scallions, sprouts, and watercress.

January Broccoli, Brussels sprouts, cabbage, Chinese cabbage, cauliflower, cherimoyas, chicory, fennel, grapefruit, uglifruit, leeks, mandarin oranges.

February Broccoli, Brussels sprouts, cauliflower, celery root, cherimoyas, grapefruit, uglifruit, leeks, sweet oranges, shallots.

March Artichokes, asparagus, avocados, beets, broccoli, cabbage, Chinese cabbage, cauliflower, celery root, chicory, chives, fennel, grapefruit, uglifruit, greens, leeks, head lettuce, leaf lettuce, okra, Seville oranges, parsnips, peas, rhubarb, shallots, spinach.

April Artichokes, asparagus, avocados, beans, beets, broccoli, cabbage, Chinese cabbage, cauliflower, celery root, chicory, chili peppers, chives, cucumbers, leeks, head lettuce, leaf lettuce, okra, sweet oranges, papaya, peas, peppers, rhubarb, shallots, spinach, summer squash, turnips.

May Artichokes, asparagus, avocados, basil, beans, beets, berries, broccoli, cabbage, Chinese cabbage, chives, cucumber, figs, head lettuce, leaf lettuce, mangoes, okra, sweet oranges, papaya, peas, peppers, rhubarb, shallots, sorrel, spinach, summer squash, turnips.

June Apricots, arugula, basil, beans, beets, berries, cabbage, cherries, chili peppers, chives, cucumbers, leaf lettuce, mangoes, okra, papaya, peppers, plums, sorrel, summer squash, watermelons.

July Apricots, arugula, basil, beans, beets, berries, cherries, chili peppers, corn, cucumber, grapes, mangoes, melons, nectarines, okra, peaches, peppers, plums, sorrel, summer squash, tomatoes, watermelons.

August Apricots, arugula, basil, beans, berries, cherries, chili peppers, corn, cucumbers, figs, grapes, mangoes, melons, okra, peaches, peppers, plums, sorrel, summer squash, tomatoes, watermelons.

September Arugula, beans, beets, berries, cabbage, Chinese cabbage, cauliflower, corn, cucumbers, dates, figs, grapes, head lettuce, leaf lettuce, mangoes, melons, wild mushrooms, okra, pears, shallots, sorrel, summer squash, tomatoes, watermelons.

Waxed and Shining

The Food and Drug Administration has registered several categories of waxes for topical use on apples, avocados, oranges, lemons, limes, grapefruit, melons, peaches, pineapples, passion fruits, cucumbers, eggplants, peppers, pumpkins, rutabagas, squash, tomatoes, sweet potatoes, turnips, and other fruits and vegetables. The produce-packing industry argues that waxes, which often contain chemical fungicides, are needed to reduce shrinkage from moisture loss and to inhibit the growth of molds and fungus. According to FDA regulations, retailers must label waxed produce. Few do, however, and the law is unenforced. The types of waxes currently in use on produce are these:

Carnauba Wax   Obtained from the wax palm of Brazil, carnauba is the hardest of the natural waxes. It is used widely in floor waxes, polishes, and lubricants.

Paraffin   A derivative of petroleum, paraffin is flammable and insoluble in water. It is used to make candles and for many industrial purposes.

Candelilla   Obtained from a reed, candelilla is a natural wax that is common in furniture polishes.

Shellac   Obtained from the bodies of the female scale insect *Tachardia lacca*, shellac is used as varnish, as a coating on wood and plaster, in electrical insulation, and in sealing wax.

Polyethylene   A plastic synthesized from petroleum, polyethylene is manufactured in sheets and films. Its many commercial uses include unbreakable bottles, shower curtains, electrical insulation, pipes, and packaging materials.

Oleic Acid   Obtained from vegetable oils, animal fats, or synthesized from petroleum, oleic acid is used in industrial lubricants.

Tallow   Obtained from the tissues and fatty deposits of animals, especially cattle and sheep, tallow is used in floor waxes, soap, and candles and as a lubricant.

Waxes cannot be washed off produce. If you want to avoid eating waxes, peel any produce that is waxed.

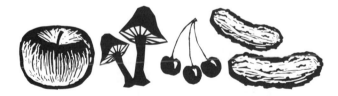

October   Apples, beets, broccoli, Brussels sprouts, cabbage, Chinese cabbage, cauliflower, celery root, chicory, chili peppers, cranberries, cucumbers, dates, fennel, figs, grapes, kumquats, leeks, head lettuce, leaf lettuce, wild mushrooms, okra, peppers, persimmons, pomegranates, prickly pears, quince, shallots, spinach, starfruit, sweet potatoes, winter squash.

November   Apples, broccoli, Brussels sprouts, cabbage, Chinese cabbage, cauliflower, celery root, chicory, cranberries, cucumbers, dates, fennel, grapes, greens, kumquats, leeks, head lettuce, leaf lettuce, wild mushrooms, mandarin oranges, sweet oranges, parsnips, pears, persimmons, pomegranates, prickly pears, quince, shallots, spinach, starfruit, sweet potatoes, winter squash.

December   Apples, broccoli, Brussels sprouts, cabbage, Chinese cabbage, cauliflower, celery root, cherimoyas, chicory, cranberries, dates, fennel, grapefruit, greens, kumquats, leeks, wild mushrooms, mandarin oranges, sweet oranges, parsnips, pears, persimmons, pomegranates, prickly pears, quince, shallots, spinach, starfruit, sweet potatoes, winter squash.

UNCOMMON VEGETABLES AND FRUITS

Thanks to better transportation, greater variety in farming, and an expanded public appetite for interesting and unusual foods, there is a growing interest in uncommon vegetables and fruits. These produce items are not necessarily more or less sprayed with pesticides than more pedestrian fare. For while there is concern that some imported produce items may contain residues or *illegal* pesticides, domestic produce often contains residues of *legal carcinogenic* pesticides. Either way, residues are potentially harmful. This is why organic produce should always be your first choice.

Pesticide caveat noted, the uncommon vegetables and fruits listed here are new tastes and are therefore worth sampling. This is not a complete list of uncommon produce but a short list of readily available uncommon items.

Uncommon Vegetables to Know and Eat

Arugula   A popular salad green in Spain, Italy, and France, arugula has dark green leaves, similar to those of the dandelion, and a pungent, hot flavor. This vegetable can make an ordinary salad special. Wash carefully to remove sand and grit, remove the root stem, and toss raw with salad greens.

Burdock Root   Native to Siberia, burdock is a long (1 to 2 feet) slender root vegetable with an earthy flavor. Scrub burdock but do not peel it, as the majority of nutrients and flavor are in or near the skin. Burdock takes about twice as long to cook as carrots. Add it to soups or stews, or cook it with grains. Burdock is a hearty winter food.

Bok Choy   Although it is mistakenly called Chinese cabbage, bok choy is in fact an entirely different vegetable. A cruciferous green, bok choy is related to the cauliflower, turnip, radish, and mustard green. A head of bok choy has pearly colored stalks with collardlike leaves. This Asian vegetable is a tasty addition to stir-fries.

Celery Root (*Celeriac*)   Used extensively in Holland, Russia, Germany, France, and Scandinavia, celery root is a tough, knobby root that comes from a variety of celery grown for its root instead of its stalks. It resembles parsley and celery in flavor and can be cooked like carrots or turnips, used in soups and purées, or grated raw into salads.

Daikon   Native to Asia, daikon is a foot-long white radish. It has a slightly hot taste that mixes well with salad greens. When cooked in soups or stews, it tastes slightly sweet. In Asia daikon is eaten shredded with sushi or sashimi, and pickled with other pungent vegetables and hot peppers.

Belgian Endive   During the 1988 presidential race, Massachusetts Governor Michael Dukakis almost ruined the reputation of Belgian endive forever when he suggested that midwestern farmers in dire straits consider planting this vegetable as a cash crop. Belgian endive, perceived to be a "yuppie food," seemed to be an elitist substitute for traditional, mainstream grain crops. Belgian endive is a member of the chicory family and looks like a cigar

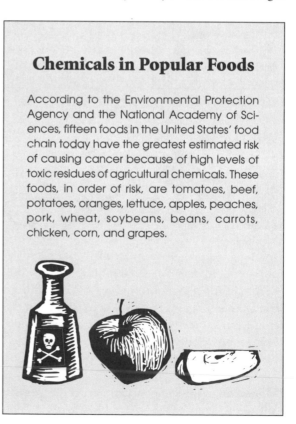

Chemicals in Popular Foods

According to the Environmental Protection Agency and the National Academy of Sciences, fifteen foods in the United States' food chain today have the greatest estimated risk of causing cancer because of high levels of toxic residues of agricultural chemicals. These foods, in order of risk, are tomatoes, beef, potatoes, oranges, lettuce, apples, peaches, pork, wheat, soybeans, beans, carrots, chicken, corn, and grapes.

made from pale yellow leaves. Its bitter flavor is a good contrast to milder-flavored lettuce in a salad.

Escarole   Another member of the chicory family, escarole has broad, coarse, flat leaves that are slightly bitter. Use it raw in salads or cook it briefly to mellow the bitter flavor.

Fennel   A compact greenish-white bulb that can be eaten raw or cooked in casseroles, salads, soups, stews, stuffings, and sausages, fennel has a unique licorice flavor and is cool, sweet, and refreshing.

Jicama   A light brown tuber grown in Mexico, jicama can be sautéed, boiled, or used raw in salads or dips. When raw, it has a crisp texture similar to that of an apple, with a somewhat sweet, refreshing flavor. It stays crisp when cooked. Peel the skin before use.

Jerusalem Artichoke   A relative of the sunflower, Jerusalem artichokes do not resemble artichokes but are brown-skinned roots that can be cooked like potatoes. They can be sautéed, boiled, baked, simmered in soups, eaten raw or in salads, or used as a substitute for water chestnuts.

Shiitake Mushroom   Originally from Asia, shiitake mushrooms have become popular in American cuisine. Shiitakes are large mushrooms with full flavor, herbaceous aroma, and meaty consistency. One or two shiitakes can impart a delicious flavor to soups, stews, and stir-fries.

Uncommon Fruits to Know and Eat

Asian Pear   The more than one hundred varieties of Asian pears are also known as nashi, apple pears, or Oriental pears. Asian pears are lightly sweet, have a granular texture, and are mild in flavor. They are crunchy, juicy, and ready to eat even though they may seem overly hard when you squeeze them. The more fragrant the Asian pear, the more flavorful it will be. Asian pears are rather expensive, but most people find the taste worth the cost.

Blood Orange   While very popular in Europe where they originate, blood oranges are still a novelty item in the United States. So named because their flesh can be scarlet or purple in color, blood oranges have a full-bodied citrus flavor with a raspberry aftertaste. A glass of blood orange juice looks like a glass of burgundy.

Carambola   Known also as starfruit, carambola is a native of Asia, where it is widely cultivated. This glossy yellow fruit has a waxy-looking exterior and five longitudinal wings that form star shapes when sliced. Sometimes it is difficult to tell on purchase whether a carambola is sweet or sour, but either way it is delicious. Look for skin that is yellow, not green, and a fruity, floral fragrance that indicates ripeness. When fully ripe, a carambola tastes like a combination of plums, grapes, and apples.

Cherimoya   Also called a custard apple, the cherimoya is native to South America and has a lizardlike leathery exterior. The flesh inside is smooth, silky, and exotically flavorful, like a combination of tropical fruits and vanilla custard.

Clementine   This sweet, seedless mandarin orange is reputed to be an accidental hybrid discovered in Algiers about 1900. Thin-skinned and easy to peel, clementines are much more succulent than standard varieties of tangerines and have a pronounced tangy flavor. Clementines are so small and tasty that you can eat ten of them before you snap out of the hypnotic spell induced by this sweet citrus.

Durian   Native to Southeast Asia, the durian is perhaps the most bizarre and enigmatic of all fruits. Although durians are not commonly available, you should know about them in the unlikely event you find one. The durian is about the size of a football, heavy, dense, and covered with sharp, hard spikes. If you are walking through a durian grove and one falls on your head, you will swiftly be relieved of your mortal fetters. Durians come into season briefly in May and are a highly coveted addicting substance to natives of Southeast Asia. Peace Corps volunteers stationed in Micronesia have been known to squander their entire month's allowance on durians when they are available. If you are lucky, you may find a durian in a large urban Chinatown during about two weeks in May. Expect to pay a fortune for it—perhaps as much as $25.

The cause of all the fuss is the durian's inner flesh. It is soft, creamy, and custardlike. The fragrance of a durian is overwhelming; it reeks of exotic tropical fruits, perfumes, onions, and rotting garbage. The taste is a creamy explosion of fruits and garbage. If you find one, buy it without hesitation, take it home, cut it open, and eat it. You may love the durian; you may not. But you will never forget the experience.

Feijoa A native of South America but cultivated in New Zealand, the feijoa, or pineapple guava, is an elongated, egg-shaped fruit with a granular, medium-soft flesh surrounding a seedy interior. The taste is tart and the scent perfumed. A feijoa can be eaten like an avocado, or cooked or puréed.

Kumquat Chinese in origin, the kumquat is about $1^1/_2$ inches long. It is thought by many to be a member of the citrus family, which it is not. It looks like a small citrus fruit and tastes like an orange, but with the kumquat you eat the skin as well as the flesh. Eating a kumquat is an amazing gustatory experience. You put the entire fruit in your mouth and bite right through it. The first sensation is a face-puckering sourness that causes rivulets of saliva to gush liberally in your mouth. As you continue to chew, the initial shock of sourness is replaced by the sweetness of the rind, which comes on stronger the longer you chew. Eating a kumquat is not just a taste treat; it is an experience. It grabs you by the ankles, turns you upside down, and shakes the change out of your pockets. Since kumquats are eaten with the skin on, select organically grown kumquats when they are available, to avoid pesticide residues.

Mango A native of Southeast Asia, the mango has been cultivated for five thousand years. The skin of the mango is smooth and is red, yellow, or green in color. The red to yellow flesh is moist and custardlike (or fibrous), with a tropical peach flavor. In India, which is the largest producer of mangoes, these fruits are eaten plain, cooked in curries, in yogurt drinks, and as spicy mango pickle, a popular condiment. A ripe mango is somewhat soft, with a pleasant fruit scent.

Papaya Native to the tropics, papayas are green or yellow skinned. The small Hawaiian papaya (the kind most frequently available in grocery stores) is

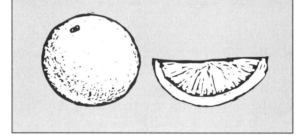

Don't Eat Citrus Peels!

Lemon peels and lime wedges add flavor to sparkling water, iced tea, and mixed drinks. Orange and lemon zests are often grated to use in dessert and other dishes. But unless you're using strictly organically grown citrus, you are advised to skip using citrus peels altogether.

Citrus crops are liberally sprayed with a wide variety of potentially carcinogenic pesticides, according to the Environmental Protection Agency. These chemicals include acephate, benomyl, chlorobenzilate, dicofol, methomyl, ophenylphenol, and parathion. Even washing the skins of citrus thoroughly will not remove all the toxic chemicals. Either buy organic or get used to drinking your sparkling water straight up.

shaped like an avocado, but the larger varieties are melon-sized and can weigh up to 20 pounds each. The flesh of a papaya can be red, orange, or yellow and is sweet, light, and refreshing. The inside cavity is filled with small edible seeds. A ripe papaya will yield to gentle pressure.

Persimmon Although the fruit is native to China, the word *persimmon* comes from the Algonquin Indians. Looking somewhat like a tomato with a lacquered orange skin, the persimmon has a mild flavor suggestive of pumpkin and plum. A ripe persimmon is a rich orange color, with no yellow. The fruit should feel very soft, as though liquid inside. Plan for a delicious but messy eating experience with a persimmon.

Plantain A staple starch in Asia, the Caribbean, and much of the Southern Hemisphere, the plantain is a green cooking banana. The light pink or yellow fruit of the plantain is fried, boiled, baked, and mashed into fritters and cakes. Plantains are versatile and delicious.

Pomegranate Believed to have originated in Persia, the pomegranate is the size of a small grapefruit, with a red, leathery skin. You do not eat a pomegranate quickly, as there is some work to do to get at the fruit. The interior contains tough, membranous compartments filled with arils, or seeds, surrounded by a succulent, scarlet-colored pulp. The taste of the pulp is sweet, sour, light, and refreshing. Look for large, heavy fruits.

Quince Another Persian fruit, the quince is similar in shape to a pear and must be cooked to be eaten. Quince has a distinctive musky, fruity perfume. The fruit contains a high amount of pectin, and so is used in jellies, jams, marmalades, and confections. Quince can be baked, stewed, or poached.

Uglifruit From Jamaica comes this strange citrus, which looks like a grapefruit with a green, loose-fitting skin. Truly ugly, it is the sharpei of citrus. Uglifruit is easy to peel and tastes like a cross between a grapefruit and a mandarin orange, with a mouth-watering acid sweetness.

DRIED FRUITS

Dried fruits are among the most popular items in natural food stores. Sweet and nutritious, with a rich, concentrated flavor, dried fruits are an excellent source of quick energy and make ideal snack foods, especially for children, who will often eat dried fruits in place of sugar-laden candies. Dried fruits store well and will last for months in airtight containers. These high-energy foods are perfect for snacking, picnics, camping, and backpacking.

Dried fruit costs far less than the same quantity of fresh fruit and thus is an excellent bargain. Nine pounds of fresh apples become 1 pound when dried. Six pounds of fresh apricots or 3 pounds of fresh plums (which become prunes) become 1 pound dried. Many types of dried fruits are available, but most of them are still conventionally grown with agricultural chemicals. Thus, dried fruits will contain pesticide residues, just like their fully hydrated counterparts. For this reason, you should purchase organically produced dried fruits whenever possible.

The Sulfur Dioxide Hazard

From a health standpoint, the biggest concern about dried fruit is whether or not it has been treated with sulfur dioxide, which keeps fruit moist and colorful. A sulfured apricot will be plump and bright orange, and an unsulfured apricot will be dry and brown. Over the past several years there has been growing concern about sulfur dioxide. This chemical compound can cause serious allergic reactions, particularly among asthmatics. In some rare cases, consuming sulfur dioxide has led to anaphylaxis, an extreme allergic reaction that can cause respiratory failure. In addition to its allergenic properties, sulfur dioxide destroys B vitamins in the body, can cause kidney malfunction, and is a suspected mutagen (a substance that causes genetic mutations, or abnormalities). Not good. As of 1987, federal law requires a label on all food products containing sulfur dioxide.

Drying Methods

Although most producers allow fruits to ripen to full maturity for maximum sugar content, size, and flavor, drying processes differ greatly between large commercial packers and smaller natural food producers. Large commercial outfits typically sun-dry or oven-dry fruit first, then soak and steam it at high temperatures in order to increase the weight and size. The fruit is then preserved. This process destroys many of the vitamins in the fruit. Smaller natural producers wash fruits and then dry them in the sun or in low-temperature dehydrators. The fruit is not steamed or preserved. This process yields a sweeter, firmer, darker, and tastier product.

In order for natural nutrients to be retained, drying should be accomplished quickly. Even though sun-drying is a natural process, it will destroy more of the vitamins in a fruit than the faster oven-drying method. The speed at which a fruit will dry depends on the amount of heat and ventilation. Fruits dry more quickly if they are on drying racks designed for fast evaporation. The trick in drying fruit is to achieve the right balance of heat, ventilation, and time.

Extra Sweetness

Some producers dip or soak dried fruits in honey for extra sweetness and to lock in more moisture. Honey-dipped dried fruits will be labeled as such. Be on the lookout, however, for mislabeled sugar-dipped dried fruits. These impostors are usually fairly easy to detect. They have a super-sweet bite to them and granular sugar crystals on the outside. There is really no need to sweeten a dried fruit with either honey or sugar, because most dried fruits contain at least 25 percent naturally occurring sugars.

Rehydration

Dried fruits are dehydrated; the water has been evaporated out of them. Dried fruits will rehydrate, or reabsorb water, as they are digested. When you eat dried fruits, be sure to drink water or juice with them. Otherwise the fruits will absorb moisture from your digestive tract. The consumption of dried fruits without adequate fluid intake can lead to stomach cramps, bloating, and gas.

Commonly Available Dried Fruits

Following are some of the most widely available dried fruits:

Apples High in magnesium, iron, potassium, and pectin, dried apples enhance digestion. Apples are peeled, cored, and sliced and then placed in a dehydrator to dry.

Apricots Known as the "aristocrat of fruits," apricots have a short harvest season and are among the most delectable of all fruits. They are a staple food in some parts of the world, including the legendary Himalayan kingdom of Hunza, north of Kashmir. The natives of Hunza, the Hunzakuts, are the longest-lived people in the world. Apricot oil is highly prized for its fineness and superb nutrient content. Dried apricots are rich in iron, phosphorous, calcium, and vitamin A.

Bananas A good dried banana is hard to find. Dried bananas come mostly in the form of chips, made from sliced green bananas, which are usually cooked in coconut oil and then dried. Banana chips aren't sweet. However, there are plenty of sugar-coated chips on the market, and a few that are honey-sweetened. Much harder to find than chips are dried whole ripe bananas. These come mostly from Costa Rica or other Central American countries and are small, rubbery, sweet, and very tasty. Dried whole bananas, especially if they are organically grown, are well worth searching for. They are quite a treat. Bananas are particularly high in potassium.

Currants Smaller and darker than raisins, but similar in appearance, currants are sweet and high in iron. Dried currants are excellent in baked goods, especially muffins.

Cherries High in vitamins A and B_1, iron, copper, and manganese, dried cherries are tangy and relatively hard to find. They are a reputed folk remedy for gout.

Coconuts This fruit has developed a bad reputation over the past few years because it contains a high concentration of saturated fat. Nonetheless, dried coconut is widely used in granolas, baked goods, and confections. Naturally dried coconut is not sweet; it has a nutlike flavor. Avoid sweetened dried coconut products that have been soaked in sugar solutions or corn syrup.

Dates Containing the highest natural sugar content of any fruit in the world, dates are also rich in vitamins A and B_1, magnesium, and phosphorous. There exist more than four hundred known varieties, from small brown dates to super-fancy jumbo Medjools. The Date Festival in Indio, California, is an annual event at which the finest specimens of hundreds of date varieties are displayed and sampled.

Figs High in iron, calcium, phosphorus, vitamin B_1, vitamin B_2, niacin, and folic acid, figs are renowned for their sweetness and flavor. There are many varieties of figs, among the most popular of which are Turkish and mission figs. Figs have more iron than spinach. This, combined with their high folic acid content, makes them an excellent food for combating anemia. They also contain isatin, a natural laxative.

Peaches Dried peaches are high in vitamins A, B_1, and C; magnesium; potassium; and iron. There are dozens of varieties, so you will find many different tastes among dried peaches.

Pears High in vitamin B_1, magnesium, and potassium, dried pears have a grainy, leathery consistency. Despite the fact that they have a texture like iguana skin, they are very tasty.

Papayas Dried papaya that has not been sweetened has very little flavor. Most alleged honey sweetened papaya is actually soaked in a sugar solution, although a few honest honey-sweetened papaya products are available. Dried papaya comes in long finger-shaped slices.

Pineapples The majority of dried pineapple comes from Taiwan and is saturated with refined white sugar. Authentic natural dried pineapple is sweetened with pineapple juice instead. The two are easy to tell apart. Sugar-sweetened pineapple is plump and firm, and coated with sugar crystals. Juice-sweetened pineapple is somewhat mottled and fibrous, with no crystals on the surface.

Raisins High in iron and minerals, raisins are the most popular of all the dried fruits. This is mainly due to their size and versatility, as they can be added to cereals, baked goods, breads, and other foods. Although almost all raisins are sun-dried, most are also fumigated with methyl bromide, which can depress the central nervous system. It is therefore wise to look for natural raisins that have not been fumigated.

These days organically grown raisins are plentiful. Most raisins are dried Thompson seedless grapes, but there are also monukka and muscat raisins, which are considerably more flavorful. Of all the foods in the world, raisins are the most cariogenic. That is, they are the No. 1 cavity-causing food, ahead of pure sugar and chocolate. This is due to their high sugar content and the fact that they are very sticky. The sugars in raisins adhere to the enamel of the teeth. When you eat raisins, be sure to brush your teeth afterward.

8

DAIRY PRODUCTS: MILK, CHEESE, AND EGGS

airy products are foods made from milk. Because eggs and margarine are stored in the grocer's dairy case, however, we have included them in this section as well. It is impossible to know when humans started to eat dairy products. Cows, goats, sheep, and yaks have been raised and kept for their milk for thousands of years. Today, the cow is the primary milk-producing animal worldwide, and the international dairy industry is built on the output of this friendly animal. Except where otherwise noted, any mention of milk here refers to cow's milk.

MILK AND MILK PRODUCTS

The U.S. Food and Drug Administration calls milk "one of the best controlled, inspected, and monitored of all food commodities." Truly, the milk industry is more carefully monitored by federal and state health authorities than any other food-related industry.

Whole milk is approximately 87 percent water and 13 percent solids, which include fat, protein, carbohydrates, vitamins, and minerals. The daily output of a dairy cow ranges from about 12 to 25 quarts of milk. Holstein cows, which are among the most prolific milk manufacturers, can produce 40 quarts daily. The most milk produced by a single cow on a regular basis is 60 quarts per day!

Unless it is certified raw, milk typically undergoes three specific processes: pasteurization, homogenization, and fortification.

Pasteurization is the heating of milk at 161°F or above for fifteen seconds to destroy any pathogenic, or harmful, bacteria that may be present. Pasteurization destroys yeasts, molds, and almost all nonpathogenic bacteria as well as enzymes that promote spoilage. Thus, pasteurization makes milk a safer product and extends its shelf life.

Ultra-pasteurization is the heating of milk at 280°F for at least two seconds to ensure the total destruction of virtually all microorganisms. Ultra-pasteurization further extends the shelf life of milk while reducing its nutritional value somewhat, as the high heat can destroy vitamins. This process is used primarily with cream products.

Homogenization is a process by which the fat

Bovine Growth Hormone: Just Say Moo!

According to the Monsanto Corporation, cows are now living better through chemistry, pumping out as much as 25 percent more milk per day. This is thanks to recombinant bovine growth hormone (rBGH, also known as recombinant bovine somatotropin or rBST). This genetically engineered hormone is similar to one secreted in the pituitary glands of cows that plays an important role in milk production.

Though Monsanto and the Food and Drug Administration insist that rBGH is not biologically active in people, there is still great concern about its safety. Milk from cows treated with rBGH has a slightly higher level of insulin-like growth factor (IGF-1), the protein responsible for growth. A study in the January 1996 issue of the *International Journal of Health Services* concluded that consuming milk from cows treated with rBGH increased one's risk of breast and colon cancer. Other studies have shown that IGF-1 is associated with glucose intolerance, hypertension, and swollen limbs. Cows given rBGH are subject to mastitis, and their milk is more likely to contain residues of antibiotics.

The National Farmers Union, several midwestern state legislatures, and many commercial dairies did not want rBGH approved. In 1988 the European Parliament recommended that

meat and milk from animals administered this drug should not be fed to people or animals. The Netherlands has banned further research on the drug, and three Canadian provinces (Ontario, British Columbia, and Alberta) have followed suit. The FDA, on the other hand, which bows constantly to commercial interests, approved the drug.

The result is big profits for Monsanto but almost certain economic homicide for many of the nation's dairy farmers. Use of the drug increases milk production, decreases milk prices, escalates veterinary costs, and may well force a large percentage of small- to medium-sized dairy farmers out of business.

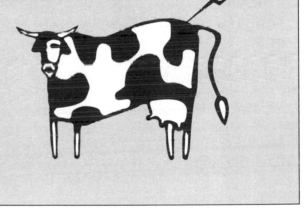

globules in milk are emulsified by mechanical means until they become so tiny that they remain suspended evenly throughout the product, thus maintaining uniform consistency. Homogenization is not required by law, but most milk sold commercially is homogenized. In nonhomogenized milk, the cream rises to form a layer on the surface.

Fortification is the addition of nutrients, notably vitamins A and D. These vitamins are added to milk in the form of concentrates. If fortified, milk must contain not less than 2,000 international units (IU) of vitamin A and 400 IU of vitamin D per quart. These amounts must be stated on the label.

The supplements used to fortify milk are synthetically manufactured and usually contain antioxidant preservatives.

Besides vitamins supplied by fortification, the primary nutritional factors in milk include protein, fat, carbohydrates, and calcium.

Protein accounts for about 38 percent of the nonfat solids of milk. The primary protein in milk, 82 percent of it, is casein, which contains all the essential amino acids. The essential amino acids are not manufactured by the body and must be obtained from dietary sources. Whey proteins make up the remaining 18 percent of milk protein. The proteins in milk are high in quality and play an important role in building and repairing body tissue and in forming antibodies, hormones, and enzymes.

Fat. Whole milk contains at least 3.25 percent milk fat. The composition of milk fat includes over five hundred various fatty acids, about 66 percent of which are saturated. These fats are a source of concentrated energy and are readily metabolized by the body. Milk fat, however, is also a source of dietary cholesterol. An eight-ounce serving of whole milk contains 33 milligrams of cholesterol as well as 150 calories. Because of its fat and cholesterol content, whole milk is to be avoided by dieters or those with a high blood cholesterol count.

Carbohydrate/Lactose. The primary carbohydrate in milk is lactose, otherwise known as milk sugar. Lactose accounts for about 55 percent of the total nonfat solids in milk. Lactose is a source of energy and promotes the growth of beneficial bacteria in the intestinal tract. About 20 percent of the U.S. population, however, is lactose intolerant. These individuals lack sufficient lactase, the enzyme that breaks lactose down into its component sugars. Common symptoms of lactose intolerance are stomach cramps, bloating, and diarrhea. The test to determine whether an individual is lactose intolerant involves measuring the amount of hydrogen expired in the breath after the person has ingested a quantity of lactose. Lactose intolerance is more common among blacks and Asians than among whites. To help with this problem, there are lactose-digesting enzyme products, in liquid and in tablet form, available in natural food stores. There are also some lactase-fortified milk products.

Storage and Handling

To keep milk products as fresh and usable as possible, observe the following guidelines:

- When shopping, pick up milk just before proceeding to the cash register.
- Store milk in a refrigerator at not more than 39°F.
- Use milk before the date code on the package.
- Keep milk products out of the direct light, as light depletes their nutritional value and alters their taste.
- Keep milk containers closed to prevent the absorption of odors from other foods.
- Serve milk cold.
- Return milk to the refrigerator immediately after use.

Categories of Milk and Milk Products

CERTIFIED RAW MILK

In many states you can buy certified raw milk, which is not pasteurized but is regulated by the stringent standards of the American Association of Medical Milk Commissions. The production of certified raw milk involves regular veterinary examination of cows, sanitary inspection of milk production facilities, and medical examination of employees working at the dairy. These standards ensure a safe, wholesome product.

Dioxin in Milk

In the summer of 1988, Canadian scientist John Ryan determined that a form of dioxin called TCDD, which is found in cardboard milk cartons, migrates into the milk. Dioxin, the most potent cancer-causing agent known, gets into paper products during the chlorine bleaching process. The EPA says that 1 part per trillion of TCDD poses an unacceptable cancer risk. Avoid cardboard cartons whenever possible.

Goat's Milk

Often preferred by health enthusiasts, goat's milk is sometimes tolerated well by those who cannot tolerate cow's milk. Goat's milk contains 165 calories and 10 grams of fat per cup, compared with whole cow's milk at 150 calories and 7.75 grams of fat per cup. The fat globules in goat's milk tend to be smaller than those in cow's milk, which may contribute to enhanced digestibility. Goat's milk is deficient in both vitamin B$_{12}$ and folic acid but contains more vitamin A and calcium than cow's milk. Goat's milk has no "goaty" odor or taste if properly refrigerated after milking.

Low-Fat Milk

Low-fat milk contains milk fat ranging from 0.5 to 2.0 percent. To be shipped interstate, low-fat milk must be pasteurized and fortified with vitamin A.

Skim Milk

Skim milk is milk that has had as much fat removed as is possible by current methods. Pasteurization and fortification requirements are identical to those of low-fat milk.

Low-Sodium Milk

This is milk that has had approximately 95 percent of its naturally occurring sodium removed by ion exchange. It is pasteurized and homogenized.

Flavored Milk

Milk can be sold flavored, colored, and sweetened. Most flavored milks are sweetened with refined sugar. Some small dairies, however, make chocolate milk with whole cocoa and Sucanat or some other unrefined sweetener. Chocolate milk naturally contains approximately 5 milligrams caffeine and as much as 99 milligrams theobromine (a caffeine-related alkaloid with diuretic and stimulant qualities) per cup.

Eggnog

Eggnog contains milk products (usually milk and cream), eggs, and some sort of sweetener. It can also

Low-Cholesterol Milk?

While whole milk contains approximately 532 milligrams of cholesterol per gallon, researchers at Cornell University have developed a process to reduce cholesterol in milk to just 40 milligrams per gallon. Dr. Syed Rizvi and his associates inject carbon dioxide into butterfat at high pressure. The butterfat, which is high in cholesterol, is removed from the milk, manipulated to extract much of the cholesterol, and then added back into the milk. The result is a much-lower-cholesterol milk with 2 percent butterfat, which tastes like any other 2 percent milk. The dairy industry is taking a serious look at low-cholesterol milk as the possible health wave of the future. Does this process destroy nutrients or otherwise harm milk? We don't yet know.

contain artificial or natural flavors, artificial colors, stabilizers, added butterfat, and salt. Some small dairies do make a "clean" eggnog at holiday time, using only milk, cream, eggs, and a natural sweetener such as honey, with a touch of vanilla. Eggnog must be pasteurized. It is absurdly high in fat and calories and typically delicious.

Evaporated Milk and Evaporated Skim Milk

Milk is evaporated by heating, stabilizing the proteins, and concentrating the product in a vacuum to remove 60 percent of the water. It is then fortified and canned. Total milk fat is not less than 7.5 percent, and milk solids are not less than 25 percent. Evaporated milk must be homogenized and must contain 25 international units of vitamin D per fluid ounce.

Evaporated skim milk is skim milk that has undergone the same process. It contains not less than 20 percent milk solids, and not more than 0.5 percent milk fat. It does not need to be homogenized, but it must contain 125 IU of vitamin A and 25 IU of vitamin D per fluid ounce. Evaporated milk is not sweetened but is highly processed.

SWEETENED CONDENSED MILK

This is evaporated milk with sugar added and is not a particularly healthy product.

BUTTERMILK

Buttermilk originally was a by-product of the arduous manual butter-churning process. Known to have been consumed for more than five thousand years, buttermilk is now a cultured milk product. Buttermilk is typically made with lowfat or skim milk, which is pasteurized at 185° to 190°F and then cooled to 70° to 72°F. After cooling, cultured bacteria are added to the milk. These include *Streptococcus lactis, Streptococcus cremoris, Leuconostoc citrovorum,* and *Leuconostoc dextranicum* bacteria. The mixture is then incubated for about twelve hours at 68° to 72°F until the bacterium has converted some of the lactose into lactic acid, which gives buttermilk its characteristic tangy taste. The milk is then stirred and cooled to halt fermentation. Buttermilk may contain salt and stabilizers. Read the label.

ACIDOPHILUS MILK

Acidophilus milk is milk cultured with *Lactobacillus acidophilus,* a friendly bacterium that helps to maintain intestinal flora. Acidophilus milk has a slightly acid flavor and is typically drunk to enhance digestion.

NONFAT DRY MILK

This is pasteurized skim milk with all the water removed. The water is removed by either jet-spraying the milk into hot air or jet-spraying hot air into the milk.

LACTASE MILK

This is milk to which lactase, the enzyme that breaks down lactose (milk sugar) into usable component sugars, is added. Lactase milk is useful for those who are lactose intolerant.

YOGURT

One of the oldest fermented milk products known, yogurt is produced by heating milk to destroy harmful bacteria, cooling the milk down, and adding the live cultures *Lactobacillus bulgaricus* and *Streptococcus thermophilus.* These cultures aid digestion, make milk more digestible for those who suffer from lactose intolerance, stimulate the immune system, and combat diarrhea.

While all yogurts are made with live bacterial cultures, some yogurts are pasteurized after being cultured, thus destroying those bacteria. The World Health Organization and the Food and Agriculture Organization specify that yogurts must contain live, active cultures. In the United States, however, a product may be called yogurt even if the bacteria have been destroyed by pasteurization. You don't want yogurt with dead cultures. Yogurt that has not been pasteurized after culturing will state on the label: "with active yogurt cultures," "living yogurt cultures," or "contains active cultures." If a yogurt label doesn't say this, then assume that the bacteria in that product are dead. Yogurt may contain additives, including nonfat dry milk, sweeteners, flavorings, fruit preservatives or purées, colorings, and stabilizers, including gelatin. If you are buying flavored yogurt, look for a product with live cultures, with a natural sweetener and fruit only. Avoid yogurts that contain artificial colors and flavors.

Yogurt with live cultures is valuable for those who have taken antibiotics. Antibiotics destroy important intestinal bacteria, and yogurt helps to replenish them.

KEFIR

Another cultured milk product, kefir has been in use for thousands of years in the Caucasus mountains in Russian Georgia, whence this marvelous drink originates. Kefir is made by inoculating heated milk with kefir grains, which are made from insoluble milk caseins removed from previous batches of kefir. Kefir is high in B vitamins, enhances digestion, and restores intestinal flora. Kefir is sold plain or flavored. As with yogurt, look for kefir that contains active cultures without artificial additives.

BUTTER

Butter is made from milk from which the cream is separated and churned, and contains not less than 80 percent milk fat by weight. It may be salted or unsalted. Butter has come under fire over the past several years because of its high fat and cholesterol content. One tablespoon of butter contains 36 milligrams of cholesterol. Although eating a lot of butter can be a direct route to a fat, cholesterol-laden body, butter is still better for you than margarine. If you want a spread for a piece of toast, use a small amount of butter. If you are used to cooking with butter, try using a very small amount of butter mixed with olive oil.

MARGARINE

This pseudo-butter was originally made from lard but is now typically made from hydrogenated vegetable oils. Hydrogenation is a process by which hydrogen is added to oils to turn them solid. This creates a saturated fat, which is the type of fat that causes the body to produce cholesterol. Margarine, which often contains artificial flavors and preservatives, offers no advantages over butter. Although heavily promoted on television as though it were healthful manna from heaven, margarine contains the same amount of calories as butter and may actually cause the body to produce more cholesterol than can be obtained from an equal amount of butter. This is because margarine is full of trans-fatty acids, which are by-products of the hydrogenation process. Recent studies have shown that trans-fatty acids raise the risk of heart disease even more than do the saturated fats in meat and dairy products. In 1994 two Harvard scientists announced that "Transfatty acids are so dangerous they should be eliminated altogether. These fats contribute to 30,000 U.S. deaths from coronary heart disease each year."

The only reason a person should select margarine over butter is if that individual is eating a strict vegetarian or kosher diet. Otherwise, margarine is a product that makes no sense.

CRÈME FRAÎCHE

This is a heavy, cultured cream with a delicate, tart flavor. Definitely not a weight-watcher's food, crème fraîche can be made at home by whisking together equal parts of heavy cream and sour cream. Chill the mixture in the refrigerator for about 24 hours or until it is thick. Crème fraîche is delightful spooned over fresh fruit, mixed into vegetables, or added to salad dressings.

CREAM

Cream is the fat layer of whole milk. Commercial cream contains not less than 18 percent milk fat. It is separated from liquid milk and may be adjusted with added milk, dry milk, skim milk, concentrated skim milk, or nonfat dry milk. Cream, in all of its various forms, is a very high-fat food and should be used (if at all) in moderation.

HALF-AND-HALF

This is a mixture of cream and milk. Half-and-half contains not less than 10.5 percent milk fat, but less than 18 percent. It must be pasteurized or ultra-pasteurized. Homogenization is optional.

LIGHT CREAM

Light cream contains between 18 and 30 percent milk fat. It is pasteurized or ultra-pasteurized. Homogenization is optional.

LIGHT WHIPPING CREAM

Containing between 30 and 36 percent milk fat, whipping cream is typically ultra-pasteurized. Homogenization is optional. Whipping cream may contain additives, so read the label.

HEAVY CREAM

Heavy cream, also used for whipping, must contain at least 36 percent milk fat. It is pasteurized or ultra-pasteurized. Homogenization is optional.

SOUR CREAM

This is cream that has been pasteurized and cultured with *Streptococcus lactis.* Cultured sour cream contains not less than 18 percent milk fat.

CREAM CHEESE

This is a pasteurized cultured cream product. At 37 percent milk fat by weight, cream cheese is so high in fat and cholesterol that you can almost feel it pumping like thick sludge into your arteries as you eat it. You can eat it on bagels or just apply it directly to your hips and abdomen. Eat it once in a blue moon, but not more often.

ICE CREAM

Containing 10 percent or more milk fat by weight, ice cream is one of America's favorite snack foods. However, many commercial brands contain artificial flavors, including some bizarre additives that are believed to cause health problems. Virtually all ice creams are loaded with refined sugar. Though you can obtain ice cream with unrefined sweeteners, from a nutritional standpoint it doesn't matter much whether your ice cream is sweetened with honey or refined sugar. In either case, the product will still be high in fat and calories. Look for brands that use all-natural ingredients for flavoring, including fruits and nuts. You should definitely steer clear of artificial additives.

FROMAGE BLANC

A fresh spreadable cheese with a flavor between cheese and yogurt, fromage blanc has 36 milligrams of sodium, 20 calories, and just 0.05 grams of fat per ounce. By government standards, fromage blanc is a non-fat food.

CHEESE

One of the most popular foods in the world, cheese comes in more than two thousand varieties, many of them named after the locale from which they originated. Roquefort, France, is the village in which a cheese with visible veins of blue-green mold was first made. Stilton, England, and Gorgonzola, Italy, are both known for their distinguished cheeses.

Cheese is a fresh or matured product made by draining whey after coagulating casein, the primary milk protein. Various kinds of milk are used in cheese making. Skim milk is used to make cottage cheese, whole milk is used to make Cheddars, and a variety of cheeses are made from goat's milk and sheep's milk. The coagulation of milk casein is accomplished with milk-clotting enzymes, or by acid from microorganisms. The resulting curd is then cut, heated, drained, and salted.

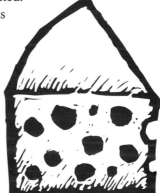

Uncured cheese, such as cottage cheese, can be eaten right away. Ripened cheeses, however, are exposed to specific temperatures and degrees of humidity for varying periods of time. They are often further modified by the action of specific enzymes, yeasts, and molds to produce the specific desired characteristics and texture of the final product. With all of its subtle manipulations, cheese making is a highly sophisticated science. Cheese is the wine of milk products.

Cheese in the Diet

It can take as much as nine or ten pints of milk to make a single pound of cheese. This makes cheese a concentrated source of calcium, protein, vitamin A, and riboflavin. Unfortunately, this also makes cheese a concentrated source of fat and cholesterol. An ounce of Cheddar cheese has about 9 grams of saturated fat and contains about 110 calories. Because cheese is cured with a great deal of salt, it is also usually a concentrated source of sodium. Just one ounce of Cheddar cheese can contain 200 milligrams of sodium. Due to the high fat, cholesterol, and sodium value of most cheeses, cheese should be eaten in moderation rather than as a staple food.

Fat Labeling

Be observant of fat claims on cheeses. Just because a cheese label says "lower fat" or "reduced fat" does not mean that the actual fat content is low. These delineations mean only that the particular cheese product at hand is lower in fat than the original version. A Havarti cheese with its fat content reduced from 60 percent to 55 percent can be labeled "lower fat," but it is still a high-fat food. Additionally, be wary of labels that read "made with part skim milk." The cheese may also contain a high quantity of cream.

Even if a cheese is "lower fat," a majority of the calories in that product will still come from fat. Gram for gram, fat contains twice the calories of protein or carbohydrates. More than 66 percent of the calories in a cheese with a 50 percent fat content will come from fat, most of which is saturated.

Look for the fat content on cheese labels whenever available, and remember that each gram of fat contains 9 calories.

Categories of Cheese

Semifirm Cheese These are dense and firm in texture. Cheddar, gruyère, and swiss are examples. These cheeses are good for melting.

Soft-ripened Cheeses These have a white crust on the exterior and ripen from the exterior to the interior. Soft-ripened cheeses should be ivory colored inside, with a smooth, buttery texture. If the crust develops an ammoniated scent, then the cheese is overripe and should be discarded. Brie and Camembert are the best known of the soft-ripened cheeses.

Semisoft Cheeses Similar to soft-ripened cheeses but firmer. Havarti, Provolone, and Edam are examples.

Double-Crèmes To qualify as a double-crème according to French law, a cheese must contain at least 60 percent butterfat. These cheeses are particularly smooth, creamy, and rich. There are many double-crème Bries.

Triple-Crèmes These cheeses contain at least 75 percent butterfat, making them the fattiest of all cheeses. Explorateur and St-André are the two best-known triple-crèmes. These cheeses are rich and creamy beyond compare, with a consistency close to that of pure butter.

Specialty and "Diet" Cheeses With an increasing awareness of fat, cholesterol, and sodium in the diet, consumers are looking for more healthful cheeses. Some lower-fat, reduced-sodium cheeses are available, including Lorraine Swiss, New Holland, and salt-free Gouda.

Grating Cheeses These are hard cheeses with a grainy texture. Romano cheese, made from sheep's milk, and Parmesan are the best-known grating cheeses.

Blue-veined Cheeses The blue-green veining of cheeses is achieved by inoculating them with *Penicillium* molds, then storing the cheeses under controlled temperature and humidity. Roquefort cheese, ripened in caves in the otherwise barren Causses area in Aveyron, France, is the original blue-veined cheese. Many cheese lovers consider Roquefort to be the finest cheese in the world. Unfortunately, Roquefort made for export has a higher salt content than the original variety. If you want a traditional Roquefort at its height of perfection, you'll have to take a trip to France. Stilton, Bleu de Bresse, and Gorgonzola are other blue-veined cheeses.

Processed Cheeses These imposters are tinkered with by the liberal addition of salt, emulsifiers, lactic acid, preservatives, colorings, sugar, and other additives. Processed cheeses are typically very high in sodium. Avoid them. There is no reason to eat processed cheeses when real cheeses exist. Processed cheese is to real cheese what pressboard is to fine hardwood lumber.

Cottage Cheese

Cottage cheese has been a traditional favorite farm cheese because it is relatively easy to make and tastes delicious. The home kitchen method involves scalding skim milk and then letting it sit at room temperature for a couple of days until it sours. As souring occurs, whey separates from the curd. Boiling water is added to the pot, and the liquid is allowed to cool. With the curd settled and the whey separated, the mixture is poured through a cheesecloth and allowed to drain. The remaining dry curds are then mixed with a little cream and salt, and voila!—cottage cheese.

Commercial cottage cheese is made in much larger batches under controlled conditions. Culturing and direct acidification are the two methods used to settle the curd. Culturing involves adding *Streptococcus lactis, Streptococcus cremoris, Leuconostoc citrovorum,* and rennet to pasteurized milk. The milk is kept at 72°F for sixteen hours until the curd settles.

Acidification involves the addition of one or more acidifying agents, sometimes with additional enzymes, to pasteurized milk, to coagulate the curd. Cottage cheese is made by mixing dry curds with a pasteurized cream mixture. The finished product contains at least 4 percent milk fat. Low-fat cottage cheese is made in the same manner but has a milk fat content ranging from 0.5 to 2 percent.

Cheese Storage and Handling

Cheese should be refrigerated between 35° and 40°F for maximum freshness. Cut cheese should be tightly wrapped with plastic, waxed paper, or aluminum foil to keep it from drying out. Containers with locking seals are also good for storage, particularly for cheeses with strong odors, such as Limburger.

Hard cheeses such as Cheddar, Parmesan, and Swiss will keep for several weeks under refrigeration. Soft cheeses, however, such as Neufchâtel, Brie,

Caloric Values of Cheese

The calories from cheese come from fat, protein, and carbohydrates. The following list shows the percentage of calories obtained from each of these sources in fifteen different cheeses. Note that the percentage of total calories obtained from a source is not the same as the percentage of that source in the product. In other words, a cheese may be 50 percent fat by weight, but almost 70 percent of its calories may come from fat.

Cheese	Fat	Protein	Carbohydrate
Blue Cheese	73%	24%	3%
Brie	75%	25%	0%
Cheddar	74%	25%	1%
Cottage Cheese	13%	71%	16%
Edam	70%	28%	2%
Farmer	58%	34%	8%
Feta	72%	22%	6%
Gouda	69%	28%	3%
Mozzarella	56%	39%	5%
Muenster	74%	25%	1%
Neufchâtel	81%	15%	4%
Parmesan	60%	37%	3%
Ricotta	52%	33%	15%
Sapsago	27%	73%	0%
Swiss	66%	30%	4%

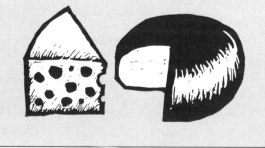

ricotta, and Camembert are highly perishable and should be used within a few days of purchase.

Most cheeses can be frozen. If you freeze cheese, seal it in a moisture-proof container to prevent dehydration. Some cheeses, especially the blue-veined cheeses, become crumbly after freezing and thawing.

With the exceptions of cottage cheese, cream cheese, and Neufchâtel, which should be served cold, cheeses are best served at room temperature. This allows for full aroma and flavor.

Eggs

Philosophers have banged their heads in vain over the age-old question: which came first, the chicken or the egg? While we may never know the answer to that brain-teaser, we do know that eggs have stirred up more than just philosophical controversy. In recent years, eggs have come under fire because of their cholesterol value, their possible contamination by salmonella bacteria, and the manner in which egg-laying chickens are raised, including the heavy use of drugs.

Taking Eggs to Heart

Eggs are concentrated nutrition. A whole egg has 6 grams of protein, 5.6 grams of fat, and about 270 milligrams of cholesterol. The amount of cholesterol in eggs has hurt the reputation of this food, for good reason. Dietary cholesterol is linked to arteriosclerosis and heart disease, including heart attack. A single egg contains more than 25 percent of the amount of cholesterol produced by the body daily. This is a significant amount of added cholesterol.

The American Egg Board has fought back against the cholesterol issue by pointing out that our bodies need cholesterol. This is true, but we manufacture as much cholesterol as we need. There is no evidence whatsoever that extra dietary cholesterol is beneficial in any way. There are many studies, however, that link dietary cholesterol to cardiovascular disease.

Bad Bacteria

In 1989 the U.S. Department of Agriculture issued a warning that eggs may contain salmonella bacte-

Low-Cholesterol Eggs?

The American Heart Association recommends that Americans consume no more than 300 milligrams of dietary cholesterol per day. That's bad news for egg producers, because a single egg can contain anywhere from 210 to 275 milligrams of cholesterol. That's over twice the amount of cholesterol in two 4-ounce pork chops.

Because of public concern about cholesterol in eggs, industry sales have plunged from $4.1 billion in 1984 to $3.1 billion in 1989. To combat the sales slump, egg producers are attempting to manipulate the dietary intake of their chickens to produce a lower-cholesterol egg. Some producers say they have already accomplished this.

The federal standard for cholesterol in a Grade A large egg is currently 274 milligrams of cholesterol. A few commercial hatcheries in Pennsylvania have been marketing their eggs as lower in cholesterol than the federal standard, claiming that their eggs contain between 185 and 210 milligrams of cholesterol. The difference, they say, is due to a secret feed formula.

But are there really low-cholesterol eggs, or is the federal standard simply higher than the average cholesterol value of most eggs? According to a year-long study conducted by the Department of Agriculture and the Egg Nutrition Center in Washington, both regular eggs and those labeled "low cholesterol" actually contain the same amount of cholesterol. The eggs sampled contained between 210 and 230 milligrams of cholesterol apiece, regardless of how they were grown.

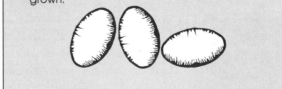

ria. The USDA urged consumers to refrain from eating raw eggs in any form and recommended the thorough cooking of all eggs. The danger was apparently due to salmonella-contaminated breeding stock. Salmonella bacteria have previously been detected on the shells of some eggs, but this poses no real health hazard. If a shell is cleaned, the egg can be cracked and used without concern. There is some evidence now, however, that a small percentage of eggs may actually contain salmonella bacteria *inside* their shells. Thus, it is important to cook eggs thoroughly, for a minimum of 3 minutes. Forget about 1-minute eggs, or eggs sunny side up with runny yolks. For safety's sake, avoid runny yolks.

Chickens on Drugs: Just Say Cock-a-Doodle-Doo

Although some chickens are raised in hen houses in which they have the run of the floor area, many egg-laying chickens are housed in cramped cages in which their movement is severely restricted. The cage system is favored for its efficiency as far as egg production is concerned, but is highly criticized as inhumane. In today's egg-laying facilities, light, temperature, and humidity are carefully controlled. The hens live in windowless, insulated, force-ventilated housing, with an artificial day/night light cycle designed to stimulate egg production. Caged birds are suspended over troughs that catch their fecal droppings. In these crowded conditions the hens exhibit cannibalistic tendencies. To combat this, their beaks are clipped by a machine that cauterizes the beak.

The egg industry claims that such housing actually protects the chickens from the elements, disease, and predators. This rationale is so thin that no further comment is needed. In these cramped, unnatural conditions the hens are fed rations that typically contain antioxidant preservatives, mold inhibitors, and antibiotics. Antibi-

otics are particularly important, because in such close living quarters chickens can easily spread disease. Chickens are fed such a high quantity of antibiotics that the drugs pass into the feces, which discourages flies from breeding in the waste. Chicken feed may be contaminated with high levels of pesticides, but these residues most often go undetected because of lack of feed testing. Some of the chemicals in chicken feed wind up in the eggs.

Making the Grade

Eggs are graded and sized according to the quality of the egg and its shell, and the size at the time of packing.

Grade AA eggs stand up tall when cracked. They have firm, stand-up yolks. The area covered by the white is small. There is more thick white than thin white. These eggs are sometimes labeled "Fresh Fancy."

Grade A eggs are just a little less firm than Grade AA. The yolk is still thick and upstanding, and there is more thick white than thin white.

Grade B eggs are thinner and spread out more. Their yolks tend to be flat, and there are about equal parts thick white and thin white.

Egg Sizes Based on Net Weight Per Dozen

Jumbo:	30 oz per dozen
Extra Large:	27 oz per dozen
Large:	24 oz per dozen
Medium:	21 oz per dozen
Small:	18 oz per dozen
Pee Wee:	15 oz per dozen

Fertile Eggs

Fertile eggs are from chickens that have had sex. So at the very least, the hens are happier than their sex-starved counterparts at most commercial hatcheries. If allowed, a fertile egg will hatch, whereas a non-fertile egg will not. Beyond this fact, there appears to be no nutritional difference between fertile and non-fertile eggs. Fertile eggs contain a small amount of male hormone.

Brown Eggs vs. White Eggs

Despite the fact that brown foods just look more natural than white foods, there is no qualitative difference between white-shelled and brown-shelled eggs. Shell color is due to different breeds of hens. If feed rations between breeds are the same, there will be no nutritional difference in the eggs.

Eggs in the Diet

Because eggs are a good source of protein, they can be of value in a healthy diet. Unless you suffer from high blood cholesterol or some form of cardiovascular disease, you can most likely eat as many as three eggs per week. With eggs, as with other high-cholesterol foods, the key is moderation.

Sunny, Runny, and Raw

Perhaps you like your eggs sunny side up with a runny yolk. Or maybe you are used to tossing a fresh, raw egg into a blender to make a protein shake. Or maybe you just like hollandaise sauce. Think again. According to the U.S. Department of Agriculture, salmonella contamination of eggs is a problem. It is unwise, and potentially unsafe, to eat raw eggs and raw egg products. Additionally, raw eggs contain avidin (part of the egg protein), which inhibits the absorption of biotin, one of the B vitamins. Cooking eggs thoroughly inactivates avidin.

9

ECO REPORT: BACTERIAL FOOD CONTAMINATION

*T*he three primary sources of food contamination common to the food chain today are toxic agricultural chemicals, harmful chemical food additives, and pathogenic (disease-causing) bacteria. Of these three, the most immediate threat to health comes from food-borne bacteria. This is not to say that agricultural chemicals and chemical food additives do not represent a serious threat to health. We know that many of these chemical agents are toxic and carcinogenic. What we do not know, however, is how many people will be adversely affected by these chemicals, what amounts of these toxins need to be consumed in order to pose a serious threat to health, and how much time is required for chemical-induced health disorders to manifest.

With pathogenic bacteria, the threat to health is fairly well understood. Only microscopic amounts of harmful bacteria are required to cause sickness. Virtually everyone is susceptible to bacterial food poisoning, the symptoms of which range from slight digestive discomfort to death. And while toxic chemicals in food may cause cancer or other health problems over a period of years or decades, the ef-

fects of harmful food-borne bacteria usually manifest within one day's time.

Moreover, while artificial chemical food contaminants can (at least in theory) be eliminated from the food chain over time, harmful bacteria occur naturally and are ubiquitous. They are found most commonly in meats, seafoods, and dairy products, and experts believe that they can never be eradicated from the food chain. Former U.S. Commissioner of Food and Drugs Dr. Frank E. Young says that "We are seeing a marked increase in microbial contamination . . . in our food supply." This increase, he says, has led to an explosion of bacterial food-borne diseases. Among health and safety experts there is universal agreement that bacterial food contamination is on the increase and that this contamination represents a major threat to public health and safety.

The Dirty Half-Dozen Bacterial Contaminants

Six pathogenic bacterial contaminants commonly occur in foods:

Salmonella   Perhaps the most common food-borne microbe, salmonella is a family of more than two thousand related bacteria, including *Salmonella typhosa,* which causes typhoid fever. Salmonella bacteria occur in the intestinal tracts of humans and animals and wind up in the food chain because of fecal contamination of meat, eggs, milk, and poultry.

The typical symptoms of salmonella poisoning are diarrhea, vomiting, and fever. Symptoms usually appear within twelve to thirty-six hours after eating and can last for a week. As with all harmful bacteria, children, the sick, and the elderly are at greater risk of serious illness from salmonella poisoning, which can result in death. Salmonella bacteria are relatively easy to control, as they are killed by thorough cooking.

Campylobacter   Similar to salmonella in its effects, campylobacter is a common cause of diarrhea and is transmitted in chicken, shellfish, mushrooms, and raw milk. This organism causes spontaneous abortion and infertility in cattle but is not known to produce the same effects in humans. Proper cooking kills campylobacter.

Staphylococcus   Found in localized suppurative infections, including pimples and boils, as well as in sputum and inside the nose, staphylococcus is an organism that grows quickly, producing a toxin that causes nausea, vomiting, and diarrhea. This microbe is transmitted to food by handling and grows rapidly at warm temperatures.

Unlike other bacteria, the toxins produced by staphylococcus are not destroyed by cooking. Staphylococcus contamination is most common in cooked and cured meats, cheese and meat salads, and starchy foods. Sanitary and hygienic food preparation and storage practices are the most effective ways to reduce the health risks associated with this organism.

Perfringens   Known as "the cafeteria germ," perfringens is found in human and animal intestines, in sewage, and soil. It is an anaerobic bacterium, which means that it thrives where there is little or no oxygen. (In contrast, staphylococcus and sal-monella bacteria require oxygen to reproduce.)

Perfringens typically occurs in food that sits for extended periods on steam tables or is left at room temperature. It is a common contaminant in stews, casseroles, gravy, dressing, and cooked turkey and beef. The symptoms of perfringens poisoning are diarrhea and gas pains. Individuals with ulcers, however, can be seriously affected by these bacteria. The best ways to prevent the proliferation of perfringens are to prepare food under sanitary conditions, refrigerate food carefully, and serve food from small dishes rather than from large containers that may sit for long periods.

Botulinum   Watch out for this one! Although contamination of food by these bacteria is rare compared with most other bacteria, botulinum causes botulism, a form of poisoning that attacks the nerves. This causes dryness of the mouth, difficulty in swallowing, impaired vision, vomiting, abdominal pain, respiratory failure, and death by suffocation. These are not friendly bacteria.

Botulinum spores come from soil and water and proliferate in foods that are not adequately cooked. Most commonly found in improperly canned or bottled foods, including canned meats and vegetables, botulinum often turns clear liquids milky. Botulinum is so toxic that it cannot be cooked out of foods. If you encounter milky-looking liquids in canned or bottled foods, loose lids, cracked jars, or swollen cans or lids, throw the food out. *Do not taste foods* to find out whether they are spoiled by these bacteria. Even the smallest taste of food contaminated with botulinum can send you to the emergency room of your local hospital, gasping for breath.

Botulism symptoms develop within twelve to forty-eight hours after eating. If you even suspect that you are suffering from this condition, call the nearest poison control center, pronto.

Yersinia   Occurring in the feces and lymph of animals and humans, and frequently transmitted by body lice, the various yersinia bacteria can survive and reproduce under refrigeration. Outbreaks of yersinia poisoning in raw vegetables, milk products, and tofu have been reported. Yersinia poisoning can

Aflatoxin

Aflatoxin is a potent carcinogen produced by the *Aspergillus flavus* and *Aspergillus parasiticus* molds, which grow commonly on field corn, peanuts, and grains. The proliferation of these molds and the resulting contamination by the poison they produce occur when crops have been weakened by insects, drought, or other adverse conditions, or have been stored improperly.

Aflatoxin, which can cause liver cancer, is transmitted to people through milk products, meats from animals fed contaminated field corn and nut meals, and peanut butter, cornmeal, and grits. In the United States, aflatoxin contamination is most common in the southeast in peanuts and corn products. Fresh, frozen, or canned sweet corn does not typically contain any aflatoxin.

Both the U.S. Department of Agriculture and the Food and Drug Administration recognize aflatoxin as a serious health risk, and the FDA has set a tolerance for aflatoxin at twenty parts per billion. These standards, however, apply only to foods that cross a state line. There is no legal limit to the amount of aflatoxin that may occur in foods grown and sold in the same state. Furthermore, the FDA allows corn and cottonseed meal contaminated with aflatoxin exceeding the twenty parts per billion level to be fed to livestock.

In 1989 federal officials discovered that high levels of aflatoxin were present in midwestern corn and grains grown during the 1988 drought. Inspectors subsequently discovered that meats and milk products also contained unacceptable levels of this toxin. While there is some government inspection of crops for aflatoxin, industry is largely responsible for ensuring that foods are not contaminated with this substance. Several companies in the natural foods industry test their nut butters, cornmeal, grits, and chips for aflatoxin, and certify them as aflatoxin-free. Unfortunately, grind-your-own peanut butter machines in particular can be contaminated with aflatoxin. The peanuts used may carry this toxin, which can increase during storage. The machines, unless thoroughly cleaned every day, can become breeding grounds for the *Aspergillus* molds. Ask your natural food store how they deal with this problem.

To protect yourself, look for certified aflatoxin-free corn and peanut products. Find out what your state health department is doing about in-state dairy and meat products from corn-fed dairy cows and livestock. Avoid nut pieces of any variety, because they are particularly susceptible to aflatoxin contamination. Last, do not eat moldy, rotten, or bitter nuts at all.

---

cause lymphadenitis, an inflammation of the lymph nodes connected to the intestines. This condition resembles acute appendicitis and can be fatal.

Government Protection?

At a time when the national debt is at an obscene high and defense spending ensures several tons of explosive power for every human being on earth, the beleaguered U.S. Department of Agriculture and the Food and Drug Administration don't have the people, money, or time to adequately protect the public against bacterial food contamination. We may have enough nuclear bombs, tanks, rocket launchers, and nerve gas to kill everyone on earth, but we don't have the resources to protect the public from bacteria in the food supply.

Government agencies have been virtually paralyzed by budget cuts and staff reductions. Meanwhile, livestock growers, slaughterhouses, and processing plants have run increasingly unsanitary operations. Cramped conditions, insects, and rodents contribute to contamination. USDA surveys show that the incidence of salmonella-contaminated chicken averages 35 percent.

We may hope for this situation to improve soon.

In 1996 higher standards and more rigorous federal inspection practices for the meat and poultry industry were announced.

A 1986 New York Department of Consumer Affairs report criticized the USDA for the increase in microbiological food-borne diseases, and identified several areas, from ranch to retail, that could be improved to reduce this epidemic. The report was particularly critical of poultry operations, which the USDA has already identified as a primary source of bacterial food contamination. In the following graphic description, the report describes chicken processing.

Chickens are cramped in crates which become filled with feces. The frightened birds defecate, and as the animals attempt to move about, their filth is spread. When birds are brought for slaughter, the feathers are taken off by a machine that literally beats them off with rubber fingers. These pluckers get covered with feces which fill up the holes of the chicken skin. As a result, some of these chickens become heavily contaminated.

Bacterial food contamination is not exclusive to the meat industry. Food service operations, including restaurants, commissary kitchens, and commercial processors, are also culprits. Much of the bacterial contamination of foods in these places is due to the poor personal hygiene of workers. Failure to wash hands after using the bathroom, sneezing and

The Chicken Evisceration Horror Story

According to health authorities, the commercial processing of chickens is causing a disease epidemic. At issue is the evisceration of chicken, a process by which the insides are removed. As first brought to public attention in 1987 by the television news program "60 Minutes," most chickens are eviscerated by machines that often do not do a thorough job. The evisceration machine disembowels the chicken, frequently tearing the intestines and spreading fecal waste inside the body cavity. Even though the chicken is washed afterward, bacteria remain on the skin.

Up until the late 1970s the U.S. Department of Agriculture would have condemned carcasses contaminated with feces. But today processors are allowed to wash the birds and sell them. They are dipped in tanks of water laden with fresh, raw feces, and are thus contaminated with harmful bacteria.

In 1987, Delmar Jones, chairman of the National Joint Council of Food Inspection Locals, wrote the *Washington Post:* "From slaughter to the shelves of your grocery store, broilers, fryers, and chicken parts go through a speedy, filthy process that practically insures contamination and disease."

According to the USDA, at least one out of every three mechanically eviscerated chickens contains harmful bacteria due to fecal contamination. Bacterial contamination is not an insubstantial problem. The federal government calculates a total of 80 million food-borne illnesses each year in this country. Two-thirds of all cases of food poisoning are caused by bacteria. The problem of fecal contamination of chicken accounts for approximately 30 percent of all cases of bacterial food poisoning.

Some stores carry poultry that has been eviscerated and washed by hand. This process allows for more careful cleaning as well as for visual inspection. Look for chicken processed in this manner. In any case, cook all chicken thoroughly, just to be safe.

coughing into food, and picking noses and skin blemishes can all transmit pathogenic bacteria to food. Unfortunately, the situation is likely to get worse before it gets better.

What You Can Do

Since the government can't really protect you against food-borne bacterial disease, you had better adopt the highest level of safe food handling practices possible, to stay healthy.

Shopping　When you purchase food, read the freshness dates on canned and packaged goods. Pay particularly close attention to the "sell by" date on labels of dairy products and prepared meats, and don't buy anything that is older than that date. Look for any signs of spoilage, and avoid dented, cracked, or swollen packages, as well as foods that are partially opened or have loose lids.

If you are buying refrigerated goods, feel the temperature of the refrigerated case. If the case or the foods in it are warm, shop somewhere else. When buying meat or fish, avoid products that appear or smell old or spoiled or look off-color. Remember that fresh fish does not smell "fishy." If you encounter such an odor, it means that the fish may be "fresh" (as opposed to frozen), but it's old. Avoid old fish.

Do not buy imported shellfish. The risk of bacterial contamination is too great because of poor handling and irregular refrigeration practices. Ask your grocer specifically where the shellfish comes from.

When shopping, pick up perishables last. In hot weather, take your food home and refrigerate it as soon as possible. Do not shop for food and then run errands. If you live more than half an hour away from where you shop, bring an ice chest for meats and dairy products.

Food Preparation　Before you prepare food, wash your hands thoroughly. Wear gloves if you have a cut or infection on your hands. Do not cough or sneeze onto food.

When you have finished preparing meat, poultry, or fish, wash all cutting boards, knives, plates, and other utensils. *Do not prepare vegetables or other foods with utensils used to prepare flesh foods until the utensils have been cleaned.* A piece of chicken may contain harmful bacteria, but if you cook that chicken thoroughly, the bacteria will most likely be completely destroyed. The utensils used to prepare the chicken, however, can carry live bacteria to salads, breads, and other foods that will not be cooked. Starchy foods and items containing dairy products are the foods most easily contaminated. This can lead to food poisoning.

Clean all cooking utensils thoroughly after use. Make sure that sponges, pot scrubbers, dishcloths, scouring pads, and drying towels are meticulously clean. All can carry bacteria.

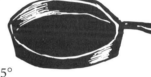

Cooking　The surest way to kill food-borne bacteria is to cook food thoroughly at temperatures between 165° and 212°F. Although you may love steak tartare or raw eggs in your protein drink, it's crazy to eat raw animal products, because the possibility of bacterial contamination is so high. Certified raw milk from certified dairies is usually safe because those dairies are carefully monitored. *Never eat raw hamburger, ever.* The risk of contamination is simply too great. Be cautious about making sushi at home. Sushi properly prepared at a high-quality restaurant is typically made with fish that is deep frozen to kill bacteria. But be careful.

If you delay serving food after cooking, keep it hot: above 140°F. Cooked food left out unheated can breed bacteria that thrive at room temperature. Don't let food sit out in a chafing dish or on a steam table for more than 2 hours. When you reheat leftovers, cook them thoroughly. Gravies, sauces, meat stews, and soups should be brought to a full boil.

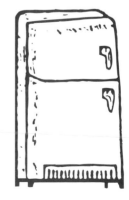

Refrigeration　Few harmful bacteria can survive in the cold. Refrigerators should be kept at no higher than 40°F, and freezers should be no higher than 0°F. Foods being refrigerated or frozen should be well wrapped or placed in tightly sealed containers. It is unwise to cool foods at room temperature before refrigerating them. Instead, put them directly into the refrigerator. Thaw frozen meats overnight inside the refrigerator, rather than at room temperature. Bacteria in meats multiply too easily at room temperature.

In summary, play it safe. Don't assume that the food you buy is bacteria free. That is highly unlikely. Select food carefully, prepare it under clean conditions, cook it thoroughly, and store it well. If you have doubts about a food, don't eat it. You certainly never want to waste good food, but neither do you want to eat bad food. At this point in time, in protecting yourself against bacterial food contamination, you're on your own.

10

MEATS

Meats of all kinds, from poultry to beef, play an important role in the human diet. Meats provide protein, B vitamins, zinc, and iron, and they represent part of the diet of virtually every culture in the world. Meats are not essential to human survival, and you can obtain virtually all the nutrients in meat from vegetarian sources. The exception to this is vitamin B_{12}, which cannot be obtained from a diet free of all dairy products and flesh foods. In moderation, meats provide concentrated nutrition and can play a nutritious role in a healthy, balanced diet.

Meats and Human Health Issues

The meat industry today, however, is fraught with serious problems and is in a period of transition. The beef producers in particular have been hard hit by negative publicity about cholesterol in red meat. Pork is now being marketed as "the other white meat," and the sales of poultry have increased enormously in the past several years. Furthermore, there are several issues related to meat production that threaten public health and safety. Three of these issues are (1) the feeding of antibiotics to livestock, (2) the administration of hormones to livestock, and

(3) inadequate inspection of meat slaughterhouses and packing operations.

Before you purchase meat products, you need to understand these critical health and safety issues. For as nutritionally viable as meats are, you are better off eating a vegetarian diet if you cannot obtain safe, wholesome, drug-free meats.

Issue No. 1: Antibiotics, Super Germs, and the Meat You Eat

In 1949, Dr. Thomas Jukes, a researcher for American Cyanamid Corporation, accidentally discovered that feeding small doses of a newly developed antibiotic, chlortetracycline, caused chickens and piglets to gain 10 to 20 percent more weight than normal. Dr. Jukes's discovery revolutionized the livestock industry, providing growers with a profitable shortcut to substantial animal weight gain. Within a few short years, growers of poultry, hogs, and cattle were feeding their animals "subtherapeutic" doses of antibiotics: doses less than the amounts needed to battle disease. Not only did the antibiotics enhance weight gain; they protected animals against infection. This meant that more animals could be kept in smaller spaces without succumbing to the diseases typical of crowding. The result of these advances was that livestock production became possible on a much greater scale than ever before. The factory farming of livestock became a major industry.

Biological Time Bomb

Today the use of antibiotics in animal feed accounts for half of the 35 million pounds of antibiotics produced each year in the United States. Despite the widespread use of these drugs, many scientists and health experts are opposed to antibiotic-driven animal husbandry. They warn that the use of penicillin and tetracycline in animal feed is a biological time bomb waiting to explode. Karim Ahmed, a senior scientist for the Natural Resources Defense Council, says that the use of antibiotics in animal feed is "perhaps one of the most serious public health problems this country faces. We're talking about rendering many of the most important antibiotics ineffective." The problem is that animals fed subtherapeutic doses of antibiotics have naturally occurring bacteria in their systems that gradually become resistant to the drugs. Even harmful bacteria like salmonella and campylobacter, which both cause food poisoning, can become resistant to antibiotics.

Super Germs

Bacteria in animals fed antibiotics don't just become resistant to the drugs. They also produce drug-resistant offspring. Just like insects that become resistant to specific pesticides, the bacteria become virtually immune to the drugs that are supposed to kill them. Opponents of antibiotic feed additives point out that these bacteria, or super germs, can be passed on to humans.

Bacteria pass on resistance not only to their own offspring but to other strains of bacteria as well. This is known as plasmid transfer. Plasmids are bits of genetic material that can go from one strain of bacteria to another. Because of plasmid transfer, a broader number of super germs are being formed.

Plasmid biology expert Stuart Levy of Tufts University opposes the use of subtherapeutic doses of antibiotics in animal feed. "This major use of antibiotics is a tremendous contributor to the environmental pool of resistant bacteria. And it's a use that could be eliminated," says Levy. Dr. Levy, Dr. Ahmed, and over three hundred other scientists have signed a statement for the Natural Resources Defense Council, urging the Food and Drug Administration to ban the feeding of tetracycline and penicillin. Though spokespeople for the livestock industry argue that their drug-feeding practices are safe, scientific studies tell another story.

Bacterial Food Poisoning

Harvard University medical researcher Thomas O'Brien and associates have discovered a method for following the transfer of antibiotic resistance from animals to humans. Their findings, which were reported in the *New England Journal of Medicine* in 1982, traced antibiotic-resistant salmonella from cattle in twenty states to twenty-six people suffering from salmonella poisoning. The conclusion that O'Brien drew was that drug-resistant plasmids passed to people from the meat they consumed.

In another study, Scott Holmberg, an epidemiologist at the Center for Disease Control in Atlanta, investigated the cases of eighteen Midwesterners who were infected with antibiotic-resistant salmonella. Holmberg traced the cases of disease back to a herd of cattle from South Dakota that had been fed regular doses of tetracycline. Yet another study, conducted by the Food and Drug Administration, says that drug-resistant bacteria may infect humans through poultry consumption. The use of antibiotic feed additives in poultry production creates drug-resistant super germs that may render food poisoning untreatable with antibiotics.

The Natural Resources Defense Council, which has been investigating the use of antibiotics in animal feed for several years, calculates that penicillin and tetracycline are implicated in more than 270,000 cases of food poisoning each year, approximately three hundred of which result in death. All meat sold in this country is now required to be labeled with instructions for safe handling to minimize the risk of food poisoning.

Inhumane Animal Husbandry

"The breeding sow should be thought of, and treated as, a valuable piece of machinery whose function is to pump out baby pigs like a sausage machine."
—*National Hog Farmer, March 1978*

If your idea of livestock production includes pictures of pastoral scenes filled with animals contentedly grazing on natural grasses in the warm sun, think again. Factory livestock production is rife with unnatural and cruel conditions that add up to a life of misery for animals.

Beef steers are castrated without anesthesia to make them more manageable. This procedure is performed by workers with no surgical or veterinary training. Veal calves are separated from their mothers at birth and are confined in the dark in cramped wooden crates. They are fed an iron-deficient diet to turn their meat white and are given massive quantities of drugs to hedge against bacterial disease.

As many as five egg-laying hens are crammed into small cages made of tight wire mesh about 1 cubic foot in size. Their beaks are clipped to prevent cannibalism, and they are fed a continuous diet of drugs to combat bacterial disease from constant contact with fecal waste.

These practices, which are typical of factory livestock production, are cruel and unnecessary. It is possible to raise animals in comfortable conditions, with plenty of room to move around and without the use of dangerous drugs. Don't accept animal products from livestock raised under inhumane conditions.

What You Can Do

Only a few meat producers currently grow livestock without antibiotic feed additives. Don't be misled by the label "naturally raised" on meat. Ask your grocer specifically whether or not the meat has been raised with antibiotic feed additives. Find out how your grocer knows one way or another. Do they know the livestock grower? Do they have affidavits that describe the growing process? Will they share that information? You can afford to be politely demanding about this issue.

In addition, you can contact the regional office of the Food and Drug Administration in your area and let them know that you want the feeding of antibiotics to livestock to stop.

Issue No. 2: Hormones—Meaty, Beefy, Big, and Burly

In December 1988 the European Community (EC) announced that it would ban the import of all meats from the United States raised with growth hormones. The U.S. Department of Agriculture cried foul, claiming that the ban was an economic ploy implemented to protect European meat prices. The EC, however, adamantly held to the claim that the ban was implemented for health reasons. The EC had for several years petitioned the United States to stop the use of growth hormones in livestock production, to no avail. Domestic drug companies, fearing serious financial losses, fought the EC request, keeping hormones in the food chain. After exhausting other avenues, the EC finally chose to initiate a ban on hormone-raised meats.

Drugs, Drugs, Drugs

Growth hormones, also known as anabolic steroids, are administered to beef, lamb, and pork to accelerate weight gain, thus cutting feed costs and increasing production profits. Growth hormones are administered through ear tags, which release small amounts of these drugs into the animal's bloodstream on a continuous basis.

The hormones used for growth promotion fall into two categories. Endogenous hormones, which are those produced naturally in animals and humans, include estradiol, testosterone, and progesterone. Exogenous hormones, which are synthetically produced, include zeranol and trenbolone acetate. All five of these hormones are used widely in livestock production. Of course, the USDA claims that the use of these drugs in livestock production is completely safe. That's what government officials said about DES, or diethylstilbestrol, another hormone that was used in livestock production, until it was proved to cause uterine cancer and other reproductive disorders. DES was subsequently banned from use in the food chain.

Inadequate Testing

The purpose of the Food Safety and Inspection Service (FSIS) is to ensure the safety of foods produced and sold in the United States. There is almost no testing, however, of meats for hormone residues. The FSIS is supposed to test foods for more than one hundred compounds, including chemical contaminants, drugs, and hormones; but serious budget cuts implemented by the Reagan administration have weakened the ability of the FSIS to protect the public food supply. Thus we cannot be certain of the level of hormone residues in meats, or the extent of the health hazards they pose.

Say No to Drugs!

When Olympic track star Ben Johnson was stripped of his gold medal in the 1988 Summer Olympics in Seoul, Korea, it was for using growth hormones. Coaches and trainers worldwide are urging athletes to keep completely away from hormones because of the risk they pose to health. Athletes frequently use these drugs to accelerate muscle gain and increase strength. Hormone supplements, however, can cause glandular disorders, tumors, reproductive damage, and other debilitating conditions. Some athletes have suffered irreversible bodily damage because of their use of anabolic steroids.

Science Fiction

The question must be asked: If growth hormones pose such a serious health risk to athletes, how can the U.S. Department of Agriculture condone their use in livestock production? The exact same growth hormones used by athletes are used to make animals big. The USDA claims that the small amounts of these hormones administered to animals are safe. This is exactly what they said about DES before several thousand women wound up with uterine cancer. The truth is, there is not one single long-term human study showing that hormones in meats are safe for human consumption. In other words, the USDA's position on hormones is science fiction.

What You Can Do

Many food retailers now are offering naturally raised meats grown without hormones. Ask your grocer for these naturally raised meats, and find out exactly how the meats in your grocery store are raised. The odds are excellent that the staff in your supermarket have no idea how their meats are raised. They can find out, however. In addition, call your regional office of the U.S. Department of Agriculture, and tell them that you want the use of growth hormones in livestock to stop.

Issue No. 3: Inspection—Whittling Down to Nothing

Certainly the worst news about meats has to do with inspection. Federal meat and poultry inspectors are engaged in a full battle to prevent unsafe food from making it to market. In 1987, vigilant food inspectors impounded 12 million pounds of meat and condemned over 60 million birds as unfit to eat. This was accomplished by conducting daily on-site inspections of the sixty-three hundred meat and poultry processing plants operating in the United States.

Good-Bye, Inspection

As a result of legislation proposed under the Reagan administration, the deregulation of meat and poultry processing in 1989 began in earnest, and the daily inspection system began to be phased out. A meat processing plant might not be visited by a federal food safety inspector more than two or three times a year. In theory, federal inspectors, whose numbers were reduced, concentrated their attention on meat processing operations known for chronic health code violations. In reality, thousands of processors went largely uninspected.

A Broken System

Over the past several years, the protective efforts of the much-beleaguered federal food safety inspectors have not been enough to defend the public against unsanitary meat products. In order to visit several meat processing plants in one day, inspectors have often spent more time in their cars than in conducting plant inspections. As a result, bacterial contamination of meats has become a major national food problem. The incidence of food poisoning due to salmonella, *E. coli*, and campylobacter contamination has radically increased in the past several years. This coincides with the reduction of the number of federal inspectors in the same period of time. Two thousand deaths annually have been attributed to bacterial food contaminants. The result has been a sharp increase in bacterial diseases from contaminated, uninspected meat products.

In response to this disgraceful situation, new federal regulations were announced in 1996. The meat and poultry industries will now be required to conduct regular testing for pathogenic bacteria and to improve their production procedures so as to minimize the risk of bacterial contamination.

Sulfa Residues in Meat and Milk

Sulfamethazine is an inexpensive, effective drug that is widely used to treat bacterial diseases in cattle, hogs, sheep, and poultry. Sulfamethazine also helps hogs to grow faster and is typically administered to them in feed and water for their entire lives. Manufactured by American Cyanamid, this drug is available without prescription. Federal residue standards for sulfamethazine in meats are enforced on the basis of voluntary compliance by livestock producers, without federal testing or inspection.

It is illegal to administer sulfamethazine to dairy cattle. Results of a study performed by the National Center for Toxicological Research show that this drug causes cancer in laboratory mice. A follow-up study by the Food and Drug Administration showed the same result with rats. Residues of sulfamethazine in meats are significantly higher than is allowed by legal residue standards. Recent samples show that 5 to 15 percent of hogs and 3 percent of veal calves contain illegal residues of sulfamethazine after slaughter. Furthermore, the FDA has disclosed that the nation's milk supply is largely contaminated by residues of this dangerous drug. In 1988, 25 percent of the U.S. milk supply contained illegal sulfamethazine residues.

In a mailing to hog farmers intended to counter revelations that sulfamethazine is a cancer-causing agent, American Cyanamid protested that the drug has "an enormous margin of safety" and that it poses no threat to human health. The pork industry, in response to a U.S. Department of Agriculture proposal to turn away shipments of pork containing illegal residues of the drug, pressured the USDA to delay implementation of that plan.

Today sulfamethazine, a suspected cancer-causing agent, is still available without prescription. The drug is still administered to livestock in excessive amounts and is fed to dairy cattle in violation of the law. Illegal residues of sulfamethazine are known to occur regularly in meat and milk, and not a damn thing is being done about it.

What Can Be Done?

The diminishing of the meat processing plant inspection system is a blow to the United States food supply. Every retailer of meats should become familiar with their meat growers, slaughterhouses, and processing plants. On a regular basis, retailers will need either to conduct visits to these outfits to ensure that food safety standards are being observed or to conduct in-store bacterial tests to ensure that meats are sanitary, uncontaminated by harmful bacteria. Ask your grocer questions. Does your grocer have direct contact with all meat growers, slaughterhouses, and processors who supply the store? Does your grocer employ someone who inspects these suppliers? How often do the inspections occur? Does your grocer test for bacteria?

The American shopper has become accustomed to feeling protected. But the deregulation of meat processing seriously jeopardizes the effort to keep food safe. Today the food shopper must be inquiring and vigilant. Each person who buys food, particularly meat products, will need to be informed about food safety issues. Write to the Secretary of Agriculture and make it known that you want the number of federal meat processing plant inspectors to be increased, and that you want the daily plant inspection system to resume.

MEAT PRODUCTION AND THE ECONOMICS OF STARVATION

One of the dimensions of eating meat that deserves attention is the energy-intensive nature of meat production. This is because meat is high up on the food chain. The food chain is the sequence of successive nutrient consumption, starting with the soil and ending with humans. Grass, for example, is low on the food chain and requires relatively little energy to grow. Grasses, such as the cereal grains, can be consumed by humans. But often the grasses are fed to animals that are grown to maturity and are then fed to humans. It takes sixteen pounds of grain to produce one pound of beef. The higher up on the food chain, the less energy-efficient food pro-

duction becomes. For the energy needed to produce one Big Mac, you could feed a bowl of grain to each of a dozen hungry children.

Deforestation for a Burger

One of the many dark sides of intensive factory livestock production is the destruction of forests in Central and South America and in the continental United States. Millions of acres of forest have been cut down and converted into land used for grazing livestock or for producing livestock feed. In the United States, forests are being destroyed at the rate of twelve acres per minute. This deforestation contributes to a rapid loss of topsoil and eliminates the natural habitat of thousands of species of wildlife. Many animals and birds are killed off during the actual deforestation process, and others die later because they have lost their habitat.

In Central and South America, millions of acres of rain forest have been destroyed to promote the meat-producing interests of major purveyors of meat products. These rain forests contain the greatest diversity of plant and animal life on earth and are treasure troves of important natural resources, including promising plant-based medicines. In addition, the rain forests produce a huge amount of this planet's oxygen while reducing the carbon dioxide content of the atmosphere. This helps to slow down the greenhouse effect, thus providing valuable protection to all living species.

Deforestation by the livestock industry accelerates world hunger, speeds up the greenhouse effect, leads to the extinction of one thousand valuable species of wildlife each year, and causes the desertification of vast tracts of previously lush, verdant land. We all must ask the question: "What on earth will it take for us to wake up to what is happening on this planet?" We are steadily killing ourselves and our home planet. All this for what—a Big Mac?

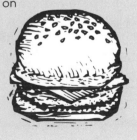

Approximately 90 percent of the grain crops grown in the United States are fed to livestock. Annually, livestock consume enough food to meet the caloric needs of over 8 billion people, or twice the world's population. Because of the energy-intensive nature of production, meat is much more expensive to produce than grains. As meat production increases, more people are priced out of being able to eat. Guatemala, for example, exports 40 million pounds of meat to the United States annually, while three out of four children in that country are malnourished. In Central America, dairy farmers have switched to raising beef for export. The result of this change is that more grains are being fed to animals, and fewer grains are available for human consumption. In addition, because of a reduction in dairy herds, there is less milk than ever before. The price of milk has increased sharply because there is greater demand than supply. Fewer families can now afford milk, and malnutrition is on the rise.

Until recently, the indigenous peoples of Central America relied on beans and corn for protein. These foods are nutritious and inexpensive. Now, with beef production draining the natural resources of that area, Central Americans are being economically squeezed out of eating. Their land is being used to grow meat for people in the United States who can afford to pay for it. While less corn and beans are being grown, the population is increasing, so there are more people to feed. Thus hunger is becoming an urgent, widespread problem. Things have gone terribly wrong.

The reason things have become so distorted has to do with the role that meat plays in a healthy diet. The belief that every meal should include meat is a recent and fundamentally American concept that disregards basic human nutritional needs. Meat is best eaten in small quantities, as a supplementary nutritional component of a diet composed primarily of grains, beans, fruits, vegetables, nuts, seeds, and dairy products. If meat were eaten in moderation, meat production would not be a cause of economic-based starvation, as it is today.

THE FOOD VALUE OF MEATS

Despite all the grim, dismal facts about modern meat production, eating meat is still a fundamentally healthy thing to do, provided the meat is grown naturally, is handled in a sanitary manner, and is part of a balanced whole-food diet. For the truth is that the human body is designed to eat flesh. We have flesh-tearing teeth as well as the digestive capacity to utilize the nutritional value of meat. Although vegetarians claim otherwise, the entire primate group eats meat. In the wild, monkeys, chimpanzees, orangutans, and gorillas are casual hunters, eating meat as the opportunity presents itself. Although the eating of meat is not essential to human life, it *is* a supportable practice.

A Few Words about Black Market Drugs

Despite Nancy Reagan's earnest "Just Say No" campaign, an increasing number of livestock producers and veterinarians are turning to illegal, untested drugs. Some livestock production operations use so many dangerous illegal drugs that they resemble

---

Meat and Cancer Prevention

There is ample evidence that a diet high in fat may increase the risk of cancers of the breast, colon, prostate, and lining of the uterus. Meats are a major source of dietary fats, which account for approximately 40 percent of the standard American diet. It is believed that reducing dietary fat intake to below 30 percent can decrease the risk of several types of cancer.

To reduce your dietary fat intake from meats, choose lean cuts of beef, lamb, and pork. Trim away any fat on the meat. Avoid meats that are "marbled," which indicates a high fat content. Reduce your intake of beef, pork, and lamb, and choose more chicken and turkey. Eat poultry with the skin removed.

crack houses. And residues of dangerous drugs are winding up on your dinner table. The Food and Drug Administration is doing what it can to combat the problem, and a number of dealers of illegal livestock drugs have been busted and convicted. Nonetheless, the problem is out of control, and public health is in jeopardy as a result.

Over the past decade, FDA tests have regularly detected illegal drugs in America's meat supply. One unapproved antibiotic, chloramphenicol, causes life-threatening human diseases, including aplastic anemia and nervous disorders. Four other common illicit livestock drugs—carbadox, nitrofurazone, dimetridazole, and ipronidazole—arc known to be cancer-causing agents.

Because there is a real illegal drug problem with meats, it is increasingly important to know your sources. You cannot assume that the meat you are buying is safe. You need documented assurances that the meat you purchase is free of harmful pharmaceutical contaminants.

Meat Storage and Handling

Meat will keep well under refrigeration for a few days if properly wrapped and stored, provided it has been handled correctly prior to purchase. Ideally, meat products should be refrigerated at temperatures between 28° and 32°F. However, most refrigerators operate between 36° and 40°F. Frozen meats will keep well for months, provided they are wrapped and sealed and frozen at 0°F or lower.

Beef

Beef sales have taken a beating since 1978, the high point in beef consumption. Nonetheless, beef is still the most popular meat in the United States. In 1988, 27 million cattle were slaughtered for human consumption in this country. Beef is sold according to a voluntary three-category U.S. Department of Agriculture grading system. Grades of beef are determined by fat content. The higher the fat content, the higher the grade.

Where the Beefalo Roam

Beefalo, a hybrid of three-eighths buffalo and five-eighths beef, is raised naturally, without growth hormones or antibiotic feed additives. It's not the exotic pedigree of beefalo that makes it so popular. The reason is its outstanding flavor, along with a superior nutritional profile. Beefalo has 95 percent less cholesterol, 85 percent less fat, and 55 percent fewer calories than the average supermarket beef. Yet it's sweet and tender and will satisfy any beef lover. Beefalo cooks in about two-thirds the time of regular beef because of its low fat content. Although it is generally hard to find, beefalo is becoming more popular across the United States.

- **Prime** The most tender beef of all, prime beef has the greatest amount of marbling, or intramuscular fat. Prime beef is regarded as superior and is the beef found at fine steakhouses and restaurants and gourmet butcher shops. Only about 2 percent of beef is graded prime.
- **Choice** Somewhat less tender, choice beef has less marbling and thus a lower fat and caloric value. About 65 percent of beef is graded as choice. Choice beef is found in most restaurants and supermarkets.
- **Select** Formerly known as "good" (a term that apparently lacked sales appeal) until 1988, select beef has even less marbling than choice. Since the name change, however, sales of select beef have soared. What a neat trick that was.

On the average, beef contains (per 3-oz. serving)
- Calories   192
- Fat   9.4 grams
- Cholesterol   73 milligrams

"Mad-Cow Disease"

"Mad-cow disease" is the sadly accurate nickname given to a fatal brain infection that has killed thousands of British cattle in the past decade. While it was believed that the disease, bovine spongiform encephalopathy (BSE), could not be transmitted through beef products, recent tragedies and scientific reports suggest otherwise. In 1996 a government-appointed scientific commission in Britain discovered a new strain of Creutzfeldt-Jakob disease, a deadly virus resulting in Alzheimer-like symptoms. At least eight people have died from this new strain of Creutzfeldt-Jakob, and it is believed that BSE is responsible for the spread of the disease. Because Creutzfeldt-Jakob has an incubation period as long as fifteen years, it can't be known when exposure to the virus occurred.

When questions about the safety of British beef were first raised in 1989, the U.S. banned imports of British beef. Now that the trail of human deaths seems to lead to BSE, nearly every European Union country has ended trade of beef with Britain.

It is uncertain whether mad-cow disease will spread beyond Britain, though strains of similar diseases have appeared in the United States recently. If you are questioning the safety of the beef you eat, the safest solution is also the healthiest—to simply eat none at all!

Pork

Pork is now marketed as "the other white meat" to distance it from beef, which has a bad cholesterol reputation these days. The campaign seems to be working: pork consumption in the United States has risen from 49 pounds per capita in 1986 to 53 pounds in 1995, while beef consumption has slipped from 79 to 68 pounds during the same time period. Yet many cuts of pork are actually higher in both fat and cholesterol than beef. Huge pork factories in the Midwest, which pose great hazards to groundwater and other aspects of the environment, are coming under greater scrutiny and regulation by state and local governments.

On the average, pork contains (per 3-oz. serving)
• Calories   198
• Fat   11.1 grams
• Cholesterol   79 milligrams

Lamb

Lamb has managed to escape the bad press suffered by beef, pork, and poultry. In general, lamb is raised more naturally, with fewer drugs, than other meats.

On the average, lamb contains (per 3-oz. serving)
• Calories   176
• Fat   8.1 grams
• Cholesterol   78 milligrams

Poultry

Because of the bad press suffered by beef, poultry products have enjoyed a meteoric rise in sales over the past decade. Truth be known, poultry actually has about as much cholesterol as beef, though its total fat content is less.

CHICKEN

On the average, chicken contains (per 3-oz. serving)
• Calories   134
• Fat   4.1 grams
• Cholesterol   76 milligrams

TURKEY

On the average, turkey contains (per 3-oz. serving)
• Calories   129
• Fat   2.6 grams
• Cholesterol   64 milligrams

Prepared Meat Products

Prepared meat products, including hot dogs, lunch meats, and sausage, typically contain additives.

Some of them, like the vinegar that is used to acidify meat products, are relatively benign. Others can be carcinogenic. Some of the common additives used in meat products are these:

- **Preservatives** BHA, BHT, TBHQ, and propyl gallate are used in pork products, beef products, and Italian sausages. BHT and BHA cause cancer in laboratory animals. The actual safety of others is not known.
- **Curing agents** Sodium nitrite and sodium ascorbate are used in salami, bacon, bologna, hot dogs, and other cured meat products. Sodium ascorbate is benign, while

sodium nitrite leads to the formation of cancer-causing nitrosamines in the body.
- **Flavoring agents** Corn syrup and dextrose are commonly used to enhance flavor in hot dogs, sausage, and canned hams. Both are refined sugars.
- **Binders** Whey, sodium caseinate, and isolated soy protein are used to bind and thicken sausages, meat loaves, soups, and stews. They're all harmless.
- **Acidifiers** Acetic acid (vinegar), citric acid, phosphoric acid, and lactic acid are used to improve both texture and flavor in sausage. They're all harmless.

Heptachlor in Chicken

In the 1970s heptachlor, a deadly pesticide and a chemical cousin of DDT manufactured by Velsicol Chemical Corporation, was found to cause malignant tumors in animals. Considered an extreme risk to infants, children, and nursing mothers, heptachlor was outlawed for use on food crops in 1978. Its illegal use continues, however.

In February 1989 the Townsend Poultry Products plant in Batesville, Arkansas, destroyed 400,000 chickens after the birds were found to contain dangerously high levels of heptachlor from contaminated feed grain. This was the fourth time since 1981 that meat or milk products from Arkansas were found to contain residues of dangerous chemicals banned in the 1970s.

A 1987 government report stated that over 1½ million bushels of seed contaminated with illegal chemical residues were coming to market each year. In the case of the chickens from Townsend Poultry Products, it is believed that heptachlor-tainted sorghum seed was sold to the company, which unwittingly used it for chicken feed. The residues eluded government inspectors but were detected in resi-

due tests conducted by the Campbell Soup Company, which operates a plant in Fayetteville, Arkansas. The company, which routinely analyzes poultry for residues of approximately three hundred pesticides, had purchased two hundred pounds of the Townsend chicken for use in test batches of a new product. Campbell's discovery of the heptachlor in the chicken led to the eventual destruction of the 400,000 birds that had consumed the contaminated seed.

Pesticide contaminated seed that is too old to germinate is often sold illegally as animal feed. This leads to residues of toxic chemicals in meat, which wind up being consumed by the public. "This is exactly what happens if you use a lot of pesticides in agriculture," notes Charles Benbrook, the executive director of the National Academy of Sciences board on agriculture. According to Lester Crawford of the U.S. Department of Agriculture's Food Safety and Inspection Service, "The public is at risk because this treated seed is not being monitored properly." As long as supplies of illegal toxic chemicals remain at large, they will be used, occasionally resulting in the contamination of foods that reach dinner tables all across the United States.

USDA Standards for Meat Product Labeling

If you pick up a can marked "Beef with Gravy," the product must contain at least 50 percent beef. But if it's labeled "Gravy with Beef," it need contain only 35 percent beef! The wording on a meat product label can make a big difference in the actual meat content of that item. Here are a few meat products and their legal meat contents:

Meat Products	Required Contents
Ham, Water Added	At least 17% meat protein
Hamburger	No more than 30% fat
Turkey Pie	At least 14% cooked turkey meat
Chicken Soup	At least 2% chicken meat
Beef Stew	At least 25% beef

If you want the U.S. Department of Agriculture standards for more than two hundred popular meat and poultry products, write away for *A Consumer Guide to Content and Labeling Requirements,* Home and Garden Bulletin No. 236, July 1981. This is available free of charge from FSIS Publications Office, USDA, Rm. 1165-S, Washington, D.C. 20250.

11

FISH AND THE FRUITS OF THE SEA

*F*ish is a general term used to describe the more than twenty thousand known species of non-vegetable aquatic creatures that inhabit the fresh and marine waters of the world. Generally categorized as freshwater fish, saltwater fish, or shellfish, they vary widely in their size and living environments. The smallest adult fish known is the half-inch long goby, found in Luzon, the Philippines. The largest fish, the whale shark, weighs several tons and may grow to a length of fifty feet. Fish live in waters as shallow as a few inches to depths exceeding thirty-five thousand feet.

The life cycles of the many species of fish vary greatly. Catadromous fish, such as eels, are those that live in fresh water but enter salt water to spawn. Anadromous fish, which include salmon, sturgeon, striped bass, shad, and smelt, are born in fresh water but spend most of their lives in salt water, returning to fresh water to spawn. While a majority of fish lay eggs that then hatch into young, some fish give birth to living young. These species, known as viviparous fish, give birth to offspring as large as one fifth their size. Sea perches of the Pacific Coast are viviparous.

For as long as history can recount, fish has been consumed by the people of all cultures. In many parts of the world, such as Japan, Norway, the Philippines, the South Pacific, Greenland, Alaska, and New England, fishing has played a major role in the development of culture.

Fish is one of the most popular foods in the world, and demand is rapidly increasing. According to the Alaska Seafood Marketing Institute, Americans consumed about 15 pounds of fish per person in 1994. When you consider that an additional yearly catch of over 700 million pounds of fish is required to increase the per capita consumption by just 1 pound, you get a sense of the magnitude of the fish industry today. There's no question about it: people are eating a lot more fish. Even McDonald's and Burger King, the quintessential beef stops, offer fish products.

Health from the Sea

From the standpoint of nutritional value, digestibility, and prophylactic benefits, fish is the most healthful flesh food in the world. Fish is an excellent source of protein. With variations according to species, fish is approximately 20 percent high-quality protein, with less than two-thirds the cholesterol of lean meats. Four ounces of fish is generally less than 100 calories, and its fat content averages about 20 percent. Fish contains a concentration of minerals, most notably iron, zinc, magnesium, and phosphorus. Fatty fish species are excellent sources of vitamins A and D. In fact, the greatest known concentration of natural vitamin A is in fish liver.

Fish flesh contains less connective tissue than other flesh foods, making fish easier to digest than meat and poultry. Thus, when we eat fish our bodies perform less work for more nutrition.

Because there is some evidence that fish may diminish the activity of the immune system, fish consumption by elderly people and anyone with reduced immune activity should probably not exceed two servings a week.

Omega 3s: Taking Fish to Heart

Greenland Eskimos eat a high-flesh, high-fat, high-cholesterol diet, yet they exhibit almost no incidence of coronary disease. Their unusually good cardiovascular health led nutritional researchers in the 1960s and 70s to explore the various components of the diet of the Greenland Eskimos. What the scientists discovered was that these people eat an abundance of a group of polyunsaturated fatty acids known as Omega 3s. Omega 3s are manufactured by marine micro-algae and are consumed right up the food chain by small fish, larger fish, marine mammals like walruses and seals, and humans.

The Omega 3 fatty acids are precursors to potent hormones in the body known as prostaglandins. The particular prostaglandins manufactured from Omega 3s regulate nerve activity, skin health, and reproduction. Omega 3s have been proved to lower blood cholesterol and triglyceride levels. They reduce platelet aggregation—the coagulation of sticky cells in the blood—thereby inhibiting arteriosclerosis, hardening of the arteries.

Omega 3s are believed to play a beneficial role in inflammatory diseases such as rheumatoid ar-

thritis, and to enhance immune function, thus improving one's resistance to certain diseases. Further research into the additional, undiscovered benefits of Omega 3 fatty acids is ongoing.

Though virtually all fish have some Omega 3s, the greatest concentration of these fatty acids is found in the oilier cold-water species such as salmon (all varieties), mackerel, and sablefish. Eating fish high in Omega 3s can greatly benefit your heart and help to keep your arteries clean and healthy.

Buying and Keeping Fish

Your fish dealer should be well informed about the products he or she sells and be able to tell you where and when various types of fish were caught. Expert fishmongers know fish the way skilled mechanics know engines. They know the best times of year for species, exactly which boats caught which fish, how long the fish have been on ice, and how they have been processed or prepared.

Did you know that many markets sell fish that has been dipped in a solution of chlorine and water to retard spoilage? This practice is fairly common, though vendors do not post signs indicating that this has been done to their fish. Nor are they legally obligated to say so. You should be sure to ask whether the fish you are buying has been chlorine-dipped. If it has been, shop elsewhere. If vendors tell you their fish has not been dipped, find out how they know for sure. Chlorine is toxic and offers no benefits to the quality of fish.

Whole fish will not smell "fishy" if it is fresh. Shark and skate are exceptions to this rule, as they naturally have a slight ammonia odor when fresh. The eyes will be clear, not cloudy, and the skin will be moist and shiny but never slimy. The scales should be intact and attached instead of dry or flaking.

Cuts of fish, whether they are steaks or fillets, should be moist, with no fishy odor, bruises, odd-colored edges, or spots. Bruised, gray, spotted, or fishy-smelling cuts of fish should be assiduously avoided, as they are either old or bad or both.

Shellfish is especially sensitive to bacterial

A Nutritional Analysis of Fish

100g (3¹/₂ oz) raw, edible portion	Calories	Protein (g)	Fat (g)	Sodium (mg)	Cholesterol (mg)	Omega 3 (g)
Albacore tuna	102	18.2	3.0	50	25	1.3
Catfish	103	17.6	3.1	60	55	.3
Clams	80	11.0	1.5	80	40	trace
Cod	70	16.7	.7	70	40	.2
Crab, Dungeness	81	17.3	1.3	266	90	.3
Crab, king	75	15.2	.8	70	60	—
Croaker	85	18.0	.8	80	50	.2
Flounder	90	18.1	1.4	56	50	.2
Grouper	87	19.3	.5	80	—	.3
Haddock	80	18.2	.5	60	60	—
Halibut	105	20.9	1.2	60	50	.4
Herring	150	18.3	8.5	75	80	1.7
Lobster	90	16.9	1.9	210	85	.2
Mackerel	160	21.9	7.3	80	40	2.5
Mahi mahi	102	21.0	1.0	130	85	—
Monkfish	70	15.5	1.0	—	35	—
Mussels	75	12.2	1.6	80	25	.5
Ocean perch	95	19.0	1.5	70	60	.2
Octopus	76	15.0	1.5	—	122	.2
Orange roughy	65	14.7	.3	—	—	—
Oysters	70	14.2	1.2	75	50	.6
Pollock	85	19.5	.8	60	50	.5
Sablefish	130	17.9	5.7	55	65	1.5
Salmon	142	20.0	7.0	50	65	1.1
Scallops	82	15.3	.2	160	50	.2
Shark, thresher	90	20.0	1.0	50	—	—
Shrimp	90	18.8	.8	140	158	.3
Skate	95	20.0	1.0	—	—	—
Sole	70	14.9	.5	55	45	—
Squid	85	16.4	.9	160	—	.3
Swordfish	120	19.4	4.4	70	50	.2
Tilefish	90	18.6	1.2	—	—	—
Trout, rainbow	195	21.5	11.4	52	50	.5
Whiting	95	21.3	1.2	50	20	.4

These figures are a general guide. The actual nutritional values of species will vary according to season, location, temperature, and other factors.

contamination, as previously described. To ensure freshness, clams, oysters, and mussels should always be purchased live. They can be stored in the refrigerator covered with a damp towel for a couple of days. Shrimp still in the shell is usually fresher than when peeled. Most peeled shrimp has been previously frozen, which is fine. Crab and lobster are best purchased live and cooked to order.

Frozen fish is appreciably harder to evaluate. Unless you notice any discoloration or a strong odor, you can only assume that the frozen fish you are buying is in edible condition. Look for intact packaging, recent date codes, and a piece of fish that feels frozen solid. Avoid pieces covered with a lot of ice crystals, an ancient date code, or rips and holes in the packaging.

Surimi, the Phony Fish

Surimi is a versatile processed fish product that is cropping up everywhere disguised as crab meat. Most surimi is made from pollock, an inexpensive fish available in huge quantities from the Bering Sea near Alaska. The surimi manufacturing process occurs in three steps. First, the oil of the pollock is removed. Next, the flavor is eliminated. Last, the color is bleached out. This renders a colorless, tasteless paste, which is then extruded into strands that can be formed to look like shellfish. Surimi is now available nationwide as imitation crab legs or flakes, with artificial flavor, wheat, egg white, and artificial color added. Yum.

Surimi is fast replacing crab, primarily because of its comparatively low price and great availability. Any time you see crab spelled with a "k" you can be sure it's surimi. An expanded assortment of surimi products is expected as other popular species of shellfish become too pricy or too rare.

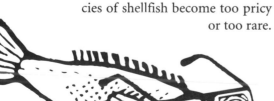

Processed Fish Products

Your grocer's frozen food case is a world of highly processed foods loaded with chemical additives and ultra-refined ingredients. Fish products are no exception. Prepared fish items such as ready-to-bake breaded items, fish sticks, and entrees are filled with artificial preservatives, hydrogenated oils, and far too much salt for health considerations.

PERILS IN THE FISH CASE

Despite the undisputed nutritional value of fish, all is not well in the marketplace. A host of contamination issues makes fish a food that must be purchased from reputable vendors who uphold the highest standards of purity and safety. Otherwise, you may succumb to serious or life-threatening illnesses by consuming unwholesome fish products. The contamination of fish is a result of improper handling, polluted waters, and naturally occurring toxins. Following are the primary issues regarding the contamination of fish products.

Issue: Fish Handling and Related Illness

The most common fish-handling conditions that result in illness are contact with polluted water, improper sanitation aboard fishing vessels, unsanitary processing plants, inadequate refrigeration, and poor hygiene in restaurants and retail establishments.

The bacteria that can contaminate fish as a result of the above conditions include salmonella, campylobacter, shigellae, staphylococci, *Clostridium botulinum,* and *Vibrio parahaemolyticus,* to name only a few. Consumption of any of these bacteria can result in illness and, in some cases, death. The most common symptoms of bacterial poisoning due to contaminated fish are vomiting, nausea, and diarrhea. More extreme allergic reactions, however, including hallucinations, severe cramping, and dangerously high fever, can occur. The severity of the illness depends on the type and quantity of bacteria consumed and the physical condition of the vic-

How Many Dolphins Died for Your Tuna Sandwich?

For a long time, an estimated twenty thousand dolphins were killed annually by tuna fishing vessels, in direct violation of the Marine Mammal Protection Act. The killing of the dolphins occurred during purse-seining of yellowfin tuna in the eastern tropical Pacific. Purse-seining involves using mile-long nets to trap yellowfin tuna, which often swim below the dolphin schools. The nets entrapped the friendly mammals and the cash crop beneath them.

The dolphins were unable to get out of the nets, and often little attempt was made to free the mammals before the tuna were harvested. As a result, several dozen at a time were killed as the tuna were hauled aboard. As many as seven hundred dolphins were killed in a single netting—not quickly or painlessly, but drowned and crushed to death as the long purse seines were hauled in.

Yellowfin tuna caught in the eastern tropical Pacific amount to only 5 percent of the total tuna catch worldwide. Other species of tuna in other waters are caught without harming dolphins. It was not necessary to continue the purse-seine yellowfin catch for the tuna industry to continue to thrive. Despite this fact, major tuna canning companies continued this practice, resulting in the needless slaughter of dolphins.

A nationwide tuna boycott initiated in 1988 finally brought the three biggest packers in the tuna industry to their knees by kicking them in their pocketbooks. In early 1990, owing to intense public outcry, H. J. Heinz Co. (Starkist) announced it would stop purchasing tuna from the eastern tropical Pacific. Bumble Bee and Van Kamp (Chicken of the Sea) soon followed.

The Dolphin Protection Consumer Information Act of 1990 requires labeling standards for all tuna harvested by ocean vessels, and established conditions for the protection of dolphins.

tim. Children, the elderly, and the sick are most susceptible to extreme reactions.

Scromboid Poisoning Scromboid fish include mackerel, tuna, and bonito. If these fish are improperly refrigerated after they are caught, bacteria in their flesh create histamine and related compounds. This "scromboid toxin" quickly produces an allergic reaction on consumption. Within as little as a few minutes of consumption, dizziness, heart palpitations, muscular paralysis, an unquenchable thirst, and itchy red welts can result. The symptoms usually go away after about twelve hours, but the experience of scromboid poisoning is uncomfortable at best and terrifying at worst.

Where's the Government? Despite weak claims to the contrary, federal food inspection officials do a completely inadequate job of ensuring the safety of fish products. In fact, fish is the only flesh food that does not have a mandatory inspection program. The National Marine Fisheries Service inspects a relatively small proportion of domestic fish. More than half of the fish consumed in the United States is imported and receives little inspection. The FDA has official jurisdiction over fish inspection.

Safety Precautions: What to Do? To ensure the purity of fish, and to reduce the potential for bacterial contamination, proper handling procedures should be observed by fishermen, fish processors, wholesalers, retailers, food service personnel, and consumers. In addition, *there should be a mandatory federal fish inspection program!*

As a consumer, you can't really influence other people along the fish-handling chain, but there are many things you *can* do to minimize the risk of bacterial contamination:

- Purchase your fish from a reputable dealer. Don't buy from outside "bargain" markets or discount fish vendors. A cheap price on a contaminated fish does not constitute a bargain.
- Avoid eating raw or undercooked seafood. Sushi is fine if you know that the fish comes from unpolluted waters and has been carefully inspected. Some sushi bars serve

fish that has been deep frozen to kill any possible parasites. Find out how your local sushi bar operates. As far as raw oysters and clams are concerned, avoid those products from polluted waters, and forget about imported shellfish entirely. Some aquacultured clams and oysters are safe to eat raw because they have been meticulously handled. But be extremely careful. If you have any condition resulting in a deficient immune system, including cancer, diabetes, liver disease, AIDS, ARC, or HIV infection, do not eat raw fish or shellfish.

• Keep all fish well refrigerated, preferably at 32°F, and not higher than 40°F. Storage at higher temperatures will result in proliferation of naturally occurring bacteria.

• Do not store fish for more than a few days unless it is frozen.
• Cook fish thoroughly before eating it, to kill any possible bacterial contaminants.

Issue: Parasites in Fish

Though the presence of parasites (also known as helminths) in fish is not contamination but a natural occurrence, it is nonetheless undesirable. The most common marine parasites are worms, including nematodes, trematodes, and cestodes. Other parasites include protozoa and copepods.

Fish become infested with parasites when they consume parasitic eggs or larvae, usually carried by small crustaceans. Larval worms burrow into the flesh or internal organs of fish, where they set up

---

Troubled Waters

Just as we are destroying the soil, air, forests, and wildlife on this delicate planet, we are also ruining the waters and killing or polluting vast numbers of fish in the process. The coastal waters of the world are choking with industrial waste, raw sewage, agricultural runoff, and garbage. Some areas are so badly polluted that the waters are unsafe to swim in, and the fish that survive are inedible.

Approximately one-third of U.S. shellfish beds have been closed because the waters where they are located are too contaminated with toxins to yield wholesome fish. Boston Harbor, one of the world's greatest seaports, is so heavily polluted that fishermen are advised to avoid fishing there at all. Mutant lobsters, fin fish with visible rot, flounder with tumors, and bacteria-laden shellfish are today's catch in Boston Harbor.

The situation is no more hopeful elsewhere. While 14.7 million pounds of striped bass were fished from New York waters in 1973, bass fishing is now banned near the city. Bass spawn in the polluted Hudson River, which for several years was a dumping ground for PCBs (polychlorinated biphenyls) by General Electric Co. As a result, the fish are inedible.

Along the Gulf, Louisiana and Florida waters are thick with sewage. Over two-thirds of Louisiana's oyster beds are closed at least six months each year as a result, and the Florida sport fishing industry has been badly hurt. Farther over on the Texas shore, oil companies still operate with permits to discharge industrial sludge and heavy metals into coastal water, killing virtually all marine life in some areas.

Although Europeans staged a moratorium on the ocean disposal of radioactive waste in 1983, decades of dumping have caused an underwater radioactive waste problem that will most likely last for thousands of years. In the Mediterranean, rampant sewage disposal has polluted some of the world's most beautiful beaches. An estimated 90 percent of the sewage in that area is still dumped into coastal waters.

The world's rivers, oceans, lakes, and other bodies of water can't take much more abuse. At the rate we are going, we will render the oceans unusable as a source of food and for recreational purposes in just a few more decades. Time is running out, and we are doing precious little to make things better.

housekeeping. If consumed, these parasites can enter the human digestive system, where they lodge in the digestive organs.

Cod and herring worms are common names for two species of anasakid nematodes, a family of roundworms. Despite their names, cod and herring worms actually live in many different species of fish. Consuming a live cod worm generally causes gastric upset, without other notable symptoms. If the head of the worm penetrates the stomach lining, however, it can cause severe abdominal pain and vomiting. If this penetration occurs, the worm must be removed by gastroscopy, a surgical procedure accomplished via the throat and esophagus. It's not particularly comfortable. Herring worms burrow into the intestinal lining. This can be a serious problem, involving a more complicated surgical procedure.

Freshwater fish can carry the larvae of *Diphyllobothrium*, or tapeworm. Tapeworm can cause weight loss, anemia, weakness, and abdominal pain. There are drugs that will treat tapeworm infection, however, so surgical removal is not necessary.

Freeze It, Cook It, Kill It The good news about parasites is that if you freeze fish to an internal temperature of approximately 0°F for 24 hours, you will kill the parasites. Likewise, if you cook fish to an internal temperature of 140°F, parasites will be destroyed. Parasites pose a health problem only when people consume raw or lightly cooked fish such as sushi, sashimi, and ceviche. Think twice before you eat raw fish.

Issue: Fecal Contamination

Oysters, clams, mussels, and scallops may be contaminated by fecal bacteria from the pollution of coastal waters, particularly near densely populated areas. Shellfish are prone to viral and bacterial contamination from sewage because of the way they feed. Shellfish constantly pump water through their digestive systems and feed on microorganisms in the water. If the water is contaminated by sewage, fecal-borne bacteria will enter the shellfish during filtration and will contaminate them.

If people eat fecal-contaminated shellfish raw or undercooked, they can contract cholera, typhoid, hepatitis, or gastroenteritis. Infectious hepatitis, an inflammation of the liver, has been associated with the consumption of contaminated shellfish. Symptoms of hepatitis manifest about three weeks after contaminated food is eaten, and include nausea, abdominal pain, and vomiting. The liver becomes enlarged and produces an abundance of yellow pigments resulting in jaundice, a yellowing of the skin and eyes.

Ask questions about where shellfish comes from. If it is obtained from waters known to be polluted with sewage, don't buy it. And in any case, be extremely careful if you are going to eat shellfish raw or undercooked. It is best to cook shellfish thoroughly to ensure safety.

Issue: Mercury and Heavy Metals

Mercury, lead, arsenic, and cadmium are heavy metals used in industry and are frequently discharged into waterways by manufacturing plants. Though these metals occur in nature in trace amounts, in greater concentration they are toxic to humans and animals. Fish can become contaminated with mercury and other heavy metals in two ways. The first is by direct contact through the gills and skin because of the presence of these metals in water. The second way is through the food chain. Microorganisms in water ingest inorganic mercury and convert it into the more toxic organic methyl mercury. Small fish feed on these microorganisms, larger fish feed on the smaller fish, and people eat the bigger fish. The toxic metal goes right up through the food chain and into the human body. Toxic metal poisoning can cause irreversible damage to the nervous system. Mercury, specifically, can impair vision and hearing and can cause severe brain damage resulting in insanity and an excruciatingly painful death. In the 1950s and 60s hundreds of Japanese people died when they consumed mercury-poisoned fish from waters polluted with mercury discharged from industrial facilities. Thus, mercury poisoning is now known as Minimata disease, a reference to the area where the deaths occurred. These tragic incidents prompted both the United States and Canada to establish federal monitoring and inspection programs to test for mercury in waters that are fished commercially. Nonetheless, businesses continue to dump mercury and other heavy metals into waterways, and the threat of poisoning is real.

Fish from the Great Lakes, the Hudson River in New York, and several rivers in Massachusetts are known to contain toxic levels of mercury and other heavy metals. Freshwater species including walleye, bass, and perch, and marine species, including swordfish, tuna, and halibut, are the fish most commonly contaminated by heavy metals. Neither thorough cooking nor any other method of preparation can remove heavy metals from fish, so know exactly where the fish you are eating comes from. Seek out fish obtained from deep, clean waters. Forget about fish from heavily populated coastal areas or from inland waterways near industrial facilities.

Issue: Naturally Occurring Poisons in Fish

Various species of fish may contain naturally occurring poisons. These poisons may be manufactured internally by the fish, may result from consuming toxic organisms such as some types of algae, may be due to pathogenic bacteria growing within the fish, or may occur as a result of bacterial growth due to improper handling. Whatever the cause, the result can be illness, and in some rare cases death.

Probably the best-known and most feared of all toxic fish is the puffer fish. This species contains a potent poison called tetrodotoxin, which is found in specific glands of the fish. If even a tiny amount of this substance is consumed, violent poisoning ensues. Tingling of the victim's lips and mouth is accompanied by convulsions, muscular paralysis, and respiratory failure. Consumption of tetrodotoxin is usually fatal.

As a game of gustatory roulette, puffer fish,

known as *fugu,* is consumed as a delicacy at some sushi bars in Japan. Highly trained sushi chefs carefully remove the deadly tetrodotoxin-laden glands from the fish. The remaining flesh is thinly sliced and served raw to daredevil gourmands. Deaths do occur as a result of this practice. As of 1988 there are some licensed *fugu* bars in the United States. The treat is expensive and may be fatal.

The tetrodotoxin in puffer fish is potent enough to be readily absorbed into the skin. Dried puffer fish powder is an essential component of a paste smeared onto selected human victims in bizarre Haitian voodoo rituals conducted to produce "zombies," or the walking dead. As a result of application of the paste, total muscular paralysis occurs. Usually the victim does not die but remains fully alert, paralyzed and unable to communicate in any manner for several days. These individuals are buried alive in caskets and are exhumed after a couple of days, fully insane as a result of their ordeal. Though muscular activity returns, victims of the "zombie" process rarely recover their mental health.

OTHER FISH POISONS

Other types of fish poisons are less exotic, and their stories are less strange:

Ciguatoxin   As many as four hundred species of fish from subtropical and tropical waters may contain this poison. Red snapper, grouper, and barracuda can contain toxic levels of ciguatoxin, which is believed to come from a particular blue-green marine algae. Ciguatoxin poisoning starts with tingling of the mouth and lips, chills, fever, and respiratory difficulty and can be fatal.

Moray Eels   Besides having a nasty bite, moray eels may consume microorganisms that produce a poison similar in activity to ciguatoxin. Tingling of the mouth, lips, hands, and feet is followed by nausea, respiratory difficulty, and loss of motor control. Moray poisoning looks like drunkenness and can result in violent convulsions and death. So, avoid eating moray eels if you possibly can.

Scromboid Fish   Mentioned previously in the section "Fish Handling and Related Illness," scromboid fish (mackerel, tuna, bonito) contain a bacteria that proliferate if the fish are not adequately chilled after being caught. These bacteria produce histamine and related compounds that can cause dizziness, heart palpitations, muscular paralysis, and an unquenchable thirst. Eat only properly handled mackerel, tuna, and bonito.

Sharks, Rays, and Skates   These fish are believed to ingest toxic microorganisms that produce poisons in their flesh. Consuming poisoned sharks, rays, and skates can result in nausea, vomiting, and diarrhea.

Shellfish   Oysters, clams, mussels, and scallops can become poisoned from ingesting microorganisms known as dinoflagellates. This poisoning usually occurs during the warmer months of the year. See "Issue: Red Tide" for further details.

KNOW YOUR SOURCES!   If these lurid tales of fish poisoning make you want to swear off marine foods forever, relax. Compared with the total volume of fish consumed, the incidence of serious poisoning is relatively rare. Nonetheless, you don't want to be an unlucky statistic. You can't cook poisons out of fish, but you can buy your fish from merchants who are experts in their field. High-quality, reputable fishmongers know about these hazards and are sensitive to issues of poisoning, dangerous exotic species, and seasonal contamination. Take time to find out exactly which vendors in your area really know their fish.

Issue: Red Tide

When environmental conditions along coastal areas are favorable, a phenomenon called red tide occurs. Calm seas, warm surface temperature, high nutrient content, and low salinity (which follows heavy rains) provide the perfect environment for a fast proliferation of dinoflagellates, a family of microscopic plankton. Though there are several different strains of dinoflagellates that cause red tide, their effect is similar. The water along coastal areas becomes reddish brown.

The organisms that cause red tide contain toxins that can be extremely dangerous to human health. Whereas fin fish do not become contaminated by these toxins, some shellfish do. For this reason, it is imperative that people do not eat oysters, mussels, clams, quahogs, scallops, and soft-shell crabs from waters affected by red tide. Shrimp, lobsters, and crabs caught during red tide, however, are safe to eat.

Consuming shellfish contaminated with dinoflagellates can result in paralytic shellfish poisoning (PSP). Tingling sensations start in the mouth and lips and spread to the feet and hands. Dizziness, nausea, and loss of motor control may also occur. Instances of respiratory failure and fatalities have been reported. Do not under any circumstances knowingly catch or eat shellfish from waters affected by red tide!

Aquaculture

Aquaculture is fish farming: the science of raising fish in controlled ocean beds or inland tanks and ponds. Practiced for more than four thousand years by the Chinese, aquaculture is being taken seriously by entrepreneurs sensitive to the increased demand for fish and to the escalating problems of marine pollution. Today aquaculture specialists are growing more than twenty species, from trout to tilapia, catfish to clams, salmon to lobsters.

Although many aquaculture operations grow their fish in ocean beds that could possibly become contaminated with pollutants, inland growers have a unique opportunity to produce fish without exposing them to PCBs, heavy metals, or other toxins. Considering the rate at which we are destroying the purity of our natural water resources, the filtered, carefully monitored tanks and ponds used by aquaculture operations may eventually prove to be the only safe waters from which we can obtain fish fit for human consumption. Just as cattle ranching has changed from grazing steers on the open prairie to factory farming, the intensive yield systems of aquaculture may eventually replace the boats, nets, and hooks of commercial fishing.

Issue: PCBs

First discovered in 1881, the more than two hundred chemical configurations of PCBs, or polychlorinated biphenyls, were used extensively in industry until they were banned in the United States in 1977. Originally manufactured by Monsanto Corporation (one of the largest toxic polluters in the world), PCBs are fire resistant, have low water solubility, and have a low boiling point. Over 1.2 billion pounds of these chemicals were produced in the United States before they were banned according to the strictures of the Toxic Substances Control Act.

PCBs settle in fresh and marine waters, where they are consumed by various microorganisms and travel up the food chain, accumulating in fatty fish. Though PCBs have been detected in hundreds of different waters, they are most concentrated near industrial areas. The waters in the United States with the greatest known PCB contamination include the Great Lakes, the Mississippi River, the Hudson River in New York, and the Acushnet and Housatonic Rivers in Massachusetts.

Although the U.S. Food and Drug Administration established a safe tolerance level for PCBs in edible fish to 2.0 parts per million, there is no reason to be reassured by this action. Fish is rarely tested for PCB contamination, so there is no way to know whether the fish you are eating is safe according to federal tolerances. Symptoms of PCB poisoning include fatigue, headache, eye irritation, nausea, vomiting, skin eruptions, and liver disorders. PCBs are carcinogenic and may cause fetal abnormalities. In other words, PCBs are heavy-duty toxins.

PROTECTING YOURSELF   Don't eat fish of any kind from waters known or believed to be contaminated with PCBs. Additionally, certain methods of fish preparation can lower the potential risk of poisoning. PCBs accumulate in the fatty tissue of fish. Older, larger, fattier fish will contain a greater quantity of PCBs, if any. When you prepare fish, remove the skin, cut off any visible fat, and broil, grill, or bake the fish on a rack so the oils can drain. Do not sauté or pan-fry the fish, as this seals in the fish oils.

Issue: Radionuclides in Fish

Radionuclides are disintegrating atoms that emit radiation. Though minute amounts of radionuclides occur naturally in the marine environment, a greater concentration of these substances is now present as a result of improper and illegal industrial dumping of radioactive waste materials. Though the Ocean Dumping Act of 1972 was established to develop safe guidelines for the disposal of radioactive waste in the ocean, violations of safe dumping practices are rampant. Contaminated land runoff and nuclear fallout are additional factors that contribute to radionuclide contamination of the marine environment. The effects of exposure to high levels of radioactivity are well documented. Radiation sickness starts with loss of appetite, vomiting, and diarrhea. There is a reduction in blood cells, increased tendency toward bleeding, and reduced defense against infection. Bone marrow, spleen, and lymph nodes are impaired, and death can result. Nothing is known, however, about the long-term effects of the human consumption of fish contaminated with radionuclides. The presence of radionuclides in fish is ostensibly monitored by the Food and Drug Administration. In reality, however, very little testing of fish for radioactivity is performed.

To safeguard yourself against radionuclide poisoning from fish, avoid consuming fish caught near nuclear reactors, from waters known or suspected to be dumping grounds for radioactive waste, or from waters near industrial areas where radioactive materials are used.

Issue: Oil Pollution

Humans are not the only species endangered by pollutants and imbalanced environmental ecology. Fish also suffer from our toxic transgressions. Petroleum hydrocarbons from oil and its various refined products enter the marine environment via ocean dumping, industrial emissions, land runoff, accidents, spills, tanker and maritime activities, and other methods of leakage.

Petroleum hydrocarbons are toxic to marine life and are particularly dangerous to fish larvae, young fish, and shellfish. In areas where petrochemical dumping or discharge occurs, the populations of many marine species can be greatly reduced.

The carcinogenic compounds of petrochemicals, known as polychlorinated aromatic hydrocarbons (PAHs), have been found in seafood. In animal feeding studies, these compounds have been proved to cause cancer. Though there is currently no research that shows a direct link between the consumption of petroleum-tainted seafood and the incidence of cancer in humans, the Food and Drug Administration warns people to refrain from eating seafood of any kind if it tastes or smells like oil or other petroleum products.

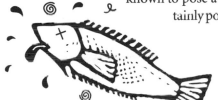

Issue: Cancer in Fish

High rates of cancer in multiple species of fish caught in waters near heavily populated or industrial areas tell a frightening story of an environment gone mad. Toxic pollutants bind to microorganisms and particulate matter, which are then consumed through the entire marine food chain. The incidence of cancer among fish has a relationship to the types of pollutants present in water, the concentration of these toxins, the motion or stillness of the water, and the species of marine life present. Bottom feeders, shellfish, and flounder seem particularly prone to cancer in polluted areas. While cancer in fish is not known to pose a health problem to humans, it certainly poses a health problem to fish, thereby threatening a major part of the world's food supply.

12

ECO REPORT: WATER

The Need for Water

There is nothing like pure water. It is called the "universal solvent," and nobody can do without it. Life as we know it is entirely dependent on water. The human body is made up mostly of water. About 55 to 65 percent of a woman's body is water, while a man's body contains from 65 to 75 percent of this life-preserving fluid. This supply must be replenished daily. Although humans can survive without food for extended periods—as long as two months—no one can go without water for more than a few days without either causing serious damage to the body, or dying. We replenish our body water by eating foods that naturally contain water and by drinking water or other beverages.

The Water Supply

There is a tremendous amount of water on our small planet. Yet, only about 1 percent of the water on earth is fresh and drinkable. The other 99 percent is either ice or brine. The earth has a water supply of about 326 trillion gallons. The supply remains constant, but the water changes form continuously. Evaporated water from lakes, rivers, and oceans becomes

rain. Much of this pours down on land and works its way to underground freshwater aquifers. From there it bubbles up through springs into other bodies of water. Fresh water from springs may wind up frozen in huge masses of ice in the polar regions. Polar ice is constantly melting. Water occurs as fresh water, salt water, snow, fog, rain, sleet, hail, and ice. A large amount of water is locked up inside vegetation, plants, trees, bushes, and grasses of all kinds.

The United States has 2 million miles of streams and over 30 million acres of lakes and reservoirs, as well as an enormous freshwater supply in underground aquifers. This supply is fifty times greater than the total amount of surface water. Over 100 million Americans obtain their drinking water from groundwater. The U.S. public water systems supply each American with approximately 160 gallons of fresh water every day, making our per capita water consumption the highest in the world.

The Problem with Water Today

Both surface water and ground water are becoming increasingly polluted. This pollution represents a major health problem for humans and the environment, because if water is contaminated it can act as a physical and environmental poison. While this is a concern worldwide, pollution is a particularly great problem in industrialized nations. From large-scale factory farming to manufacturing, the production of goods uses a vast amount of water, which is typically contaminated with by-products of the production process. This report focuses on polluted water as it relates to human consumption and does not address the impact that polluted water has on the environment at large. Water pollution can occur at three different stages prior to human consumption. These stages are before treatment, during treatment, and after treatment.

Before treatment, water can be polluted by human and animal waste; agricultural chemicals from runoff; minerals and salts; decay products of radon, radium, and uranium; leaking storage tanks; leaking hazardous waste landfills, ponds, and pits; underground injection of industrial waste; and surface runoff from sewers or rainwater from oil-slicked or salt-treated highways.

Human and Animal Waste   Approximately 25 percent of the homes in the United States use septic systems that may contaminate groundwater with fecal bacteria. In addition, much raw sewage is poorly handled and is introduced into waterways, thereby contaminating both surface water and groundwater supplies. Microbiological organisms of concern in water supplies include coliform bacteria, fecal coliform, and streptococcal and other bacteria. Water contaminated with these microorganisms can cause dysentery, hepatitis, gastrointestinal inflammation, typhoid, cholera, and several other life-threatening diseases. One water-borne bacterial contaminant, *Giardia lamblia,* is chlorine resistant and is known to have infected a minimum of twenty thousand Americans since 1972. Giardia can be sexually transmitted, is hard to detect, and is difficult to treat.

Agricultural Chemicals from Runoff   Millions of tons of pesticides, herbicides, fungicides, fertilizers, and other agricultural chemicals are spread on the

ground annually, primarily in rural areas. Many of these are known carcinogens or mutagens. These chemicals sink into the ground, thereby contaminating underground aquifers. Or they run off land during rainstorms, into streams, rivers, lakes, and ponds, polluting surface water supplies and ultimately leading to the contamination of groundwater. The end result is widespread water pollution. Since the mid-1940s, agricultural chemical use in the United States has increased 1,000 percent. The impact that this has had on human health and on the environment is virtually incalculable. But we do know that agricultural contaminants occur in drinking water and that these contaminants are associated with a variety of diseases and health problems, including leukemia and several forms of cancer.

Minerals and Salts   Depleted aquifers near coastal areas may be invaded by salt water, thus contaminating the water supply with brine. Particles of sulfates, chlorides, and nitrates frequently show up suspended in untreated water and are also found in water that is not adequately treated. These particles can be allergenic and carcinogenic. Arsenic, a toxic metal, occurs as an impurity in minerals and ores of various commercially mined metals. Arsenic can occur in water that is inadequately treated, and can cause liver and kidney damage if consumed by humans. The inorganic chemical fluoride, which is often abundantly present in water, can cause skeletal damage as well as fluorosis, a brownish discoloration of the teeth.

Decay Products of Radon, Radium, and Uranium Radionuclides are radioactive substances that emit radiation as they decay, a process that can last for tens of thousands of years. These radionuclides include uranium, radium, and radon. Uranium and radium are ingested in drinking water and are associated with bone cancer and kidney cancer. Radon, now recognized as an environmental pollutant of serious proportions, is a gas that occurs naturally as a result of the radioactive decay of radium-226. Radon is colorless, odorless, and tasteless and occurs naturally in various types of rock and soil found in many regions of the United States. Radon gas is inhaled after being released into the air during or after water use, such as taking showers or baths and washing dishes or clothes. Radon gas inhalation is estimated to cause as many as twenty thousand deaths in the United States annually.

Leaking Storage Tanks   There are approximately 6 million underground storage tanks in the United States, several hundred thousand of which are believed to be leaking. These storage tanks are filled with waste materials, toxic chemicals, paints, solvents, and petroleum products. Waste from storage tanks seeps into the ground, where it contaminates freshwater aquifers, many of which are primary public water supply sources.

Leaking Hazardous Waste Landfills, Ponds, and Pits   In the United States, there are approximately 29,000 hazardous waste sites that are potential clean-up sites for the Superfund National Priorities List. There are also 500 known hazardous-waste land-disposal facilities, and an additional 16,000 legal landfills, not to mention tens of thousands of illegal dumping sites, all of which can contaminate ground and surface waters. There are also almost 200,000 lagoons, pits, and ponds that are believed to be contaminated with microbial and chemical pollutants.

Underground Injection of Industrial Waste   Industrial wastes are routinely injected into underground deep disposal wells that directly contaminate groundwater. These wastes, which can be solid or liquid, include degreasing agents, solvents, paints, thinners, glues, dyes, pesticides, and other highly toxic compounds.

Surface Runoff from Sewers or Rainwater from Oil-slicked or Salt-treated Highways   The salting of roads is a major water problem, as it increases the sodium content of municipal drinking water supplies to (in some cases) hazardous levels. Individuals with restricted sodium diets frequently must abstain from consuming public water. Rec-

ognizing this problem, many communities in snow regions throughout the United States are voluntarily restricting or eliminating the use of salt on roadways. Oil and other petrochemical residues on roads and highways also find their way into the water system.

Disinfection By-Products   During treatment, water can be contaminated by disinfection by-products and other additives. Chlorine is the major disinfectant used in U.S. water-treatment facilities. Environmental Protection Agency scientists have discovered that chlorine can react with other naturally occurring compounds in water to create a group of chemicals known as trihalomethanes (THMs). One of these chemicals is chloroform, a cancer-causing agent.

Other Additives   Copper sulfate, alum, and other chemical additives typically used in the water-treatment process may remain in water after treatment is complete, because of faulty filtration methods. The result is that drinking water may actually contain toxic additives introduced solely for the purpose of making water safer to drink. Copper poisoning is a concern 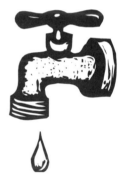 among children in particular. Excess levels of copper in the body can adversely affect the immune system and are believed to be associated with some behavioral disorders.

After treatment, water can be contaminated by lead and asbestos from pipe materials, dirt and bacteria from leaky pipes, and polluted water that enters pipes instead of leaving them.

Lead and Asbestos from Pipe Materials   Lead from pipes and solder can leach into water supplies in the home, thereby causing lead poisoning. Consumption of lead can cause damage to the central and peripheral nervous systems and to the kidneys. Lead is particularly toxic to infants and pregnant women. Asbestos is a cancer-causing agent.

Dirt and Bacteria from Leaky Pipes   Any and all microbiological contaminants, including the entire coliform group of bacteria, can enter pipes through breaks and cracks. The same is the case with all chemicals and compounds that may occur in the soil around piping.

Water and Methods of Water Purification and Treatment

The alarming condition of our public water supplies has led an increasing number of people to turn to bottled and purified water products. Of course, not everyone who purchases these products does so because of concern about public water safety. Many water products, especially those that are carbonated and flavored, appeal to people who want good-tasting, sparkling beverages but don't want the chemicals and sweeteners found in most sodas and colas.

At present there are no uniform regulations governing the purity and quality of bottled water. This means that bottled water can come directly from a tap, or it can be the result of extensive and complex filtration. In food stores you will be confronted by a variety of water products, from spring water to distilled to carbonated and flavored varieties. Some products will list the methods by which they are purified (if they are), while natural spring waters will typically identify their sources.

If you are in doubt about the purity of a bottled water product, write or call the bottler and ask which methods of purification it uses, or how it otherwise determines product purity. Any reputable water vendor will provide you with a detailed laboratory analysis of its water. If the vendor is not willing to do so, drink another brand.

Following is a list and brief explanation of the methods by which water can be purified, and the results typically obtained by these methods.

Activated Charcoal Adsorption   Widely used in home filtration systems, carbon adsorption removes disagreeable chlorine taste and fishy or musky odors. Activated carbon can be made from nut

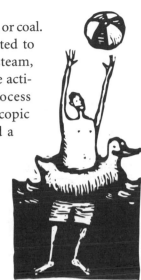

shells, petroleum, fruit pits, or coal. These ingredients are heated to high temperatures with steam, without oxygen (this is the activation process). This process leaves millions of microscopic pores on the material and a huge surface area. Just one pound of activated carbon provides over 125 acres of surface area. The tiny pores capture microscopic particles as well as larger organic molecules. The activated surface areas cling to, or "adsorb," smaller organic molecules.

When carbon filters are fresh, they remove almost all impurities in water. However, carbon filters accumulate organic impurities, which then become breeding grounds for bacteria that can multiply greatly. Another problem with carbon filters is chemical recontamination. Once the surface area of the activated filter is covered with particulate matter, then those particles may be released back into the water, thus negating the value of the filter.

If activated carbon filters are used, they should be kept clean, and water should be flushed through them if they have not been used for several hours or overnight. This flushing may purge the filter of built-up bacteria.

Bacteriostatic Carbon, Silver Impregnated, or Oligodynamic Filters   These filters are impregnated with silver compounds designed to inhibit the growth of bacteria in the carbon bed. Environmental Protection Agency testing of these filters does not support this claim. The EPA says that such filters are "neither effective nor dependable in meeting their claims."

Carbon Block Filters   Very fine pulverized carbon, fused into a solid block, creates an intricate maze that more effectively traps and removes organic impurities from water. Some carbon block filters (not all) have such a fine porous structure that they actually filter coliform and other disease bacteria from water. Carbon block filters plug up easily, however, because of their fine porous nature, and some of these filters actually give off toxic chemicals of their own.

Distillation   Certainly one of the finest ways of purifying water, distillation is a process by which water is heated until it turns to steam. This steam is captured and cooled back into water again, leaving behind toxic metals, sediments, total dissolved solids, nitrates, and microorganisms. The result is, or should be, pure water.

Unfortunately, though, there are now organic contaminants in water (like trihalomethanes) that have a lower boiling point than water itself. Because of this, these contaminants wind up in the distilled water. In addition, distilled water often tastes flat. This can be easily remedied by aerating the water: literally shaking it so that it can accumulate additional dissolved oxygen.

Reverse Osmosis Ultrafiltration   This technology is probably the state of the art as far as water purification is concerned. Originally developed by the U.S. government for desalinization, reverse osmosis ultrafiltration (RO) uses a semipermeable membrane to purify water.

RO strains out bacteria, particulate matter, asbestos, microorganisms, turbidity, and even single molecules of heavy organic compounds. This is due to its unique membranes, the superfine pores of which are approximately 2 ten-millionths of an inch in diameter. That's incredibly tiny! But RO ultrafilters are more than just mechanical screens. Reverse osmosis is a phenomenon by which impurities in water are actually repelled from the surface of the filter membrane. The filter, however, is permeable to water, which accumulates on the other side of the membrane in a pure state. Almost. Unfortunately, RO technology is ineffective in filtering low–molecular-weight volatile organic compounds such as carbon tetrachloride, vinyl car-

bon, and trihalomethanes. This is because these substances are small enough to pass through the micro-pores of the membrane and are not repelled from the filter surface.

Reverse osmosis technology is becoming more widely used for industrial purposes, and we will see an increasing number of beverage companies using this type of filtration over the next decade. Some companies are now using a combination of carbon and RO filtration in an attempt to purify water to the greatest extent possible.

At this time, it is unlikely that we can obtain absolutely pure water, without any pollutants whatsoever. This is because humans have done such an effective job of contaminating the planet's water supply. Even waters from very deep springs in remote rural areas may contain traces of chemical contaminants that cannot be removed from water by present filtration and purification methods. Nonetheless, purification and filtration can make water appreciably safer to drink. The impact that we have had on the world's water supply most likely will not be fully understood for a long time to come. But one thing is certain. We have altered the basic nature of water in our world, perhaps forever.

Water Products

As a product category, water has had a meteoric rise in sales over the past few years. This is indicative of both an increased concern about public water sources and a desire to consume more healthful beverages. As more is known about the damaging effects of drinking sodas and colas, more consumers are switching to water products. As far as the human body is concerned, water, not Coca-Cola, is the real thing.

Just because water is in a bottle, however, does not mean that it is pure. It is perfectly

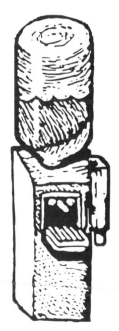

legal to pour tapwater from any municipal source and sell it in a bottle. The only thing that is not legal is to mislabel water as far as its source or method of purification is concerned. Be aware of what you are buying. Water, like any other product, requires label reading.

Distilled Water   As previously described, distilled water has been purified by a process that involves heating water and evaporating the steam, leaving behind many, though not necessarily all, impurities. Those compounds that have a boiling point as low as water, or lower, will remain in the final distilled product. Despite possible residues, distillation is still one of the best ways to purify water.

Mineral Water   This is simply nonpurified water containing minerals that occur in water from a variety of natural sources. Higher-quality mineral waters will state their sources, which are typically specific springs known for their purity. Some brands have particularly high amounts of calcium, magnesium, potassium, and other minerals, which give flavor to the water obtained from these sources.

Seltzer   Nothing more than tapwater with bubbles in it, seltzer is far better for you than most sodas but is usually less free of contaminants than most spring waters. The bubbles in seltzer are formed when harmless carbon dioxide gas is pumped into water, a process that also occurs in nature.

Sparkling Water   This can be either carbonated tapwater or carbonated spring water. Read the product label to determine what you are buying. Many sparkling waters today are made with high-quality spring water to which carbon dioxide gas is added. Still other waters bubble up from the ground already carbonated and are bottled that way. Some waters are carbonated naturally, and as they bubble up from the ground the carbon dioxide gas escapes from the water, is captured, and is mechanically reintroduced into the water.

Sparkling Water (Flavored)   Many sparkling waters now come flavored with fruit essences, which are made from oils obtained from the skin of various fruits. The majority of these are not sweetened. Beware of sweetened versions, which usually contain fructose, corn syrup, or some other highly refined sugar.

Spring Water   Plain spring water is water obtained from natural springs that bubble up from the ground. Spring water may be run through a screen to remove any undesirable particles, but it is otherwise untinkered with. Beware of "springlike" rip-off products. If a products says "spring pure" on the label, it really means "straight from the tap." Read the label. Any real spring water will proudly label its source. An example of this is Poland Spring Water, from Poland Spring, Maine. The label doesn't allow you to miss the source of the water.

13

OILS

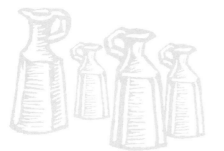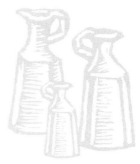

BASIC FACTS ABOUT OILS

Vegetable oils play a more significant role in our health than most people realize. Vegetable oils are *lipids,* or fats. They are a primary source of dietary fats, which provide calories for energy as well as essential nutrients. Thus, their nutritive value and the manner in which they are processed are important to understand.

Vegetable oils are made up of *fatty acids,* which are the essential components of all dietary fats. There are basically three kinds of dietary fats, distinguished by their levels of *saturation.* All fats, including vegetable oils, are made up of a combination of saturated and unsaturated fatty acids. Saturation refers to the number of hydrogen molecules a fat can accept. This determines the hardness of that fat. Beef fat or butter, for example, will be solid at room temperature, whereas corn oil will be liquid, because of differences in saturation. The saturation of a fat has a lot to do with whether that fat will contribute to an increase or a decrease in blood cholesterol levels. The following categories of fats include a partial list of their sources.

Saturated fats are found in milk, eggs, cheese, meat, poultry, chocolate, vegetable shortening, and some vegetable oils, including coconut and palm oils. The consumption of saturated fats causes your body to produce excess amounts of cholesterol. For this reason, palm and coconut oils have come under fire in recent years. They are more highly saturated than lard, and are the two most saturated fats known. When you see a product that claims to be cholesterol-free, check the label. If the product contains palm or coconuts oils, it may wind up causing your body to manufacture more cholesterol anyway. Saturated fats and foods that contain them are best eaten in moderation.

Monounsaturated fats are found in almond oil, peanut oil, sesame oil, avocados, high-oleic safflower oil (from hybrid strains that yield high amounts of heart-healthy oleic acid, a nutritious fatty acid), high-oleic sunflower oil, canola oil, and olive oil. Monounsaturated fats have been shown to help decrease blood cholesterol levels. Olive oil, for example, is widely cited by medical experts as an ideal oil for cooking and for salad dressings because of its cholesterol-lowering properties. In Mediterranean regions olive oil is widely consumed, and there the rate of coronary disease is typically low. If olive oil is kept refrigerated, it will harden. This does not mean that the oil is bad in any way. Monounsaturates will harden or partially harden at cold temperatures.

Polyunsaturated fats are found in corn oil, safflower oil, sunflower oil, soybean oil, walnuts, pecans, and filberts. Polyunsaturated fats have been touted as heart healthy for years. One significant difference between polyunsaturated and monounsaturated fats, however, is that polyunsaturated fats tend to go rancid more easily. This means that polyunsaturated fats require more careful storage and handling.

Approximately twenty fatty acids are commonly found in the human diet. Of these, the human body can synthesize all but three fatty acids: arachidonic, linoleic, and linolenic acids. These fatty acids are essential to life and can be obtained only from the diet. Thus, they are known as the *essential fatty acids.* The essential fatty acids are referred to collectively as vitamin F.

Vitamin F is found in nuts, seeds, whole grains, beans, and some oil-bearing fruits such as avocados and olives. Vitamin F promotes growth and is essential for healthy skin, hair, glands, mucous membranes, nerves, and arteries. It functions in cholesterol regulation, menstruation, the regulation of blood pressure, the absorption of calcium, and body lubrication and resilience. An inadequate dietary intake of vitamin F can lead to acne, dandruff, dry hair, diarrhea, weak nails, allergies, menstrual disorders, eczema, and below-average weight.

Fatty Acid Composition of Oils

The saturated or unsaturated fatty acid composition of a vegetable oil, along with its essential fatty acid content, is due to the source of the oil and how

Percentage of Fatty Acid Composition

Oil	Saturated	Monounsaturated	Polyunsaturated
Almond	9	65	26
Used for salad dressings, sauces, sautéing			
Avocado	20	70	10
Used for salad dressings, sauces, sautéing			
Canola	6	60	34
Used for baking, frying, salad dressings, sauces, sautéing			
Corn	13	27	60
Used for baking, salad dressings			
Olive	10	82	8
Used for salad dressings, sauces, sautéing			
Peanut	19	51	30
Used for baking, frying, sauces, sautéing			
Safflower	8	13	79
Used for baking, salad dressings, sautéing			
Sesame	13	46	41
Used for baking, salad dressings, sauces, sautéing			
Soy	14	28	58
Used for baking, salad dressings			
Sunflower	12	19	69
Used for baking, salad dressings, sautéing			
Walnut	16	28	56
Used for baking, salad dressings, sautéing			

that oil is processed. Vegetable oils are commonly obtained from these foods:

- *Seeds*   Safflower, sunflower, sesame, flax
- *Nuts*   Almond, walnut, filbert, palm, coconut
- *Grains*   Corn, wheat
- *Beans*   Peanut, soy
- *Fruits*   Olive, avocado

The table on this page lists vegetable oils and describes their fatty acid composition and primary dietary uses.

Oils and Health

A full 40 percent of the calories in the American diet comes from fats. Excessive consumption of dietary fats is the primary cause of obesity. Consumption of saturated fats leads to high cholesterol. The higher the percentage of calories obtained from fats, the lower the proportion of nutrient-rich foods in the diet, such as fruits, vegetables, grains, and beans.

Processed foods are typically loaded with added fats to create a rich, satisfying flavor. The Surgeon General's *Report on Diet and Health* recommends a reduction in fat intake as the single most urgent dietary change required today. We are becoming an increasingly overweight population, living on calorie-rich fatty foods.

Oils and other processed fats appear in a multitude of items, from cookies to pie crusts, burgers, fries, potato chips, dessert toppings, baked goods, and virtually all varieties of snacks and fast foods. This is one more reason why it is most healthful to eat a diet of nutritious whole foods. You can obtain all the fats and oils your body needs from whole grains, nuts, seeds, and beans, fresh meats, and dairy products.

Which Oils to Use?

If you are going to use vegetable oils for baking, cooking, salad dressings, or other purposes, choose unrefined oils whenever possible. For everything but baking (because of flavor considerations and low smoking point), extra-virgin olive oil is the ideal oil. Olive oil is particularly high in monounsaturated fatty acids (82 percent), which actually help to lower blood cholesterol. Another oil that is ideal for all purposes, including baking, is canola oil, which is also high in monounsaturates (60 percent). Canola oil has a high smoking point and thus is good for sautéing.

Learn to use only a small amount of oil, whatever the purpose. Instead of frying or sautéing foods, broil, stew, poach, steam, or bake them. Remember that fats contain twice as many calories as carbohydrates or proteins. Once you get used to a healthy low-fat whole-foods diet, you'll find it easier to maintain an ideal weight. Additionally, you'll reduce the risk of heart disease, arthritis, and gastrointestinal disorders.

VEGETABLE OILS AND MANUFACTURING

When you face a shelf full of vegetable oils and read the labels, you will quickly realize that you don't really know how to determine what distinguishes a healthful, high-quality oil from a nutritionally inferior product. This is because manufacturers either say little on their products or litter their labels with terms like "polyunsaturated!" and "cholesterol free!" and "cold pressed!" So let's sort out a few facts.

To say that oil manufacturing is big business is an understatement. Large commercial extractors crush several million pounds of raw materials every day. To do so, they use the quickest, most cost-effective means possible. Many of the steps used in oil manufacturing expedite the finishing of the product while harming the nutritional value and flavor of the oil. There are three methods of extracting vegetable oils from their sources: expeller pressing, solvent extraction, and cold pressing. Additionally, oils may be refined or unrefined. The following describes the processes by which these methods are performed:

Expeller Pressed (Unrefined)

1. The materials (seeds, nuts, grains, or beans) are **cleaned** and hulled. This is performed mechanically, without chemicals or heat.
2. The materials are **cooked** at low temperature, between 110° and 160° F, to warm the oils, thus making them easier to extract.
3. An auger or screw press is used to crush the materials, **pressing** out the oil. If this is the sole process used to extract the oil, then that product can be labeled "100% expeller pressed." The result of this process is an unrefined, nutrient-rich oil. If an oil is bottled at this point with no further processing, it may be additionally labeled "unrefined." Brands of expeller-pressed, unrefined oils are available in natural food stores today.

Phony Fats

If you'd like to sit down to a big, gloppy dessert with little or no calories or cholesterol, or sink yourself into a pile of greasy, low-calorie French fries, then Procter & Gamble's Olestra and NutraSweet's Simplesse are for you. These two phony fats are a tribute to the marvels of food technology, and insulting to both human health and nature itself.

Olestra is a combination of soybean oil and sucrose that has been manipulated into molecules too large to be absorbed or digested by the human body. Thus Olestra passes untouched through the digestive system and therefore contains no calories or cholesterol. It is seen as having huge potential to replace fat in the chips and crackers market. Test-marketing of Olestra products, under the brand name Olean, began in the Midwest in the summer of 1996. It is reported to have all the flavor and "mouth-feel" of regular fat.

Preliminary studies suggested that Olestra causes tumors in laboratory animals. According to Procter & Gamble, however, subsequent studies do not show that effect. Even if Olestra is not carcinogenic, it does interfere with the body's absorption of vitamin E. Vitamin E is fat-soluble, which means it is carried into the blood stream by hitching a ride on fat molecules. But Olestra never reaches the bloodstream; it is a non-stop train carrying its vitamin E passengers with it straight to Eliminationville. To counteract this effect, Proctor & Gamble has promised to add vitamin supplements to its Olestra products.

Other possible side effects of the large, undigestible Olestra molecules include intestinal cramping, flatulence, and loose stool. Proctor & Gamble states that at "normal levels of consumption" consumers should not experience unusual digestive problems. But the temptation to binge on tasty, fat-free snack foods may be too much for some people. And when that first bag of low-cal Olestra chips gets wolfed down, things could get ugly.

Simplesse is made from scientifically engineered milk protein or egg white. Simplesse is actually absorbed by the body but is very low in calories. Those who are allergic to milk or eggs will react adversely to this synthetic fat. Look for Simplesse in ice cream, yogurt, mayonnaise, sour cream, salad dressing, and other foods.

Phony fats are being promoted as the means to curb obesity. But these nonfoods are more likely to encourage overeating of nutritionally barren foods, while dumping dollars into the coffers of large corporations.

Refined

After extraction according to the previous steps, most oils will proceed through the following methods of refinement:

4. The oil is **degummed,** a process that removes the lecithin (which is essential to every cell in the human body), the chlorophyll, the vitamin E, and any minerals.
5. An alkaline solution is added to the oil to **refine** it by separating any and all unwanted substances (primarily nutrients).
6. Diatomaceous earth is added to the oil to **bleach** it. When the diatomaceous earth is filtered back out of the oil, it takes with it carotenes (natural vitamin A), chlorophyll, and other nutritive factors. This renders the oil clear.
7. The oil is then **deodorized** by steam distillation at very high temperatures, over 450°F.
8. Further clarification, or **winterizing,** is achieved by cooling and filtering the oil. Any waxes and stearines present (which can cloud the oil under refrigeration) are removed. The finished product is a colorless, odorless, tasteless, nutritionally inferior oil, with only the fatty acids remaining.

Only truly honest oil manufacturers will label their oil "refined." The truth is, they don't have to say anything about the process of manufacture.

Solvent Extraction

Most commercially processed oils are solvent extracted, rather than expeller pressed, because solvent extraction removes more oil from the raw material. In solvent extraction, materials are also **cleaned** and **hulled.** Then they are **flaked** by mechanical rollers that crush the materials. Following flaking, a petrochemical solvent (hexane is most commonly used) is added to the raw material. This **extracts** the oil from the solids. After extraction, the solvent is boiled off. There is valid concern, however, that not all of the solvent is extracted. Even a small amount of hexane, which is extremely toxic, can pose a threat to health.

After solvent extraction, oils proceed through the refining steps.

You'll never see "solvent extracted" on an oil label. That degree of honesty is a little too much.

Cold Pressing

The term "cold-pressed" is fundamentally a misnomer coined by Columbia University professor Henry Sherman in his book *Food Products,* in 1933. As Sherman used it, the term referred to expeller pressing. He distinguished expeller pressing from other methods that could involve greater heating of oil-bearing materials. To the casual reader, the term "cold-pressed" would seem to describe oil extraction achieved without heat. There is really no such process, except for the pressing of virgin olive oil. In the 1950s a few enterprising vegetable oil manufacturers slapped the term "cold-pressed" on their bottles as a marketing gimmick to appeal to the health food customer. Even though these oils were as heated, degummed, bleached, refined, and abused as any others, the trick worked, and those companies sold boxcar loads of their oils. In fact, the ploy worked for decades. Today, however, the ruse has been exposed. If you encounter any oil

---

Grades of Olive Oil

Olive oil comes in different grades, ranging from "extra virgin" to "pure." The following are the grades and what they signify.

Extra Virgin The natural acidity of extra-virgin olive oil cannot exceed 1 percent. Ripe, high-quality olives are picked or shaken from the trees and are immediately mechanically pressed, without solvents or chemicals of any kind. This is the highest quality of olive oil. Some extra-virgin oils are like fine wines, with distinctive aroma, color, and flavor.

Virgin The natural acidity of virgin olive oil can be from 1 to 3.3 percent. Virgin olive oil is more acidic than extra-virgin, because it usually comes from the second and third pressings of the olives. Or the olives may be somewhat inferior, thus yielding a more acidic oil even on the first pressing. Virgin olive oil is mechanically pressed without solvents or chemicals. This oil is generally good tasting, but it lacks the unique flavor of extra-virgin varieties.

Pure This is the lowest grade of olive oil, with the highest acidity. Because pure olive oil is acidic and may vary greatly in color, solvents and high heat are used to remove acidity, odor, and color. The result is a bland olive oil with less nutritional value.

(other than olive) that claims to be "cold-pressed," know that you are being insulted by an unscrupulous oil manufacturer. Buy a more honest brand. *The only real cold-pressed oil* is olive oil bottled by small producers. These companies use small presses that squeeze the oil out of olive mash at just a little above room temperature. The result is an unrefined, truly cold-pressed oil.

Unrefined Oils: Their Color, Aroma, and Flavor

Probably the first thing that you will notice about unrefined vegetable oils is that they do not look like baby oil. Instead, they have color, ranging from a golden yellow (corn oil), to a dark green (some olive oils), to a nutty brown (peanut or toasted sesame oils). When you open these oils, you will be further surprised, because they also have pleasing aroma and flavor. For a culture that has grown up on flavorless products like Wesson Oil, this may first come as a shock. But stop and think for a moment. Don't all other whole foods have color, aroma, and flavor?

Some of the color, aroma, and flavor components in oil include

Lecithin Particularly important to nerve tissue and the liver, lecithin is also valuable to healthy brain function and has been proved to enhance memory.

Chlorophyll The "blood" of plant life, chlorophyll is an internal disinfectant that is useful in digestive and urinary disorders. Chlorophyll reduces body odor and bad breath as well.

Carotenes These yellow or red pigments found in vegetation are the precursors to vitamin A in the body. They nourish mucous membranes, are useful for vision, enhance immunity, and maintain healthy teeth, nails, hair, bones, and glands.

Vitamin E This nutrient helps prevent sterility, improves circulation, promotes longevity, prevents blood clots, strengthens capillary walls, maintains the integrity of cell membranes, and contributes to healthy skin and hair.

The main point about oils is this: why would anyone choose a refined, nutritionally devoid oil? When you shop for vegetable oils, select an unrefined product. From a nutritional standpoint, this is the only kind that makes any sense at all.

CHOLESTEROL AND A HEALTHY DIET

Over the past several years people have become increasingly aware of the need to consume a low-cholesterol diet. A known factor in coronary dis-

ease, cholesterol is generally misunderstood. So here's some straightforward information on the subject:

- *Your body needs cholesterol.*
- *Your body produces all the cholesterol it needs.*
- *Too much cholesterol in the diet can lead to clogged arteries and heart disease.*
- *Only animal foods contain cholesterol!*
- *Some nonanimal foods can cause your body to produce more cholesterol than it needs.*
- *Healthy eating habits can help you to maintain a healthy cholesterol level.*
- *Some foods can help you to reduce your blood cholesterol.*

What is Cholesterol, Anyway?

Cholesterol is a fatty substance manufactured in the liver and small intestines. Our bodies use cholesterol to strengthen cell membranes, to produce the myelin sheaths that cover and protect nerves, and to produce sex hormones. The adult body manufactures about one gram (1,000 milligrams) of cholesterol daily.

More Than We Need

The body doesn't need any more cholesterol than the amount it manufactures, but we get extra cholesterol in our diets just the same. In fact, the average American consumes about 600 milligrams of cholesterol every day. This is much more cholesterol than the body needs or can handle. It is important to note that cholesterol can be found only in animal foods. This includes meats, seafood, dairy products, and any foods that contain these ingredients. There is absolutely no cholesterol at all in any vegetation. This means that fruits, vegetables, nuts, seeds, grains, beans, and any other kind of plant food do not contain cholesterol.

Note: The next time you see a television ad telling you that a particular brand of vegetable oil is "cholesterol free," be aware that the manufacturer of that product is insulting your intelligence and hoping to prey on your ignorance.

The Good, the Bad, and the Oily

Three types of cholesterol are found in the blood. Each one is distinguished by the particular fatty protein (or lipoprotein) envelope in which it travels. HDLs, or high-density lipoproteins, are referred to as "good" cholesterol. HDLs seem to protect against arteriosclerosis, or hardening of the arteries. The two other forms, LDL and VLDL (low-density and very–low-density lipoproteins), are the "bad" types of cholesterol that need to be kept under control. Elevated levels of LDL and VLDL cholesterol can lead to clogged arteries and heart attacks.

Dietary fats play an enormous role in the body's levels of cholesterol. Even though vegetable-source fats and oils do not contain cholesterol, they can contribute to either the production or the reduction of blood cholesterol.

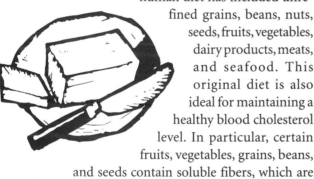

For hundreds of thousands of years, the natural human diet has included unrefined grains, beans, nuts, seeds, fruits, vegetables, dairy products, meats, and seafood. This original diet is also ideal for maintaining a healthy blood cholesterol level. In particular, certain fruits, vegetables, grains, beans, and seeds contain soluble fibers, which are now known to help reduce blood cholesterol. Soluble fibers lower cholesterol by increasing bile acid secretions, which break down the fats in cholesterol. The soluble fibers include pectin, gums, and mucilages.

- **Pectin** can be found in apples, carrots, and citrus.
- **Gums** can be found in oat bran, oatmeal, barley, and dried beans.

- **Mucilages** can be found in flaxseeds, chia seeds, and psyllium seeds.

From a cholesterol standpoint, the ideal diet will be richer in vegetable-source foods than animal-source foods, with an emphasis on grains and beans, which were the staple foods of most cultures in the world until the advent of factory food production and large-scale animal farming.

High Media Foods

Though many foods help to reduce blood cholesterol, a few have achieved superstar status in magazines and on broadcast media. Omega 3 fatty acids (components of oils), found primarily in cold-water seafoods, have been clinically proved to reduce blood cholesterol levels. Salmon, mackerel, sardines, tuna, rainbow trout, and eel are rich in Omega 3s. Flaxseed oil is also a source of these fatty acids. A diet high in Omega 3s can keep cholesterol at healthy levels.

Oat bran, the latest wonder food, has also been shown to reduce blood cholesterol because of the soluble fibers present in that grain product.

Avoiding Fast Fads and Miracle Cures

Although there are high-profile foods that can reduce cholesterol, Americans rely too much on treatment and not enough on prevention. By reducing your overall fat intake, reducing your consumption of refined sugars (which have been implicated in cholesterol production), being moderate with your intake of animal foods, and eating more whole foods, your body will be better able to maintain a healthy cholesterol level. Remember, the diet that is healthy from a cholesterol standpoint is healthy overall. A diet based on whole foods also benefits weight, energy level, sex life, mental function, immunity, disease prevention, and longevity.

14

SWEETENERS

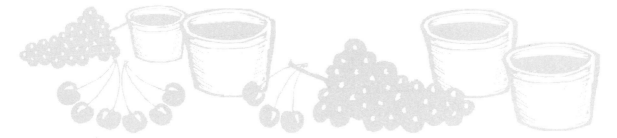

A Tempest in the Sugar Bowl

Few dietary controversies rage as intensely as the never-ending battle over sweeteners, their dietary value, and their safety. The $8 billion sweetener industry is a multinational high-stakes game. At the center of this dietary cyclone are sugars, which occur in and are refined from natural sources such as sugar beets and cane, corn, and sweet fruits including grapes and dates. Side by side with the natural-source sugars are artificial sugar substitutes, promoted for their low caloric values. In recent years new, phony sweeteners have burst forth on the food scene. Advocates of natural-source sugars say that they are safe when eaten in moderation, despite their caloric value. Advocates of phony sweeteners say their products pose no threat to human health and contain little or no calories—a presumed advantage.

Yet, even among the advocates of natural sweeteners there are splinter groups. Many natural foods enthusiasts, for example, eschew table sugar, labeling it unsafe in any amount, while embracing honey and maple syrup, which also contain sucrose (the sweetness in table sugar) and can contribute to den-tal caries and obesity. Meanwhile, back in the artificial camp, advocates are careful to distinguish exactly which of the phony sweeteners they endorse, denouncing others as unsafe and possibly carcinogenic. If all this sounds terribly confusing to you, rest assured that it is. Even the so-called experts are divided on this issue.

The First Sweet Tooth?

No one knows exactly who had the first sweet tooth, but prehistoric humans discovered sweet foods such as fruits, berries, and honey and apparently liked them a lot. Archaeological excavations show that these foods were consumed tens of thousands of years ago. Concentrated sweets such as dates and honey became highly prized. At least five thousand years ago, honey hunters in both Africa and Nepal risked life and limb by hanging from high rock cliffs with rope ladders to obtain the honey of wild bees. It seems that people have long gone to extraordinary lengths to satisfy their craving for sweets.

Phony Sweeteners

As technology battles the calorie, more innovative sweetening additives are being manufactured. Meet today's phony sweeteners:

Acesulfame K This sweetener will be appearing in an increasing number of packaged foods, including dessert mixes, baked goods, and sodas. Acesulfame K has been approved, but tests suggest that it may cause cancer. The Food and Drug Administration is reevaluating this chemical.

Alitame There are currently insufficient safety data on this new all-purpose sweetener. Alitame is a powerfully concentrated sweetener and could possibly upstage NutraSweet because of the comparatively tiny amount needed.

Aspartame The most successful sweetener since sugar, aspartame (trade names NutraSweet and Equal) is in just about everything. Because it loses its sweetness at high temperatures, aspartame cannot be used for cooking. Allegedly the most exhaustively tested food additive in history, aspartame remains controversial. The FDA gives it a clean bill of health, while brain researchers believe that it may cause seizure disorders in a small percentage of the population.

Cyclamate This all-purpose sweetener was yanked off the shelves nationwide when the FDA banned it because of its carcinogenic effects.

Saccharin Despite the fact that saccharin has been shown to cause cancer in laboratory animals, this phony sweetener is still sold legally for food purposes. The sale of saccharin violates the Delaney Amendment of the Food, Drug and Cosmetic Act, which is supposed to protect the public from cancer-causing agents in the food chain.

Sorbitol A sugar alcohol, sorbitol is a synthetic sugar used as a softener in confections. Sorbitol has been implicated in cataract formation.

Sucralose This new all-purpose sweetener is under FDA review, and there are currently insufficient safety data on the product.

A Nation of Sugar Junkies

In the United States, the consumption of sweets is an obsession. We seem to consume sweeteners in everything. Breakfast cereals have turned into sticky, gooey sugar candies. Count Chocula, for example, contains a whopping 3.3 teaspoons of sugar per ounce, yet is exceeded by Apple Jacks at 3.5 teaspoons of sugar per ounce, and Honey Smacks at 4 teaspoons of sugar per ounce. So much for a hearty breakfast! Even Life and All-Bran, which are marketed as healthy and pure as the driven snow, each contain 1.3 teaspoons of added sugar per ounce of cereal—don't be fooled by bucolic TV commercials. Cereals aren't the only category of food laden with sugar. Dannon fruit-flavored low-fat yogurt, for example, contains 6 teaspoons of sugar per 8-ounce serving. Just 2 tablespoons of Skippy Peanut Butter contains 1.3 teaspoons of sugar. Canada Dry tonic water contains 8.4 teaspoons of sugar per 12-ounce serving. One tablespoon of ketchup contains 6 teaspoons of sugar. Sugar is everywhere.

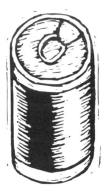

The Need for Sugar

The human body is equipped to consume sugar. Sugar, in fact, is essential to human life. Our bodies are fueled by glucose, a simple sugar, which is maintained at a constant level in our blood. Without blood sugar, we die. We can also die with too much blood sugar, however.

At issue is how to maintain a healthy blood sugar level. Complex carbohydrates, obtainable from whole grains, fruits, and vegetables, offer enough naturally occurring sugars to satisfy our need to maintain a healthy blood sugar level. Our bodies are built to eat a whole food, such as a grain, and break down the carbohydrates of that grain into simple sugars, which are converted into glucose, which is released in a controlled manner into the bloodstream. The truth is, we don't need any added sweeteners at all. But what we need and what we want are two different things.

The reality of the situation is that we crave sweets in excess of what we actually need. So why not just eat refined sugar? It's easy to obtain, it's relatively inexpensive, it's naturally derived, and it doesn't really contain that many calories. Not so fast.

The Sugar Story

There are many refined sugars, which are described below. What is commonly known as ordinary table sugar is white crystalline sucrose, refined from both sugarcane and sugar beets. Sucrose is actually a complex sugar made up of equal parts fructose and glucose, which are simple sugars. This means that fructose and glucose cannot be broken down further into other sugars.

Sugar by Any Other Name . . .

Sugar manufacturers are devilishly clever when it comes to making up new names for sugar. But it's still sugar. Here are a few clever sweet ploys:

Fructose Refined from corn syrup, not fruit as the name implies, fructose breaks down slightly more slowly in the body than sucrose. Otherwise, it's just another ultra-refined sugar, offering nothing but empty calories.

Brown Sugar Nothing more than white sugar with the faintest dab of molasses added to it, brown sugar has been touted as a "health food." It's not.

Raw Sugar There's nothing raw about it. So-called "raw" sugar, as it is marketed in the United States, is simply coarse white sugar. It's nothing special or healthful.

Turbinado Sugar Perhaps the cleverest rip-off of all, turbinado sugar appears in many brands of "natural" cookies and confections. Turbinado sugar, however, is nothing more than coarse white sugar named after the turbine in which it is refined!

Sugar Farming and Refining The farming of sugarcane, the primary source of sugar, is usually accomplished with massive quantities of chemical fertilizers and pesticides. In addition, cane is a mineral-hungry plant that depletes the mineral reserves of the soil in which it is grown. For these reasons, cane farming is notorious for destroying fertile soil.

When mature sugarcane is cut and sent to refining plants, it is rich in vitamins and minerals and contains only 10 to 14 percent sucrose. The subsequent steps of the refining process separate the sucrose from the rest of the plant material, including the nutrients. At the refining plant, the cane is shredded, then put into large hydraulic rollers that apply two hundred to five hundred tons of pressure, rupturing every cell of the cane and releasing as much liquid as possible. Cane is very juicy. This liquid is acidic, green, and turbid. It contains 10 to 18 percent sucrose, plus minerals, organic acids, pectin, and gums. Sugarcane juice is actually a highly nutritious drink. In many Third World nations you will see street vendors juicing cane with heavy-duty juicing machines and selling the cane juice by the glass. It is surprisingly refreshing, and not overly sweet.

After the cane is crushed the liquid is strained through a fine screen to remove large particles. Then lime in the form of calcium hydroxide is added to neutralize the organic acids. The juice is boiled at 210° to 238°F, and a precipitate, which includes the lime salts, is removed. The liquid is no longer acidic but has a balanced pH of 7. Mud and scum precipitate out, leaving a clarified juice that is brownish-yellow and free of turbidity.

The liquid, which is about 80 percent water, is boiled in a vacuum, which speeds up the evaporation of the water. The liquid is put through the evaporator as many as five times. After evaporation, the liquid is 55 to 70 percent solids, of which 75 to 85 percent is sucrose. The mixture is poured into trays, and more water is removed by heat and vacuum evaporation. As soon as the right amount of water has been evaporated, the liquid is quick-cooled, and the crystals form.

The liquid, including the sugar crystals, is put into a centrifuge, a large cylindrical device with a basket inside that spins at fifteen hundred to two thousand revolutions per minute. A cloth bag or fine mesh inside the basket catches the sugar crystals and lets the liquid pass through. The liquid is pushed out by the force created by the revolving basket. The sugar crystals are then dried and go through a bleaching process before being packaged. The result is 99 percent pure white sucrose. What was once a nutritious whole food is now totally devoid of nutrients. Sugar contains "empty" calories, without any vitamins, minerals, protein, or fats.

Sugar Hazards: Fact and Speculation Depending on whom you ask, sugar is either relatively benign or a great evil. At this point sugar is believed to be associated with so many potential health problems that nobody actually knows the real story.

- One thing is certain: sugar absolutely does cause cavities. Sugar interacts with bacteria in the mouth and produces acids that create holes in the enamel surface of the teeth.
- Obesity is often blamed on sugar, but the link between sugar consumption and obesity is questionable. At 16 calories per teaspoon, sugar is not a high-calorie food. The real culprit in obesity is dietary fat, which contains more than twice the calories of sugar and is consumed in much greater quantities.
- Sugar can be very dangerous to diabetics (it can kill them), but there is no evidence yet that eating sugar actually causes diabetes, a claim made by many dietary faddists. Diabetes is a disease in which the pancreas does not produce sufficient quantities of insulin, an important hormone that regulates the level of sugar in the blood. Diabetics must regulate their diets and watch carbohydrate intake carefully. Many diabetics must inject themselves daily with supplementary insulin.
- A broad variety of behavioral disorders are blamed on sugar consumption, and this entire field of study is a boiling pot of controversy. Some authorities assert that

sugar is a primary cause of hyperactivity in children, a claim supported by voluminous anecdotal evidence. The exact mechanism for this phenomenon remains unknown, however.

The most celebrated instance of a possible link between sugar and mental health is that of Dan White, who killed San Francisco Mayor George Moscone and Supervisor Harvey Milk. Convicted of manslaughter, not murder, White's famous "Twinkie defense" was based on the premise that a serious addiction to sweet junk foods had diminished his mental capacity and had caused White to kill the two officials in a fit of sugar-induced mania. This verdict has been hotly disputed, and to date there is still no conclusive evidence that sugar causes serious mental problems.

Perhaps the most compelling reason to eliminate or greatly restrict the intake of refined sugar is that it has no nutritional value. There is absolutely no known reason to consume something that offers no nutritional benefits other than energy. All natural foods, of all categories, contain at least some nutrients. The human body is designed to derive energy from nutritious foods.

Natural Sweeteners

The following natural sweeteners contain calories, can elevate blood sugar levels higher than normal if consumed in excess, and can cause cavities. In other words, there is no such thing as a free ride with natural sweeteners. They do contain at least some nutritional value, however, as found in their original whole natural source. This is an important distinction.

Barley Malt Syrup Sprouted, roasted barley, or barley malt, has a naturally sweet, nutty flavor. Barley malt in granular form is slow cooked with water to make a thick syrup. Barley malt syrup is a mild, pleasant sweetener that can be used in baked goods. The reason it is called "malt" is that maltose is the sugar that occurs when the starch in barley is

If You've Eaten Bananas and Milk

A television ad for NutraSweet (the trade name for the phony sweetener aspartame) starts out with the words, "If you've eaten bananas and milk, you've eaten everything that's in NutraSweet." That may be true, but NutraSweet itself does not exist anywhere in nature. NutraSweet is an artificial sweetener 180 times sweeter than sugar and is a methyl ester of the two amino acids phenylalanine and aspartic acid.

Manufactured by the drug company G. D. Searle & Co. of Skokie, Illinois, NutraSweet is used to mimic the taste of sugar, without the calories, in a wide variety of foods. In 1981 the Food and Drug Administration approved the use of the artificial sweetener in cereals, diet beverages, desserts, and ice creams. The FDA has received more than three thousand complaints about NutraSweet. Consumers have reported headaches, dizziness, and nausea after eating or drinking products containing the sweet chemical compound.

Foods containing aspartame must be labeled to protect babies who suffer from phenylketonuria, or PKU, a condition that renders them unable to metabolize phenylalanine, a principal ingredient of the sweetener. Consumption of NutraSweet by babies suffering from PKU can lead to mental retardation. Many brain researchers worldwide continue to question the safety of Nutra-Sweet, which they believe may produce seizures among a very small percentage of consumers. How sweet it is.

Brown Rice Syrup   Cook brown rice for what seems like an infinity, and you'll have brown rice syrup, which is impossibly thick and fairly sweet. Nobody makes brown rice syrup at home, because no one has that much time. The syrup is used in baking and is available in bottles.

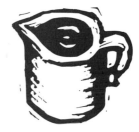

Date Sugar   This is dried pulverized dates, which contain lots of naturally occurring sugars. Date sugar doesn't dissolve well, but it is fine for cooking and baking. Date sugar usually comes in plastic bags.

Honey   By far the favorite sweetener of the natural foods set, honey is made by bees, which gather nectar from flowers and bring it back to the hive. By a laborious, painstaking process, this nectar is turned into honey, which is stolen from the bees, who simply go out and make more. There are few harder-working creatures on earth! Honey is rich in enzymes, contains some minerals, and usually contains some B vitamins and vitamin C. The primary sugars in honey are glucose and fructose, though other sugars are present. The best honey available is unfiltered raw honey, which will be labeled as such. Unfiltered honey will contain small amounts of bee pollen, which is nutrient-rich and contains live enzymes.

Most honeys are heated and the pollen is filtered out. Unfortunately, many honeys are also adulterated with either sugar or (more commonly) corn syrup, which is not easy to detect. As much as possible, avoid the commercial brands found in most supermarkets. They are often adulterated.

There are many types of honey made from the nectars of different flowers. You will find clover, wildflower, tupelo, buckwheat, sage, orange blossom, jungle, and other honeys, each with its own distinct flavor. Experiment until you find your favorite. Honey can be used as a substitute for sugar in most instances, but it should not be consumed by infants because of its bacterial content. Unlike sugar, honey does have a flavor. You may not enjoy it in your coffee.

sprouted. Barley malt may be made with some corn added, the starch of which converts to maltose. Be sure of the brand you are purchasing, because many barley malt vendors make their products with corn syrup, a cheap, refined sugar. Barley malt syrup comes in bottles.

Maple Syrup and Sugar A wonderful sweetener made from the sap of maple trees, maple syrup is high in minerals. It is the result of a boiling process that reduces forty gallons of maple sap down to just one gallon of syrup. Syrup is graded according to color and strength of flavor. Light amber is light in color, with a delicate flavor. Medium amber is darker in color with a stronger flavor. Dark amber is thicker and darker still, and has a strong flavor and some sediment. Choosing one grade over another is a matter of taste, not quality.

Maple sugar is maple syrup that is boiled down until it is a soft, granular sugar, which is typically pressed into cute little molds in the shape of maple leaves. It is very, very sweet. Some maple sugar is sold in granular form in bottles, but it tends to cake, and you'll wind up digging at it with a sharp knife to get any on your cereal. Beware of "maple-flavored" table syrups. These contain as little as 3 percent maple syrup, if any. The rest is corn syrup, and artificial everything else.

Molasses The liquid that was spun out of the centrifuge during sugar refining is boiled and crystallized several more times to yield as much sugar as possible. The healthful nutrients of the sugar remain in the liquid, and this is sold as molasses, which contains 20 to 25 percent water, 50 percent sugar (sucrose and invert sugar), 10 percent ash, and some protein, organic acids, and gums. Molasses has a very strong flavor and is usually used only in baking (it's great in gingerbread), though some health enthusiasts like to eat it right off the spoon for its mineral value.

Sorghum Sorghum is a member of the millet family. The stalks of the sorghum plant are crushed to render a sweet juice that is filtered and then evaporated down to a thick syrup. Sorghum syrup is usually lighter than molasses and has a milder flavor. It's used primarily in cooking and comes in bottles.

Sucanat The niftiest thing to happen in the sweetener world in a long time, Sucanat (a trade name that stands for *sugar cane natural*) is the dehydrated juice of organically grown sugarcane in granular form. Sucanat is what sugar should be, complete with vitamins, minerals, and a great sweet flavor. It is used just like sugar, and it actually pours well if kept in a container away from excess humidity. Sucanat exploits the nutritional richness of sugarcane very well.

Sugar Substitutes for Baking

Sweetener	Amount to replace 1 cup sugar	Liquid Reduction Needed
Honey	1/2 cup	1/4 cup
Maple syrup	1/2–1/3 cup	1/4 cup
Molasses	1/2 cup	1/4 cup
Malt syrup	1–1 1/4 cups	1/4 cup
Date sugar	2/3 cup	—
Sucanat	1 cup	—

15

SALT, HERBS, AND SPICES

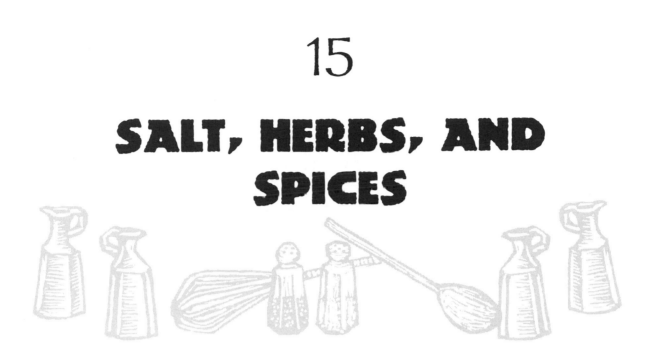

ABOUT SALT

Common table salt, or sodium chloride (NaCl), is 40 percent sodium and 60 percent chloride. Though all salt came originally from the sea, less than 15 percent of the food-grade salt in the United States is evaporated from seawater. The rest is mined land salt from ancient sea beds. Prior to refinement, salt contains over seventy different elements. Natural whole salt is a composite of *all* these elements as they occur in seawater. The process of commercial salt refining, which is typically accomplished with the use of chemicals and extremely high heat, reduces salt from a whole food to an ultra-refined sodium chloride compound. This is definitely not salt as nature originally created it. According to the standards of the Food Chemicals Codex, salt must be 97.5 percent pure sodium chloride to qualify for food use. Despite this regulation, there are still a few small salt companies that sell natural salt from evaporated seawater, with mineral values higher than those actually allowed by law (around 4 percent). Ironically, those companies cannot be identified here, despite the fact that they are selling a

nutritionally superior product, for they are in violation of federal standards. Most sea salt is over 97.5 percent sodium chloride.

Salt and Health

Salt plays an important role in human health. The sodium in salt is an essential nutrient that works with potassium to equalize the acid-alkaline balance of blood and helps regulate the balance of water in the body. Sodium is also important for proper muscle function. An inadequate intake of sodium leads to dehydration, poor muscle function, an imbalance of blood pH, and, eventually, death. Although no recommended dietary allowance has been established for sodium, the National Research Council recommends as safe and adequate a sodium intake of 1,100 to 3,300 milligrams per day.

In the United States an inadequate intake of sodium is virtually unheard of. The average daily sodium consumption of Americans is between 4,000 and 6,000 milligrams, though even double that consumption is not uncommon. Salt is heavily consumed in the standard American diet, primarily in

111

processed foods, in which it is used to compensate for the loss of natural flavors.

Salt is added to vegetables during freezing and canning and is used in meat processing, especially smoking and curing. Most ketchups, soups, sauces, salad dressings, mixes, mustard, cheeses, and breakfast cereals are typically high in salt.

Sodium-related Health Risks

Salt poses a potential threat to health because of its sodium content. Excessive sodium intake is associated with hypertension, or high blood pressure. High blood pressure, which increases the risk of heart attack and stroke, is common, affecting an estimated one out of every four adult Americans. Because high blood pressure does not usually cause any pain or discomfort, however, many people with high blood pressure don't know they have it. Excessive sodium in the diet can also aggravate kidney problems and can greatly increase water retention, thus causing swelling (edema).

Researchers at the Framingham Heart study in Massachusetts are adamant that sodium intake is a significant factor in cardiovascular health and that it should be restricted. Their conclusions are in line with those of the American Heart Association, which advises everyone to restrict salt consumption, citing a relationship with hypertension. A study reaffirming the direct relationship between sodium consumption and hypertension was published in the July 30, 1988, issue of *The British Medical Journal*. The study was the largest of its kind, involving over ten thousand people from fifty-two countries.

Cutting Back on Sodium

The Surgeon General's *Report on Diet and Health* says: "Reduce intake of sodium by choosing foods relatively low in sodium and limiting the amount

Have You Read a Salt Label Lately?

Most commercial brands of salt are iodized, which means that they contain potassium iodide. This is because iodine, an essential nutrient, is stripped from salt during the refining process. Salt that is iodine-fortified will state on the label: "This salt supplies iodine, a necessary nutrient." If a salt is not iodine-fortified, the label will read "This salt does not supply iodine, a necessary nutrient."

But there is more to salt than just added iodine. Pick up a salt container and read the ingredients sometime. You'll find sodium silicoaluminate, dextrose, potassium iodide, sodium bicarbonate, magnesium carbonate, and other additives. These substances are used to absorb moisture and to make the salt flow freely. Who needs them? You don't.

of salt in food preparation and at the table." The first way to reduce sodium intake is to choose foods that are naturally low in sodium. These foods include fresh fruits and vegetables, whole grains, beans, nuts and seeds, fresh meats, poultry, and seafood. Additionally, you can do the following:

- Throw out your salt shaker. You don't need any added salt on your food. Instead, try using various herbs and spices for enhanced flavor. Look out for herbal and spice blends that also contain salt.
- Substitute vinegar and lemon juice for high-salt products such as sauces, salad dressings, and seasonings. For salad dressings, try olive oil and an herb vinegar. Use little or no salt in cooking and baking. If you use salt at all, use half the amount called for.
- Read food labels for sodium content. Use products that contain not more than 120 milligrams of sodium per serving.
- Drain and rinse sodium from processed foods like canned tuna and canned or frozen vegetables.

- Watch out for sneaky sodium. Always check food labels.
- Give yourself time to adjust to a low-sodium diet. Within about a month, you won't even miss the extra salt.

CULINARY HERBS AND SPICES

Allspice Tastes like a combination of cinnamon, nutmeg, and cloves. Use it to flavor pumpkin pies, pickled foods, carrots, eggplant, cookies, cakes, and relishes.

Anise Good sprinkled whole on Danish pastries, cookies, and coffee cakes before baking. Use ground anise in salads and in shrimp and crab dishes.

Basil Use in soups, stews, tomato dishes, sauces, and salads.

Bay Leaf Fragrant and pungent. Use in soups and stews, and with fish. Adds flavor to steamed vegetables and stuffings.

Caraway Seed Use to flavor rye bread, crackers, cottage cheese, sauerkraut, and baked apples.

Sodium in Water

Sodium is commonly found in drinking water. In northern climates, public works trucks often salt roads to reduce hazardous driving conditions during times of ice and snow. This salt—tons of it annually—eventually drains into municipal drinking supplies. The result is high-sodium drinking water.

Water softeners also raise the sodium content of drinking water. If you are on a sodium-restricted diet, you should avoid softened water and become familiar with the sodium content of the water coming out of your tap. You may choose to drink either distilled water or spring water that you know is sodium free.

Cardamom Seed Lends a sweet flavor to breads, cookies, pastries, pickles, and curried dishes.

Cayenne Hot. Use in spicy foods, curries, chili, and anything that needs zing.

Celery Seed Adds flavor to fish, salads, soups, stews, tomatoes, salad dressings, and potatoes.

Chervil Adds pungent flavor to salads, soups, fish, sauces, egg dishes, and greens. Blend with cream cheese; use like parsley.

Chives Use for salads, cottage cheese, eggs, and sauces when a mild onion flavor is called for.

Cinnamon A sweet, aromatic seasoning for apple pie, applesauce, Danish, coffee cakes, French toast, fruit salads, baked squash, and sauces for game. Used in some curries. Whole sticks are used in hot cider and for sweet pickling.

Cloves Sweet and pungent. Use to flavor soups, stews, fruit dishes, ham, spice cake, and gingerbread.

Coriander Tastes like a combination of lemon peel and sage. Use it in gingerbread, spice cakes, Danish, roast pork, soups, sauces, lentil dishes, and poultry dishes.

Cumin Gives an aromatic taste to stews, roasts, and vegetables. It has a strong flavor; use sparingly.

Dill Seed Use for pickling, soups, sauces, eggs, and fried potatoes.

Dill Weed Use for creamed dishes, potatoes, salads, and soups.

Fennel Seed Use in Spanish and Italian dishes and as a bitter in soups and fish dishes. Gives a sweet taste to pickles.

Garlic Use for virtually any meat, fish, soup, salad, and stew.

Ginger Use in Chinese, Japanese, and Indian cooking, and in chutneys, pickles, conserves, and applesauce. Excellent in cookies, pies, and cakes.

Mace Sweet and aromatic. Use in pastries and cakes.

Marjoram　Use for stuffings, stews, soups, salad dressings, and egg dishes.

Mint　Use for drinks, vegetables, pea soup, fruit salad, and anywhere an aromatic mint flavor is desired.

Nutmeg　Use in custards, puddings, pumpkin and fruit pies, and eggnog. Has an aromatic odor and a slightly bitter taste.

Oregano　Use in soups, chili, tomato sauce, and marinades for meats or game.

Paprika　A mild cayenne; use as a garnish in broiled fish and game.

Is Garlic a Cure-all?

Garlic, *Allium sativum,* has been used for medicinal purposes for thousands of years, and in many parts of the world such uses persist right down to the present day. Manuscripts from antiquity and from medieval times relate its use for an astonishing variety of ailments ranging from coughs and colds to weak digestion, worms, tuberculosis, menstrual problems, and leprosy. Can these claims be substantiated?

Apparently many of them can be. In more recent times, a surprising number of scientific investigations into garlic's medicinal properties have been conducted. Added to the profusion of anecdotal reports, these studies provide an impressive array of solid evidence.

Garlic's traditional uses against colds, dysentery, bronchitis, and infected wounds have a sound scientific base. In studies beginning in Louis Pasteur's laboratory in 1858 and continuing well into the twentieth century, garlic has time and again been shown to be effective against a wide range of bacteria, viruses, fungi, protozoa, and parasites. Dr. Albert Schweitzer used it in Africa to treat amebic dysentery. In many cases, garlic is more effective than antibiotics. It does not encourage the development of drug-resistant bacteria, as antibiotics do, nor does it produce toxic side effects. Of vital interest these days, garlic is effective against many of the opportunistic infections that occur in AIDS patients, including candidal, mycobacterial, salmonellal, cryptococcal, and pyogenic infections.

Present-day scientists have also investigated the traditional claims that garlic is good for the circulation, and have found that garlic can indeed lower blood cholesterol and relieve hypertension. furthermore, garlic seems to discourage the formation of clots in the blood vessels, and therefore can be thought of as a preventive against stroke and some forms of coronary disease.

What about cancer? Intriguing news comes from a small town in Italy, where high garlic consumption is the rule, and the occurrence of stomach cancer is extremely low. Similarly, among garlic-eaters in a particular area of China, stomach cancer is quite rare, whereas residents of another area where garlic is not eaten have a much higher rate of stomach cancer. To bear out these observations, laboratory studies have shown garlic to have a direct cytotoxic effect on two kinds of stomach cancer cells.

Other studies have produced data to support garlic not only as a nutritional supplement with high trace mineral content but also as an immune system enhancer, an antioxidant, and a detoxifier in heavy metal poisoning. Few if any other substances, whether synthetic or natural, can match this versatility.

Which is best for health: raw garlic or cooked garlic? So far, the evidence seems to show that heat destroys many of the therapeutic properties of garlic. Raw garlic therefore appears to be best. If you are concerned about smelling like an Italian restaurant, however, cold-aged, whole-clove garlic preparations have the same medicinal properties—and the added advantage of being odorless.

Parsley   An all-purpose herb for salads, vegetables, meat, cheese and eggs, soups, baked fish, and potatoes. Also used as a garnish.

Pepper, black   Sharp, pungent, hot to the taste. Use with meats, game, sauces, and salads.

Pepper, white   More delicate and less pungent than black pepper, it is ground from peppercorns with the black outer shells removed and is not visible in foods.

Poppy Seed   Nutlike flavor. Use for toppings of cakes, rolls, and breads.

Rosemary   Delicate, slightly bitter flavor for meats, fish, soups, and salads.

Saffron   Gives flavor to rice, chicken, fancy rolls, coffee cakes, and curry sauces.

Sage   Spicy aroma and taste; use in soups, stuffings, vegetables, and game.

Savory   Use for green beans, eggs, salads, stuffings, cabbage, and soups.

Sorrel   Eaten fresh in salads and to season soups, omelettes, casseroles.

Tarragon   Use to flavor vinegars, tartar sauce, hollandaise sauce, turtle soup, salad greens, eggs, and vegetables.

Thyme   Fresh, aromatic odor. Use in pea soup, sauces, meats, rabbit and poultry dishes, soups, gumbo, and stuffings.

Turmeric   Adds a slight flavor and a yellow color to curries, cakes, breads, cookies, and rice dishes.

Vanilla   Use in baking, desserts, and syrups.

16

ECO REPORT: CHEMICAL FOOD ADDITIVES

*C*hemical food additives include preservatives, artificial colors and flavors, flavor enhancers like MSG, artificial sweeteners like NutraSweet, stabilizers, thickeners, conditioners, emulsifiers, humectants, and other non-natural agents. Though chemical food additives are ostensibly used to enhance food, they add no nutritional value and in many cases may be harmful.

Up Against the Law, Above the Law

Food additives are subject to the strictures of the Food, Drug and Cosmetic Act (FDCA), including the famous Delaney Amendment, named after New York Congressman James Delaney. This amendment reads "no additive shall be deemed to be safe if it is found to induce cancer when ingested by man or animal." Flagrant disregard of the Delaney Amendment is widespread throughout the U.S. food production system.

The legal status of the artificial sweetener saccharin is a case in point. A Canadian government study of saccharin showed that it causes bladder tumors in rats. According to the Delaney Amendment, saccharin should be banned from all food uses. However, the carcinogenic sugar substitute is widely used, thereby putting saccharin above the law. The Food and Drug Administration actually did attempt to ban saccharin in 1977, but the effort was derailed by lobbying efforts on the part of chemical manufacturers. As a feeble consolation, any product containing saccharin must be labeled as follows: "Use of this product may be hazardous to your health. This product contains saccharin, which has been determined to cause cancer in laboratory animals." Despite the presence of such a warning, the fact that saccharin remains in the food system implies that it is safe for human consumption, which it is not. Saccharin is yet one more case of public safety laws compromised by commercial interests.

Shelf Life Versus Human Life

Though many chemical additives, including cyclamates and some artificial colors have been banned, other proven carcinogens remain in use in foods.

BHA (butylated hydroxanisole) and BHT (butylated hydroxytoluene) are two common antioxidant preservatives used in breads and baked foods, cereals, potato chips, and vegetable oils. In a 1982 Japanese study, BHA was shown to cause cancer in rats, while BHT has increased the incidence of cancer in laboratory animals as well. Yet, no governmental move has been made to protect the public by eliminating these toxic agents from the food chain.

Another carcinogen in the food chain is sodium nitrite, which is used as a preservative in processed meats, including bacon, hot dogs, lunch meats, and smoked fish products. Sodium nitrite inhibits the growth of the bacteria that causes botulism poisoning. It also keeps red meats red. Sodium nitrite combines with amino acids (the basic building blocks of protein) to form cancer-causing chemicals called nitrosamines. Laboratory tests performed on bacon preserved with sodium nitrite have revealed the presence of nitrosamines. Because sodium nitrite serves a useful function, however, it remains on the market today, despite the potential danger it poses to human health. Once again, the FDA, its activities thwarted by commercial interests, allows the use of carcinogenic additives to continue, in violation of a law enacted to protect public safety.

Drug Company Cashes In on America's Sweet Tooth

In 1981 the Food and Drug Administration approved the use of the artificial sweetener aspartame, manufactured by G. D. Searle, an international drug company. Produced under the trade name NutraSweet, aspartame is used in cereals, diet beverages, desserts, and ice creams. The FDA has received more than three thousand complaints about NutraSweet. Consumers have reported headaches, dizziness, and nausea after eating or drinking products containing the sweet chemical compound.

Foods containing aspartame must be labeled to protect babies who suffer from PKU, phenylketonuria, which renders them unable to metabo-

Chinese Restaurant Syndrome

MSG, or monosodium glutamate, is a so-called flavor enhancer, used widely in restaurants and in prepared foods. Studies have shown that mice fed large amounts of MSG suffer destruction of brain cells. MSG is most famous for producing "Chinese restaurant syndrome," which causes headaches, tightness in the chest, and a burning sensation in the neck and forearms. Several years ago, baby food manufacturers stopped using MSG under intense public pressure. MSG remains otherwise in popular use, however.

lize phenylalanine, a principal ingredient of the sweetener. Consumption of NutraSweet by babies suffering from PKU can lead to mental retardation. Many brain researchers worldwide continue to question the safety of NutraSweet, which they believe may produce seizures among a very small percentage of consumers.

The Color Purple, Blue, Yellow

Each year, Americans consume more than 6 million pounds of seven artificial coal-tar based dyes in food. Of these seven dyes, four have been shown to cause cancer in laboratory animals. These carcinogenic colorings include Red 3, Yellow 5, Yellow 6, and Blue 2. Though the FDA has banned seventeen food dyes since 1918, the process of eliminating these from the food chain is slow and is accomplished with extreme difficulty. Six of the seven food dyes now in use in the United States have been banned in other nations. Artificial colors offer considerable health risk, with absolutely no known health or nutritional benefits.

What You Can Do

Today it is becoming somewhat easier to find foods without chemical additives. Many natural food stores allow no artificial preservatives, colors, flavors, refined or synthetic sugars, or MSG in the food they sell, yet manage to fill full-size supermarkets with food. What is required of the shopper is assiduous label reading. Look for foods with labels that list only recognizable food ingredients. If a food label reads like a high-school chemistry book, leave it alone.

Besides label reading, talk with your grocer. Make him or her aware that you want more additive-free foods. Direct requests from customers do make an impression. After all, customers fund the entire multibillion dollar food industry in this country. In addition, you can call or write your senator and congressperson, and tell them that you want the Delaney Amendment upheld, and you want to know what they're doing about it.

17

READING A FOOD LABEL

*S*ince 1938 the Food and Drug Administration has overseen standards of product labeling, including product identity, quantity of product, quality, and source of manufacture. These standards have been adopted and enforced to provide consumers with accurate product information and to protect the public from deceptive or fraudulent label claims. Despite the simple, straightforward intent of FDA labeling standards, the world of food labels is a labyrinth. Today's consumers must be educated about food labels just to understand what they are reading.

Not all foods have labels. Fresh fruits, vegetables, meat (except for safe-handling instructions), and fish, for example, do not need to be labeled unless they are sold prewrapped or otherwise packaged. The same is true for bulk foods such as grains, beans, nuts, seeds, coffee, oils, and nut butters. Packaged foods, however, must be labeled with the following information:

The name of the product must be prominent on the package and must be true and accurate according to the ingredients in the food. A bean dip, for example, must be labeled as such instead of being labeled "turkey spread." If fruit salad is canned in heavy syrup, the label should read "Fruit Salad in Heavy Syrup."

The net contents, or weight, should include the total quantity by weight, not volume, of the food inside the package. You will see on some cereal boxes the statement "This package is sold by weight, not by volume. It contains full net weight indicated. If it does not appear full when opened, it is because contents have settled during shipping and handling." The net weight of the cereal may be one pound, yet when you open the box, it may appear only half to two-thirds full.

The name and address of the manufacturer/ distributor must be listed. The full address does not need to be given if it can be found through directory information. An address can read "Farquhar Foods, St. Paul, MN." Since many food companies have products made for them by other manufacturers, the product can list just the distributor of the food. You will see food labels reading "Manufactured for Bon Temps Foods, Memphis, TN," or "Distributed by Grandma's Finest Foods, Berkeley, CA." This labeling indicates that the product was made for, not by, that company. Any inquiries about the product should be directed to the company.

From here, the road gets tricky. The more than three hundred FDA labeling standards are by no means uniform. Some food labels must contain certain information, while others are exempt. Since a comprehensive guide to labeling would take up about two hundred pages, the following information covers only some of the basics about food label information.

Food product ingredients must be listed clearly by their common names, in descending order according to weight. The ingredient that weighs the most must be listed first, and the ingredient that weighs the least must be listed last. If the primary ingredient by weight in a granola is rolled oats, that is the first ingredient listed on the package. If pure vanilla flavoring weighs less than any other ingredient in the product, it will be listed last. The good news is that you can look at the ingredients listed on a food label and determine whether you want to eat that product. Using the example of breakfast cereals, you will find that some cereals list sugar as the first ingredient, and many list it as the second. Do you really want to sit down to a bowl of cereal that contains more sugar than anything else? Label information helps you choose. The bad news is that labels do not have to list some ingredients, and they can be vague about some others.

Flavors A product must list that it is flavored, but does not have to list exactly what that flavoring may be. A label can simply read "artificial flavors" or "natural flavors" without providing further information. This is because manufacturers feel that the flavorings they use are proprietary to their recipes for certain foods. To list the flavors would constitute giving away trade secrets. Spices can simply be labeled "spices" and do not have to be further identified.

Colors If a food contains natural colors, it must at least list "coloring" on the label, without further identification. If artificial colors are present, the label must list "artificial colors."

Preservatives In contrast with flavors and colors, these additives must be listed, with their functions given. For example, if BHT is added to a bread the label will read "BHT added to retard spoilage."

Remember, though, that just because an ingredient is listed on a label does not mean that it is safe. Many food additives are suspected or known carcinogens.

Standardized foods are another can of worms. Standardized foods are those for which the FDA has created very specific criteria for labeling. A product that is less than 100 percent orange juice, for example, cannot be labeled "orange juice." There are hundreds of standardized foods, from condiments to juices, dairy products to canned goods. Standards for these foods are based on recipes and/or nutritional value. A ketchup, for example, must contain tomatoes. A similar-looking product that contains lettuce pulp and red food coloring instead cannot be labeled "ketchup." It can, however, be labeled "imitation ketchup."

Of course, few people know which foods are standardized. If you happen to browse through Title 21 of the Code of Federal Regulations you can find out. Otherwise, you are expected to have a general idea of which foods are which. In other words, you are expected to possess a certain level of food literacy.

As ingredients, standardized foods do not need to be described in detail. A spicy table source that contains some ketchup as an ingredient could simply list "ketchup" on the label instead of listing all ingredients of that ketchup.

Incidental additives include a host of chemicals that do not have to be listed on a product. A manufacturer must list which ingredients are in a product but is not required to list all the ingredients in each ingredient. This is a loophole as wide as the Pan American Highway. For example, if a manufacturer uses as an ingredient an oil that contains preservatives, only the oil must be listed on the label of the finished product. The preservatives in that oil do not need to be listed. If the manufacturer uses a spice blend that contains several artificial flavors, only "spice blend" need appear on the label. Added nutrients also contain preservatives (see "Nutritional Information"), which are not listed on product labels.

Product Dates/Codes

Five kinds of dates or codes are commonly used on

packaged foods:

- **Packing Date** This is the date on which the food was manufactured or packaged. It tells you how old a product is.
- **Sell Date** This is the last date on which a product should be sold in order to assure freshness. Dairy products, packaged meats, and some other refrigerated products have sell dates. After the sell date has expired, the product is pulled from the shelves.
- **Expiration Date/Freshness Date** This is the last date on which the product should be eaten.
- **Shelf Life Date Code** You probably need to decipher this code if it appears on a package, as it is used primarily by manufacturers and distributors. The shelf life date code gives an indication of when and where a product was made and how long it has been sitting around. It also identifies specific lot numbers of products in the event of a manufacturer's or FDA product recall.
- **UPC** The Universal Product Code is a block of parallel lines of varying widths. Each product has its own UPC code, which is used for scanning at checkout counters in supermarkets as well as for computerized inventory purposes.

Nutritional Information

According to Food and Drug Administration regulations, the amount of specific nutrients must be listed according to serving size. A product's serving size is a totally arbitrary measure that is not based on how much of a product is typically eaten. If $1/2$ cup is the serving size for a cereal, then the nutritional information on the label will be for $1/2$ cup of that product. Nutritional information will include calories, protein, fat, and carbohydrate content. In addition, percentages of the U.S. Recommended Dietary Allowances (U.S. RDAs) for protein, vitamins A and C, thiamin, riboflavin, niacin, calcium, and iron must be given.

Nutrients are added to products to restore nutrients lost in processing or to correct dietary defi-ciencies in the general population. Nutrients are added to white bread, for example, because it is an inferior product that has been stripped of its natural nutritional value. Adding some synthetic vitamins to white bread gives it at least some meager nutritional worth. Adding vitamin D to milk, on the other hand, is done simply to prevent rickets in children.

Many of the synthetic nutrients added to foods contain several preservatives. These will never be listed on a product label. Vitamin A added to milk may contain as many as ten or more preservatives. Despite this, the milk container needs only to say "vitamin A added" without mention of the preservatives.

Here's a typical nutrition panel:

Nutrition Facts

Serving Size 12 oz. (340g)
Servings Per Container 1

Amount Per Serving

Calories 340   Calories from Fat 45

	% Daily Value*
Total Fat 5g	**8%**
Saturated Fat 2g	**10%**
Cholesterol 30mg	**10%**
Sodium 470mg	**20%**
Total Carbohydrate 61g	**20%**
Dietary Fiber 5g	**20%**
Sugars 2–3g	
Protein 14g	

Vitamin A 10%	Vitamin C 35%
Calcium 15%	Iron 10%

* Percent Daily Values are based on a 2,000 calorie diet. Your daily values may be higher or lower depending on your calorie needs:

	Calories:	2,000	2,500
Total Fat	Less than	65g	80g
Sat Fat	Less than	20g	25g
Cholesterol	Less than	300mg	300mg
Sodium	Less than	2,400mg	2,400mg
Total Carbohydrate		300g	375g
Dietary Fiber		25g	30g

Calories per gram:
Fat 9 • Carbohydrate 4 • Protein 4

Knowing Metric Units

Since nutritional information is listed according to metric units of measurement, it is useful to know what these units mean.

1 kilogram	=	1,000 grams (g)
1 gram	=	1,000 milligrams (mg)
1 milligram	=	1/1,000 of a gram
1 microgram	=	1/1,000 of a milligram
28.35 grams	=	1 ounce
454 grams	=	1 pound

Marketing Lingo

As you read food labels, you will notice descriptive terms like "country-pure," or "kitchen fresh," or "Southwestern style." These are purely promotional descriptions, designed to evoke a mood or feeling about a product, and have no particular relationship to the actual contents of the item. Even the once-sacred term "natural" means little these days. A "natural" meat product, for example, may have no chemicals added after slaughter but may nevertheless come from an animal pumped up with enough drugs to enter a weight-lifting contest. Recognize promotional descriptions for what they are: marketing lingo.

As of July 1994, however, when the USDA's new food label regulations went into effect, some promotional claims actually do mean something. "Healthy," for example, on the package of a frozen dinner means that the product must contain at least 10 percent of the recommended daily value of at least three of the following nutrients: vitamins A or C, iron, calcium, protein, or fiber. In addition, the product must contain no more than 90 mg of cholesterol per serving, 3 grams of fat, 1 gram of saturated fat, and 600 milligrams of sodium (the sodium content must go down to 480 milligrams as of November 1997).

Here is a list of the terms that can be used on a food label and what they mean:

- Free—The product contains only a tiny or insignificant amount of fat, cholesterol, sodium, sugar, and/or calories. For example, a "fat-free" product will contain less than 0.5 grams of fat per serving.
- Low—A food described as "low" in fat, saturated fat, cholesterol, sodium and/or calories could be eaten fairly often without exceeding dietary guidelines. So "low in fat" means no more than 3 grams of fat per serving.
- Lean—"Lean" and "Extra Lean" are USDA terms for use on meat and poultry products. "Lean" means the product contains less than 10 grams of fat, 4 grams of saturated fat, and 95 milligrams of cholesterol per serving. "Lean" is not as lean as "Low."
- Extra Lean—"Extra Lean" means the product has less than 5 grams of fat, 2 grams of saturated fat, and 95 milligrams of cholesterol per serving. Leaner than "Lean," "Extra Lean" is still not as lean as "Low."
- Reduced, Less, Fewer— Means a diet product contains less of a nutrient or calories. For example, hotdogs might be labeled "25% less fat than our regular hotdogs."
- Light/Lite—Means a diet product with 1/3 fewer calories or 1/2 the fat of the original. "Light in Sodium" means a product with 1/2 the usual sodium.
- More—A food in which 1 serving has at least 10% more of the Daily Value of a vitamin, mineral, or fiber than usual.
- Good Source Of—One serving contains 10–19% of the Daily Value for a particular vitamin, mineral, or fiber.

Product labels are useful tools that can help you to make informed choices about the foods you eat. Become a label reader. Look for whole-food ingredients and avoid preservatives, artificial colors or flavors, refined sugars, MSG, and other undesirable additives.

18

FLOURS AND BAKING PRODUCTS

Because whole grains have been the primary staple foods for thousands of years, breads, baked goods, and other flour products truly are the staff of life. From thin Middle Eastern pocket breads to hearty Austrian sprouted-grain loaves, bread comes in myriad forms, shapes, and sizes. Yet, important to all breads and flour products are a few common factors: the quality of the grain, the manner of milling, the preparation and baking process, and the wholesomeness of added ingredients.

As discussed previously, an increasing number of farmers are growing grains by sustainable organic methods. As a result, there are many organically produced flour products on the market, grown by farmers who share a high regard for the health of the soil, water, air, and people. Whenever possible, choose organically grown flours over those that are conventionally produced. Although most supermarkets do not sell organically grown flours, any good natural food store will.

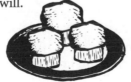

Milling

The milling of grains into flour is among the most influential factors in creating nutritionally viable breads and flour products. Millers agree that the highest-quality flours are made by slow, cool grinding with stone mills. Expert stone milling requires both experience and artistry. The miller must ensure that the temperature, fineness of grind, sifting, and mixing of flours are all optimal to deliver the most nutritious flour possible.

Stone milling is rare these days. Most flour milling is performed by high-speed, high-volume steel cylinders or hammer mills. Cylinder mills grind grains with ridged or smooth pairs of cylinders that rotate at high speed. Grains are forced between the cylinders, which grind and tear the kernels instantly. In the grinding process, a great deal of heat is generated. While stone mills can grind grains at temperatures below 90°F, cylinder mills heat grains to 150°F. At just 119°F, most of the healthful live enzymes in the flour are eliminated. At higher temperatures, many of the nutrients in the flour are destroyed. In addition, cylinder milling overexposes flour to air. This causes oxidation, which leads to the rancidity of oils in the grain. Thus, the grain spoils quickly, losing its freshness, flavor, and aroma. Hammer mills, the most widely used flour mills in operation today, are even hotter and faster than cylinder mills. High-velocity steel hammer heads smash and powder whole grains at ultra-high speed. This method destroys more nutrients, thus producing a nutritionally inferior flour.

By contrast, stone milling is accomplished with two ridged grinding stones. The stones crush and grind the whole grains slowly and progressively, without oxidizing the flour or destroying the nutrients with heat. After grinding, the flour is sifted through a screen that catches larger particles of bran and germ. These are reground in a smaller, finer mill and are then remixed with the rest of the flour to produce a uniform, fully nutritious milled-grain product.

White vs. Whole-Grain Flours

Most cylinder and hammer mills are used to transform whole nutritious grains into nutritionally devoid white flour. In the milling process, the bran and germ layers of the grains are stripped away, leaving only the white, pulpy interior kernel, or endosperm. When whole wheat is milled into white flour, 83 percent of the nutrients are removed, with mostly starch remaining. The fiber is gone, and the vitamin E content is reduced, along with twenty-one other nutrients. The flour that is produced is so useless as a food that it must be fortified with synthetically manufactured thiamin, riboflavin, and niacin, as well as iron.

In addition to nutritional abuse and synthetic vitamin fortification, flour often suffers further adulteration with chemicals used to age, bleach, whiten, and preserve the product. Chlorine dioxide, an irritant to both the skin and the respiratory tract, is used to bleach flour. Benzoyl peroxide, another bleaching agent, is also a skin irritant. Other additives include methyl bromide, nitrogen trichloride, alum, chalk, nitrogen peroxide, and ammonium carbonate. This is not the staff of life.

Whole-grain flour, when milled properly, does not lose its nutritional value. No synthetic nutrients or chemical additives are necessary. High-quality whole-grain flours smell sweet and fresh and deliver plenty of flavor when they are eaten. Unlike white flour, however, which rarely becomes infested because it cannot support life, whole-grain flour can sometimes become infested with insects. For this reason, some stone millers put their flour through pest-destroying machines containing steel disks and rods that smash insect larvae or eggs.

Storage and Handling

As with many other foods, the four enemies of whole-grain flour are heat, light, moisture, and time. Flour should be kept at a cool temperature during and after the milling process. Ideally, it is refrigerated after it is ground. For maximum nutrition, flour should be used within five days after milling. But most flours have not been shipped to retail stores by that time. Flours will retain much of their nutritional value if used within sixty days after they were ground. Select flours that have been refrigerated since they were milled, if you can find any.

Flour sold in paper bags is preferable to products packed in polyethylene. Paper bags keep flour reasonably fresh and dry. Polyethylene, however, sweats on the inside, thus promoting spoilage.

Flour

Every grain, and some beans, can be ground finely into flour. The most popular bread flour worldwide, however, is made from wheat. Though refined white flour is widely used in baking today, it is not considered here because it is a nonfood. Instead, the various varieties of whole-grain flour are described.

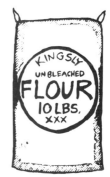

Whole-Wheat Bread Flour   As described in the "Grains" chapter, there are hard and soft varieties of spring and winter wheat. Harder wheat flours are most popular for baking bread because they contain the highest amount of gluten. Gluten is a protein with elastic properties, which enables breads to hold together and rise. Coarse whole-wheat bread flour, sometimes called graham flour, is popular for making graham crackers.

Whole-Wheat Pastry Flour Soft spring and winter wheats have a light, starchy core, with low gluten. Pastry flour is made from these varieties and is ideal for baking pie crusts, cookies, biscuits, cakes, and light rolls.

Durum Flour A variety of hard spring wheat, durum has hard, dense, starchy kernels. You can't make bread with durum flour. Any attempt to do so will yield a bricklike loaf as hard as a flagstone. Durum is used to make pasta. It holds various macaronis and pastas together very well, keeping the shape of the noodle intact during boiling, baking, and cooking in sauces. If you are going to make pasta, use whole durum flour. Avoid semolina, which is refined durum flour stripped of the bran and germ layers. Most commercial pasta is made with semolina.

Gluten Flour This is made from whole-wheat flour that has had most of the starch removed. Gluten flour increases the protein value of bread and makes the dough rise higher and more quickly.

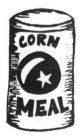

Cornmeal Made not from sweet corn, which is a table vegetable, but from flint or dent varieties, whole cornmeal contains both the outer hull and the germ of the grain. Much of the cornmeal on the market today is refined, with the hull and germ removed. As with wheat refining, this strips most of the nutrients from the grain. Cornmeal is used in corn bread and muffins. It adds a coarse, crumbly consistency to baked goods. Look for products labeled "whole yellow" or "whole white" cornmeal. If the product is labeled "bolted," this means that the fiber has been removed.

Blue Corn Also ground into meal. Because of its high protein value, distinctive flavor, and novel blue color, blue cornmeal is popular in muffins, chips, tortillas, baking mixes, and pancakes.

Buckwheat Imparting a strong grainy flavor, whole-buckwheat flour is used in pancakes, waffles, noodles, breads, and cakes. Dark buckwheat flour comes from unhulled whole groats. Light buckwheat flour comes from the whole grain minus the hard outer hull. Dark buckwheat flour contains more fiber and nutrients and is more flavorful and aromatic. In baking, buckwheat is combined with either wheat or rye flour.

Barley Flour From unhulled barley, barley flour is used in cookies, cakes, pies, and pastries. Soft, sweet, and hearty, it combines well with wheat flour.

Brown Rice Flour Used in breads, cakes, cookies, and crackers, brown rice flour has a sweet, earthy flavor. Rice has no gluten; thus, rice flour is combined with wheat flour when used in breads.

Oat Flour Chewy and sweet, oat flour is a welcome addition to cookies, cakes, pie crusts, muffins, and breads. Because oats have little gluten, the flour is combined with whole-wheat flour for baking.

Oat Bran The big nutritional story of 1988 was oat bran, which contains soluble fibers that reduce cholesterol. More recently, however, the popularity of oat bran has diminished.

Many products promoted for their oat bran content contain too little to do you any good. Additionally, much of the oat bran on the market is just whole-oat flour, as opposed to the outside bran layer of the grain. Rolled oats contain only half the amount of cholesterol-lowering soluble fiber found in oat bran. Furthermore, some oat bran products contain saturated and hydrogenated oils, which contribute to your body's production of cholesterol. Read labels carefully, and choose products that list oat bran as the first ingredient and that do not contain saturated or hydrogenated oils.

Millet Flour This light, delicate flour is always combined with wheat flour before baking and is used in sauces, cookies, cakes, croquettes, and flat breads.

Amaranth Flour This light, sweet, high-protein flour is used in cookies, crackers, baking mixes, and cereals. Amaranth flour is usually very expensive, because the harvesting of amaranth is a labor-intensive process.

Rye Flour Whole rye has a low gluten content and so is usually mixed with wheat flour in breads. Though true dark-rye flour is made from the whole grain, much of the dark-rye bread available today is made from refined rye without the bran, with caramel color added. Rye flour has a rich, hearty, satisfying flavor and is good in breads, waffles, and pancakes.

Soy Flour High in protein and bitter tasting, soy flour is used to boost the nutritional profile of baked goods. Whole-soy flour has a beany flavor. A little goes a long way. Use a ratio of about 8 parts whole wheat to 1 part soy flour in breads, muffins, cookies, cakes, pancakes, and waffles. Avoid defatted soy flour, which has had the oils removed with solvents.

Carob Powder This ground roasted pod of a Mediterranean evergreen tree is touted as a satisfactory substitute for chocolate, which it is not. Carob is used in place of cocoa in baked goods. It is naturally sweet and low in fats, and contains 8 percent protein, B vitamins, calcium, magnesium, and pectin. Carob is also used in papermaking, for stabilizing foods, and for curing tobacco. Legend has it that the carob pod, also called the locust bean, was the "locust" eaten by John the Baptist in the wilderness.

About Leavening

Leavening is a process by which batters of various baked goods are made to lighten and rise. There are basically two kinds of leavening: chemical and biological. The principle of chemical leavening is that an acid compound (an ingredient in the batter) and an alkaline compound such as baking soda or baking powder (the leavening agent) react with each other through interaction with liquid, producing carbon dioxide gas as a result. This carbon dioxide gas causes batter to lighten and rise. The principle of biological leavening is that a culture, such as sourdough or an added yeast, feeds upon starches in batter, producing carbon dioxide gas as a result of fermentation, thus causing the product to rise.

Baking Soda Typically sodium bicarbonate, but sometimes potassium bicarbonate, baking soda is a leavening agent with no known deleterious health effects. Keep in mind, however, that sodium bicarbonate does contain sodium, which should be considered if you are assessing your total dietary sodium intake. Baking soda is an alkaline agent that reacts with such acid substances in batter as fruits, dairy products, and sweeteners.

Baking Powder Unlike baking soda, which reacts with an acid ingredient in batter to produce carbon dioxide gas, baking powder contains an acid, an alkali, and a starch. Upon contact with a liquid, baking powders begins to react right away.

From a health and flavor standpoint, the most preferable type of baking powder is cream of tartar. Cream of tartar is a sediment deposited in wine casks as a result of the wine fermentation process. This sediment contains compounds from the juice of grapes, as well as yeast. Because cream of tartar acts quickly, it should be mixed into batter and baked right away.

Slower than cream of tartar is phosphate baking soda, made from various forms of calcium and sodium phosphates. Except for their sodium value, these baking powders pose no health problem. Watch out for double-acting baking powders, however, which contain sodium aluminum sulfate. Dietary aluminum is believed to play a role in neurological disorders. Research has shown that dietary aluminum collects in the brain stem. No matter how fast you think you want your batter to rise, avoid baking powders that contain aluminum compounds.

Yeasts Baking yeasts are microscopic fungi of the family *Saccharomycetaceae*, which feed on starches in batter, producing carbon dioxide gas as a result. Active dry yeasts, compressed yeast cakes, and rapid yeasts all contain similar strains of yeast. The most important thing to look for is a product that does not contain added preservatives. The use of BHA, a preservative that causes cancer in laboratory animals, is common and unnecessary. If you do a lot of baking, experiment with various types of preservative-free yeast products, and discover the one that performs best for your needs.

19

PACKAGED FOODS

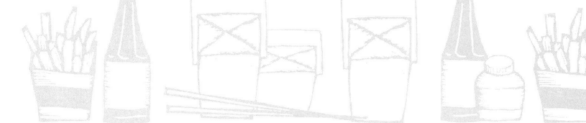

The world of packaged foods is diverse, filled with tens of thousands of national, regional, and local brands of foods in all categories. It is also a labyrinth of nutritionally devoid processed foods, chemical additives, deceptive labeling, and marketing hype. Separating the wheat from the chaff, so to speak, requires vigilant label reading and knowing what you are looking at. No matter how much a full-color front panel on a food product may grab you, go right to the ingredients panel. That's where you will learn what's actually in the food. Is the product a whole food or a whole-food look-alike?

The following categories of packaged foods include only those not covered in other chapters of this book. In most cases these foods are not as highly perishable as fresh fruits and vegetables, meats, fish, or dairy products. Although some packaged foods require refrigeration, most do not. Some will keep on the shelf for extended periods. All are made with whole-food ingredients.

Breads and Baked Goods

As discussed in the "Grains" chapter, whole-grain breads and baked goods are staple foods worldwide.

Whole-grain breads are a far cry from Wonder Bread, a well-marketed nutritionally impoverished product. Wonder Bread and brands like it are made with white flour that has been stripped of both its fiber and over 80 percent of its essential nutrients. Wonder Bread is such a nutritionally devoid product that it has to be pumped up with synthetic vitamins to achieve even a marginal nutritional profile. It is this "enrichment" with pharmaceutical nutrients that is at the heart of the claim that Wonder Bread builds strong bodies twelve ways. Actually, Wonder Bread is little more than a doughy delivery system for low-potency doses of synthetic vitamins.

People have eaten whole-grain breads and baked goods for thousands of years because these foods contain the natural fiber, oils, vitamins, and minerals that are essential to healthy, strong bodies. You need to understand what you are looking at when you encounter a bread label, in order to determine whether the bread is a wholesome, whole-grain product. The very first ingredient should be a whole-grain flour. The term "wheat flour" means white flour. Look for *whole* wheat, whole rye, or some other whole-grain flour as the first ingredient of any bread you buy. Breads do not need many

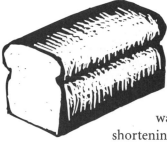

ingredients. If you are on a sodium-restricted diet, avoid breads that contain salt or any other additive with sodium in its name. Additionally, watch out for margarine, shortening, hydrogenated or partially hydrogenated oils, and palm, coconut, or cottonseed oils. These are all low-grade oils, highly saturated and/or sprayed, and deleterious to health.

Most commercial breads contain antioxidant preservatives, including BHA and BHT. You do not need these chemicals, which may cause cancer in humans. So avoid them, along with added refined sugar, dough conditioners, and coloring. The very same quality-ingredient standards apply to rolls, muffins, croissants, cakes, cookies, brownies, pies, and other baked goods. These products should be sweetened as needed with honey, maple syrup, Sucanat, molasses, barley malt, or fruit juice concentrate. Avoid refined sugar, fructose, or corn syrup.

Sprouted multigrain baked goods offer the maximum in nutrition and fiber and are among the heartiest of baked products, with a nutty flavor and chewy consistency. One increasingly popular form of sprouted grain bread is Essene-style bread, named after a bread made by a monastic brotherhood of Jews in Palestine between 200 B.C. and A.D. 200. Essene bread is made of ground sprouted grains that are patted into loaves and then partially baked. The result is a dense, moist, chewy loaf that is also quite sweet because of the natural sugars in the sprouted grains.

Another popular style of bread is pita, a Middle Eastern flat bread that forms a natural inside "pocket" when it is baked. This pocket can be filled with any kind of food, from hummus to sandwich meats. The pita has found its way into many supermarkets. Most pita breads today, however, are inauthentic, made from white flour. Look for whole-grain pita bread without preservatives.

For those who are allergic to wheat and must avoid gluten, some rice breads are available in natural food stores. The texture of rice bread is markedly different from that of wheat bread. It is porous, chewy, and delightfully flavorful. Sometimes rice breads are made with millet flour as well. Make sure the rice bread you select is made from whole brown rice, not polished white rice. All the above rules about additives and sweeteners apply here as well.

Nut Butters

Besides peanut butter there are other nut butters made from ground whole nuts and seeds. Sesame tahini and almond, sunflower, macadamia, and pecan butters offer the unique flavors of the nuts and seeds from which they are made. Nut butters are good in sandwiches, in dips or spreads, and baked into cookies. Natural nut butters are much more flavorful than commercial brands and are made without unnecessary additives. Commercial brands frequently contain added sugar, plenty of salt, and hydrogenated oils, which "stabilize" the nut butter.

You will notice when you look at natural nut butters that there is a layer of oil on the top of the nut butter. This is normal. The oil naturally separates out when no emulsifiers or stabilizers are added to keep the oils and solids together. When you open a jar of nut butter, just stir it with a knife for a minute until it is blended back together. Or you can pour off the oil, which will leave an appreciably thicker nut butter.

Though you will find salted and unsalted nut butters, unsalted ones are your best bet. You simply don't need the extra dietary sodium of a salted brand. Once nut butters are opened, you should keep them refrigerated. Exposure to oxygen on opening initiates the spoilage process, which is retarded by cold temperatures. If a nut butter ever tastes bitter or stale, throw it out. These are two indications of rancidity. As with all other foods, choose nut butters made from organically produced nuts and seeds whenever you have that option.

Jams, Jellies, Preserves

Almost everyone has a fondness for some type of jam or jelly, and most of us have our favorites. The primary issue regarding jams, jellies, and preserves is in regard to the sweeteners used. Major commercial brands are typically over 50 percent refined sugars, including cane and beet sugar, corn syrup, and fructose. A spoonful of one of these products is like a spoonful of sugar. Additionally, commercial brands may contain preservatives, artificial colors, and flavors. Again, start with the label. The very first ingredient of a jam, jelly, or preserve should be fruit. If it's not, pick another brand.

Natural jams, jellies, and preserves have stormed the grocery market and are becoming increasingly popular among traditional grocery shoppers. The basic ingredients are fruit, a sweetener, and pectin, a natural-fiber thickener that gives any fruit spread a smooth consistency. Several natural food manufacturers are now sweetening their products with fruit juice concentrate, which also naturally enhances flavor. As always, avoid all chemical additives.

Cereals

Cereals are among the most popular breakfast foods. They are an excellent food to start the day, providing protein, carbohydrates, vitamins, and minerals. The slow-digesting complex carbohydrates of whole-grain cereals provide our bodies with sustained-release energy that lasts for hours.

Commercial brands of breakfast cereals are a rogue's gallery of refined grains, high amounts of refined sugars, artificial colors, artificial flavors, and preservatives. Some popular brands of cereal on the market today, especially those marketed to children, contain over 50 percent refined sugar. But it is not just the children's brands that are nutritionally compromised. Several so-called "natural" cereals are also loaded with refined sugar, which has been conveniently dubbed "natural" by consensus among companies such as Quaker, General Mills, Post, and Kellogg. But don't be fooled by the packaging of these cereals. The boxes may show bucolic country scenes, with lavish color photographs of whole grains, fruits, nuts, and pitchers of creamy, farm-fresh milk. The labels may display colorful call-outs that read "with oat bran" or "high fiber." Forget all that, and turn your attention to the ingredients panel, which tells the real story.

If one and only one message about food is apparent, it should be that reading a label is your first act of self-protection against nutritionally inferior or harmful products. The very first ingredient of a cereal should be a whole grain. Scrutinize the ingredient panel to avoid refined grains (they will not say "whole" in front of them), refined sugars, hydrogenated oils, or any chemical additives. You will notice that most commercial brands of cereal contain added salt. The reason for this is that refined grains possess relatively little flavor, and salt helps to accent what little flavor remains.

As with so many other products, popular commercial brands of cereal are nutritionally deficient and are therefore often "fortified" with minerals and synthetic vitamins. The vitamins and minerals that are added to the cereal make up for only a fraction of what has been taken away, which includes vitamins, minerals, fiber, and trace elements. If a cereal is fortified, this is a tip-off that it is a nutritionally inferior product and has suffered extensive refining.

Whatever Happened to Granola? Undisputedly the quintessential health breakfast of the 1960s, crunchy granola was originally a blend of whole grains, nuts, seeds, dried fruits, and natural sweeteners such as honey and maple syrup. Today's mass-market cereal producers have a very different vision of what granola should be. Many brands of granola contain as much as 30 percent refined sugar, along with hydrogenated oils and dried fruits treated with sulfur dioxide. In natural food stores you can readily obtain whole-grain granolas made with natural ingredients, many of which are organically produced.

Wonders of Wheat Germ The germ layer of whole-wheat kernels, wheat germ is one of the most nutritious foods in the world. Rich in insoluble fiber, B vitamins, vitamin E, minerals, and calories, wheat germ also contains octacosanol, "the stamina factor." Octacosanol is a naturally occurring, oily, ergogenic (promotes utilization of oxygen) nutrient that has been proven to quicken reaction time, improve respiration, increase strength, reduce fatigue, boost utilization of oxygen, and enhance overall stamina and endurance.

All this nutritional power makes wheat germ a wonderful addition to your cereal bowl. Wheat germ goes rancid very quickly, however, because of its high oil content. When you buy wheat germ, look for either vacuum-packed bottles or nitrogen-flushed soft plastic or foil packages. Either type of packaging preserves the freshness of the wheat germ oil without chemical additives. Once wheat germ is opened, keep it refrigerated and use it within 2 weeks for maximum freshness. Keep wheat germ in a sealed container to retain moisture and to prevent it from absorbing odors.

Fiber, Fiber Everywhere   Now that the major cereal producers have discovered that the fiber they have always removed from their grains is highly nutritious and desirable, they are flooding the market with a plethora of fiber-rich bran cereals. Some fiber cereal packages display a message to suggest that the cereal prevents cancer or cardiovascular disease. Others simply show bucolic scenes. All of them, however, are positioned to cash in on the fiber-starved American public's recent realization that we all need more insoluble and soluble fibers in our systems. *Fiber* is the buzzword of the day.

There's nothing actually wrong with a fiber cereal, provided the ingredients do not include hydrogenated or tropical oils, refined sugars, or chemical additives. By contrast, however, a whole-grain cereal will also give you a tremendous amount of dietary fiber, along with other nutrients that you won't get in a cereal that's mostly (or all) bran. The best way to get fiber is not in one rock-em, sock-em bowl of bran every morning, but over the course of the day from fruits, vegetables, cereal grains, beans, and whole-grain breads and baked goods. If these foods make up a majority of your dietary intake, you will not need one purging bowl of bran in the morning. Nutritionally it makes sense to eat whole-grain cereals instead.

The major dietary fiber craze of 1988 and 1989 was oat bran, which insinuated itself like a persistent fungus into practically every food product except coffee creamers. Despite the fact that you have to eat two fist-size piles of it every day to bring your cholesterol level down by as much as 19 percent, everyone seemed bonkers about oat bran. Actually, this was a positive development. The public discovered in oat bran the truth that foods contain the keys to the prevention of serious and sometimes fatal diseases. The oat bran craze was a good spring board for people to jump off of into an even greater awareness of the nutritional and preventive benefits of a whole-food diet. Oat bran cereals are fine, but you're better off eating whole oats, which contain fiber, vitamins, minerals, and complex carbohydrates for sustained energy.

There are many brands of natural whole-grain cereals, from granolas to puffed grains to crispy varieties, to various shapes including O's and animals. Many cereal producers in the natural foods industry are using traditional grains like amaranth, blue corn, and quinoa in their products. This makes available a diversely flavorful and nutritious selection of whole-grain cereals. Experiment with different brands of hot and cold whole-grain cereals and discover the ones you like the most. Observe standard label-reading rules and caveats, and enjoy cereals as they should be enjoyed.

Crackers and Rice Cakes

Crackers are a pretty straightforward food category. The traditional recipe for crackers calls for unleavened ground grains to be prepared with a little water and a pinch of salt and baked. What could be simpler? But old-world cracker recipes have given way to alleged advances in food technology. Most crackers on the market today are made with refined flour, sugar, too much salt, hydrogenated oils, artificial colors and flavors, dough conditioners, and antioxidant preservatives.

As a result, buying a cracker requires careful

label reading. Look for crackers made with whole grains such as wheat, corn, oats, barley, rice, amaranth, and rye. Choose organically produced crackers when you can find them. Avoid hydrogenated oils, refined sugars, and artificial additives. Check the nutrition panels of various brands to determine their sodium content.

Whole-grain crackers contain natural oils and thus do not last forever. Once you have opened crackers, put them in an airtight container to keep them fresh, and use them within a few weeks. Observe manufacturing dates and expiration codes on packages.

Rice cakes used to be esoteric natural foods but are now found in virtually all conventional supermarkets throughout the United States. They are round and light and look a little like Styrofoam. Nothing could be simpler than a plain rice cake, which consists of popped brown rice and absolutely nothing else. Rice cakes can be made with added grains or seeds and salt. They are very low in calories, go well with just about everything, and are just plain good for you. As with all other foods, choose organically produced rice cakes whenever you can.

Chips and Pretzels

Americans love snack foods, especially chips and pretzels. Chips are made from either potatoes or refined grains and are deep-fried and salted for maximum calories and sodium value. Chips may contain hydrogenated oils, sugar, artificial colors and flavors, and preservatives. Pretzels are usually made from refined grains and are typically studded with large crystals of coarse salt. They may also contain preservatives.

In the natural chip and pretzel category, look for whole-grain products with reduced salt. Chips can be made of whole corn and other grains. They can also be made with nutritious vegetable oils instead of hydrogenated or partially hydrogenated oils, palm, coconut, or cottonseed oils. Some manufacturers now make chips with reduced quantities of high-quality oils, sea salt, and organically grown grains, with no chemical additives. You can feel

pretty good about eating these products. Because they're cooked in oil they are still relatively high in fats, but they are otherwise wholesome, provided they are fresh. The biggest difference between a "natural" potato chip and a commercial chip is in the quality of the oil used. In reality though, potato chips are not a wholesome food. They are very high in fat no matter how they are made, and they have little flavor unless they're salted.

Natural brands of pretzels, salted or unsalted, are made with ground whole grains and are about as healthful a snack as you will find. You will notice that pretzels made with whole grains are naturally sweet and crunchy. Observe all label-reading rules, and be aware that some commercial chip manufacturers are putting their chips in healthy-looking packaging. Read carefully.

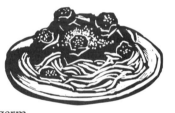

Pasta

Traditional white pasta is made from semolina flour, which is ground refined durum wheat with the bran and germ layers removed. Semolina is unique in that it holds the shape of whatever pasta it is made into, even when boiled in water and baked in sauces. Because semolina is a refined flour, it is missing important vitamins, minerals, protein, and fiber. For this reason, white pasta is sometimes fortified with extra vitamins and minerals. In your supermarket you will find an almost dizzying array of dried pastas, from spaghetti to macaroni to lasagna, as well as fresh refrigerated varieties. These products are not typically made with chemical additives, because pasta keeps well.

White pasta is not a whole food, and is thus not recommended here. There are many brands of whole-grain pasta available, made with whole durum wheat and other grains. Differences in color and flavor from one whole-grain pasta to another are due to the inclusion of buckwheat, Jerusalem artichoke, soy and rice flours, or powdered dried vegetables.

Whole-grain pasta takes getting used to, and

some brands are appreciably better than others. Overall, whole-grain pasta is heavier than white pasta. If it is not very well made, it can have a gritty or coarse texture. But well-made whole-grain pasta is a wonderful thing. It is smooth, not overly heavy, and flavorful. From a nutritional standpoint, these products offer the benefits of eating whole grains, with minimal preparation time. For those who are allergic to wheat products, whole-corn pasta is available in all shapes. Corn pasta doesn't taste or behave much like wheat pasta and will turn mushy if overcooked. However, it is an alternative for those who cannot tolerate wheat.

In addition to being particularly adept at making soy foods, the Japanese are accomplished noodle makers. Their noodles are usually made with both hard and soft wheats and often include buckwheat flour, brown rice flour, and *jinenjo,* a starchy wild mountain tuber. The three most popular Japanese noodles are soba, udon, and ramen.

Soba is made either of buckwheat flour or a mixture of buckwheat and wheat flours, and cooks faster than Western-style pasta, in only 3 to 5 minutes. Soba noodles are long and thin and are delicious eaten hot or cold. Thicker and flatter than soba, **udon** noodles are made with whole-wheat flour that is sometimes combined with brown rice flour to make a lighter pasta with a delicate flavor. Also excellent cold, udon noodles take from 5 to 15 minutes to cook.

Ramen noodles are thin spiral noodles that are usually made of whole wheat and sometimes with buckwheat, sesame, or brown rice flours. Ramen typically comes in packets with a small foil pouch of seasoned broth powder, which may contain dried mushrooms, scallions, herbs, and spices. Ramen noodles have become popular in the United States. This is not surprising, as they are inexpensive, cook quickly (in 5 minutes), and taste great.

There are also some brands of refrigerated fresh whole-grain pasta. These are not yet as commonly available as dried whole-grain pasta. Fresh whole-grain pasta is preferred whenever you can find it, because it is usually considerably more flavorful than dried varieties.

With all pasta products, read the label. Most pasta does not contain chemical additives, but look to be sure. Ramen products may contain MSG or other additives in the broth powder. Furthermore, do not think that just because a pasta is dark means that it is made from whole grains. A very small amount of spinach powder will make any white pasta look like an earthy whole food. Check to be sure that the product is made with whole grains. Pasta made from organically grown grains is always your best buy.

Salsa and Pasta Sauces

Salsa is a Mexican sauce usually (not always) containing tomatoes, along with chopped onions, vinegar, cumin, and hot peppers. There are many kinds of salsa, with a heat range from mild to blistering hot. Salsa is the quintessential dip for corn tortilla chips and is also excellent on fish, in casseroles, as a side condiment with meals, and on practically any Mexican entree. Some salsa is made with sodium benzoate, a preservative. But an increasing number of brands contain no chemical additives, and a few are made with organically grown ingredients.

Pasta sauces are usually tomato based, and from there the choices are many. Pasta sauces typically contain onions, garlic, olive oil, and spices and may also include mushrooms and ground meats. Commercial brands of pasta sauce generally contain sugar or corn syrup, though both are inauthentic and unnecessary. These sauces are sometimes preserved with sodium benzoate and may contain added corn starch, gums, and stabilizers. With pasta sauce, look for products that do not contain refined sweeteners, chemical additives, or added starches. Several natural brands are made without these ingredients. A couple of brands of pasta sauce available in natural food stores are made with organically produced ingredients.

If a pasta sauce contains meat, it is likely that the meat was raised with drugs, unless the label explicitly states otherwise. You may choose to make your own meat sauce with drug-free meats when you can.

Salsa and pasta sauces are sometimes canned, more often bottled, and increasingly available fresh.

From a nutritional and flavor standpoint, refrigerated fresh products are best, when you can get them.

Soy Foods

After corn, the second largest crop grown in the United States is soybeans. Primarily used for their oil, over 4 million pounds of soybeans are extracted every day. The remaining soy meal is used as animal fodder, in the manufacturing of paints and pharmaceutical products, and in flour, cereals, beverages, and dozens of processed foods. Despite their high protein content and low fat and carbohydrate value, less than 2 percent of the soybeans produced in the United States is used for human consumption.

This differs radically from the extent to which soybeans are eaten in other lands. In Asia, soybeans are used extensively in the human diet. One of the world's three major protein sources, along with fish and beef, soybeans can replace animal products in the human diet provided they are combined with whole grains. Four popular Eastern soy foods—tofu, tempeh, miso, and shoyu—have gained popularity among whole-foods enthusiasts and are finding their way into restaurant menus and mainstream supermarkets.

Tofu   Known as bean curd or soybean cake, tofu is regularly eaten by an estimated 25 percent of the world's population. In Japan alone there are almost forty thousand tofu shops. Tofu consists of soybeans, water, and a coagulant that is used to form the soy curd. It is made by soaking whole soybeans, puréeing them in water, and cooking the purée in boiling water. The purée is then strained, and the remaining soy milk is curdled with a coagulant. The three natural mineral coagulants that are used to make tofu are nigari, calcium chloride, and calcium sulfate. Nigari is a combination of magnesium chloride and other trace elements extracted from seawater. Many tofu makers assert that only nigari should be used as a coagulant, because it produces a superior tofu. Most commercially available calcium chloride is a by-product of the soda-ash manufacturing process and has been treated with acids. However, some high-quality tofu producers have located a source of pure calcium chloride that is mined from naturally occurring underground deposits. This coagulant, they say, produces a tofu at least as good as, if not superior to, that made with nigari. By contrast, calcium sulfate, though a natural mineral compound, produces a comparatively inferior tofu, with a chalky flavor and rubbery texture.

The coagulant in tofu making acts in the same manner as rennet in cheese making, separating the soy milk into curds and whey. The soy curds are then pressed in cloth-lined containers, resulting in bricks of tofu.

In the United States, no chemical additives are used in making tofu, because none are needed. You will want to choose tofu made with nigari or calcium chloride when you can, and you should look for brands made with organically grown soybeans. An increasing number of midwestern bean farmers are producing soybeans organically, meeting the needs of an expanding organic tofu market. Because soybeans are inexpensive anyway, you don't really pay much of a premium for organic tofu. You do, however, get a superior product, with greater flavor and lower or undetectable levels of chemical residues.

There are four types of tofu according to firmness: extra firm, firm, soft, and extra soft, or silken. These are differentiated by the amount of water and coagulant remaining in the tofu, and lend themselves to different uses. Silken and soft tofu are generally used for spreads, dressings, beverages, or desserts.

Tofu is rich in protein, containing half as much by weight as steak. Tofu yields even more protein when combined with whole grains, which balance out the amino acid profile of soybeans. Unlike animal sources of protein, tofu contains no cholesterol. It is naturally low in saturated fats and sodium and contains only 120 calories per four-ounce serving. Tofu is also easier to digest than animal protein, though some people do experience flatulence when they eat soy foods.

Most tofu is sold fresh in the refrigerated section of your supermarket or natural food store. You will also find dried tofu and unrefrigerated tofu in an aseptic brick pack. There is nothing wrong with either of these products. Neither compares, however, with fresh tofu for flavor and consistency. Tofu is very versatile. It can be baked, stir-fried, grilled, and used in soups, stews, salads, sandwiches, dips, and desserts.

Tempeh   Indonesia is the home of tempeh, a pressed fermented soybean cake. Tempeh is possibly the single best source of complete protein, roughly equaling the percentage of usable protein in beef and chicken without their saturated fat or cholesterol. Tempeh contains 19.5 percent protein and is a good source of fiber, B vitamins, and calcium. It is low in fat and sodium and contains no cholesterol. Tempeh is neutral in flavor and absorbs the seasoning with which it is prepared.

Tempeh is produced by exposing soybeans to *Rhizopus oligosporous*, a friendly bacterial culture. Hulled soybeans are cooked, cooled, and inoculated with the culture. The beans are then bound in a porous wrap and stored briefly until they are transformed into firm cakes by a network of white fibers produced by the bacteria. Black or gray spots in tempeh are normal, indicating the production of harmless spores by the culture. The bacterial fermentation of tempeh creates its unique flavor, makes the soybeans easier to digest, and enhances digestion in general.

A nutritional red herring was dragged across tempeh's path in 1977 when researchers at Cornell University's New York State Agricultural Experiment Station discovered nutritionally significant amounts of vitamin B_{12} in tempeh. News of this discovery quickly spread, and tempeh was used to vindicate vegetarian claims that all nutrients, even vitamin B_{12}, can be obtained from a diet free of animal products. Subsequent studies have shown however, that the B_{12} in tempeh is not assimilated into the human body, for reasons that are not understood. Thus, the search for an assimilable vegetarian source of vitamin B_{12} continues.

In Indonesia tempeh enjoys the same status as a mealtime staple that tofu does in Japan. This is because tempeh is a versatile culinary ingredient that can be baked, broiled, stir- or deep-fried, and used in casseroles, salads, sandwiches, sauces, soups, dips, and an endless variety of Eastern and Western recipes.

Tempeh is found fresh in the refrigerator section of your supermarket. It is not produced with chemical additives, and it may be made from organically grown soybeans. Buy organic tempeh whenever possible.

Miso   A staple of the Japanese diet for over thirteen hundred years, miso is a fermented soybean paste that is reputed to enhance health and longevity. Miso is made by cooking soybeans in water with sea salt, then inoculating them with koji, a live culture of the *Aspergillus oryzae* bacteria. The koji culture breaks down the soybeans and various grains that may be added to the miso for additional flavor and food value. After it is inoculated, the mixture is then aged under pressure in wooden kegs for as little as two months or as long as three years. Japan's dwindling number of traditional miso masters pile a ton or more of heavy stones atop a single wooden keg of miso to achieve the right pressure. Most miso makers use modern machinery and temperature-controlled environments instead of the more labor-intensive traditional methods.

Health claims about miso are not spurious. Miso is rich in protein, minerals, and B vitamins; is low in fat; and contains no cholesterol. It is high in sodium, however, because it is heavily salted. For this reason miso should be used sparingly in an otherwise salt-free diet. If you are on a sodium-restricted diet, miso is not for you, despite its nutritional value. The bacterial culture in miso additionally enhances overall digestion, and may contain nutritional factors that enhance immunity against some bacterial diseases.

All good brands of miso are aged naturally, but many brands are pasteurized prior to packaging. Pasteurization kills the healthful *Aspergillus* bacteria that are key to the value of miso. However, you can obtain unpasteurized, fresh miso in the refrigerated section of many natural food stores.

Miso varies considerably in color and flavor. Light, or white, miso is aged from two to six months. It is sweet and mild in taste and is well suited for use in sauces, soups and salad dressings. Dark, or red, miso is aged for six months to three years. It is stronger and saltier and is ideal for heavier dishes such as hearty soups, gravies, stews, and cold-weather recipes.

Shoyu (Soy Sauce)   The by-product of miso making, traditional shoyu is a dark soy sauce pressed out of fully aged miso. After it is pressed the shoyu sits to clarify until the sediment sinks to the bottom. It is heated to stop the ongoing bacterial fermentation process initiated by koji culture in the miso, and is then bottled. Traditional shoyu has a rich flavor that is the result of careful fermentation. From beginning to end, the shoyu-making process takes about two years. Its four ingredients are soybeans, wheat, water, and sea salt. You can obtain traditional shoyu in natural food stores. There you will also find tamari, which is shoyu from soybeans, water, and salt, without the wheat. True shoyu is superior to tamari in flavor because of the slow process by which it is made.

There are many soy sauces on the market that look like shoyu but are in fact inferior. Some of these are made with defatted, solvent-extracted soybeans and are quick-fermented to produce a liquid that looks like shoyu but tastes sharp and salty, with no rich flavor. Some other soy sauces are made with hydrolyzed vegetable protein, alcohol, soy extract, caramel coloring, salt, water, and corn syrup, and are not fermented at all. These look similar to traditional shoyu but taste nothing like it.

When you buy shoyu or tamari, read the label carefully. There are some pretty slick-looking soy sauces on the market that are made with inferior ingredients. You will also find "low sodium" shoyu and tamari. These products still contain a high amount of sodium, though lesser amounts than their regular counterparts. Shoyu, the primary seasoning in Asian cooking, enhances the flavor of grains, beans, vegetables, soups, stews, meat, and

fish. Because it contains sodium (about 285 milligrams per teaspoon), it should be used sparingly.

Soy Milk   Soy milk is a versatile beverage that enjoys some dietary advantages over dairy milk. People attempting to cut down their intake of saturated fats and cholesterol, or who suffer lactose intolerance or milk allergies, will find soy milk a surprisingly tasty alternative. Soy milk is made by puréeing soybeans with water, straining off the liquid, and cooking it. The soy milk is filtered to remove sediment, giving it a smooth, milky consistency with little or no bean taste. Some soy milks are flavored with barley malt or other unrefined sweeteners. A plain unfortified soy milk with the same amount of water will contain more protein and iron, less fat, fewer calories, no cholesterol, and about one-fifth the calcium of cow's milk. Soy milk can be used as a beverage, on cereal, and in many recipes that call for milk. It should not, however, be used as a milk substitute for infants, as it is lacking in nutrients that are essential to growth and development.

Sea Vegetables: Not Just Weeds

Sea vegetables, more commonly known as seaweed, have been popular foods among the Japanese, Chinese, and aboriginal Australians for as long as ten thousand years. Later, sea vegetables found their way into the diets of Scandinavians and Native Americans. Today, sea vegetables are popular among health-conscious consumers, who are ever on the lookout for highly nutritious foods.

Sea vegetables are among the most nutrient-rich foods in the world; yet, they are extremely low in calories. In fact, it probably would not be possible to gain weight by eating seaweed, no matter what the quantity. Almost all whole seaweeds contain large amounts of minerals and trace elements, including iron, calcium, and iodine. Many are rich in vitamins A, C, and the B complex.

Not a Source of Dietary B_{12}   Sea vegetables have been promoted by some dietary exponents as an excellent vegetarian source of vitamin B_{12}. Sea vegetables *do* contain ample amounts of this vitamin, which is otherwise found only in milk, eggs, meat, and fish. However, studies conducted by the Cincinnati Medical Center, the Harvard School of Public Health, and Vanderbilt and Brandeis universities show that the B_{12} in sea vegetables is not absorbed and utilized by the human body. The reasons for this are not yet understood, but people on a strict vegetarian diet who are relying on sea vegetables for B_{12} are not actually getting this essential nutrient.

Vitamin B_{12} is essential to the synthesis of hemoglobin, as well as the construction and regeneration of red blood cells. It is an antianemia factor and is involved in the metabolism of all foods, a healthy nervous system, a normal appetite, and growth in children. Dutch studies have shown that the children of vegans (who eschew all animal products) are deficient in vitamin B_{12} and have abnormal red blood cells, slower growth, and delayed motor skills compared with the children of parents who eat animal products.

A Strong Nuclear Defense? Whoever would suspect that seaweeds could be a strong nuclear deterrent? Studies conducted at Canada's McGill University show that some seaweeds can help to remove radioactive strontium from our bodies. Kombu, arame, hijiki, and other brown seaweeds contain alginic acid, which binds with strontium in the blood and carries it out of our systems. Strontium is a hazardous nuclear pollutant that is increasingly present in our environment because of nuclear accidents and the illegal dumping of radioactive materials.

Cholesterol-lowering Effects Not only are seaweeds loaded with nutrients and effective against radioactive strontium—some of them also help to lower blood cholesterol. In animal studies, carrageenan (from Irish moss), kombu, and other seaweeds have demonstrated a cholesterol-lowering effect. Sitosterol, a naturally occurring plant sterol in seaweeds, appears to play a significant role in cholesterol reduction. Animals fed daily servings of several seaweeds show an increase in fecal cholesterol, which suggests that seaweeds inhibit cholesterol absorption in the digestive tract. Additionally, quantities of thyroxin are found in brown seaweeds. Thyroxin, a hormone manufactured by the thyroid gland, is known to reduce both cholesterol and lipids in the blood.

Storage and Handling The storage and handling of seaweeds couldn't be simpler. Store them in dark, dry places. Keep them in airtight containers for maximum nutrition and freshness. Following are the most popular seaweeds:

Agar is a mucilaginous component of the cell walls of various red algae, including the *Gracilaria* and *Gelidium* species. A naturally occurring polymer of components of the sugar galactose, agar has unique properties that are valuable in food preparation. When dissolved in boiling water and then cooled, agar becomes gelatinous. In scientific laboratories worldwide, agar is used as a culture medium for bacterial experiments. In the food industry agar is a common stabilizer in jellies, jams, confections, and canned meat products. Its most noteworthy nutritional value is its high calcium content. In cooking, this sea gelatin is used in desserts and salad molds, or in any dish that needs a neutral-tasting thickener. Try making a fruit dessert with agar.

Agar is also known as *kanten* and may be labeled as such. It comes in packets of flakes or as a dry, spongy bar. Though agar grows abundantly in Japan, which is the world leader of the agar industry, it also grows off the coast of California and along the Atlantic seaboard.

Alaria is harvested from the colder waters of the Atlantic and Pacific. Though similar to Japanese wakame, alaria has a more delicate flavor. Alaria is 16 percent protein and is used in soups, salads, and marinated dishes.

Arame is harvested in Japan, the Pacific North American coast, and off Peru. Tough and fibrous, it must be boiled and softened. Arame is used in salads, casseroles, and other vegetable dishes.

Dulse comes from the cold waters of the Atlantic and Pacific. Eaten plain or in salads, sandwiches, or soups, dulse is thin and leafy and can be moistened in seconds by soaking it to make it more tender and less salty. Dulse makes an excellent snack when eaten plain.

Hijiki is a thin, spaghetti-like seaweed that grows abundantly in Japan, where it has been eaten for thousands of years. It also grows along the coast of China. Hijiki is delicious sautéed in oil with other vegetables. It is unusually high in calcium, iron, phosphorus, and potassium.

Kelp grows in huge underwater forests off the coasts of California, Norway, Japan, and other parts of the world. Kelp is both a food and a food supplement. In Asia kelp is a vegetable used in soups, stews, and salads and as a snack. As a seasoning, kelp is dried, powdered, and served from a shaker as a replacement for table salt. Because kelp grows in seawater, it is rich in minerals and trace elements. At least seventy-two of these are found in kelp, which is particularly rich in iodine. Iodine is necessary for proper thyroid function. Kelp is an excellent mineral and trace-element food. It is of value to digestion, healthy hair, skin, nails, bones, teeth, and overall health and vitality.

Kombu is from Hokkaido in northern Japan and is used to make subtle-tasting soup stocks and stews. It is high in calcium, phosphorus, and potassium and has a sweet, delicate flavor.

Nori is a name for a variety of seaweeds, most notably red and purple laver, from the northern Atlantic and Pacific. The seaweed is washed, chopped, and sun-dried into thin sheets. Nori is the delicate seaweed wrapping used to make sushi. It can also be crushed and used as a seasoning. Nori is high in calcium, iron, phosphorus, and vitamin A. In Japan, nori is rolled into balls and chewed instead of gum.

Wakame is a thick sea vegetable that is soaked and then cut into strips used in salads, soups, or stews. Grown along the coasts of Japan, China, and Korea, wakame is high in calcium, iron, phosphorus, potassium, and vitamin C. Chewy and substantial, this seaweed is particularly hearty.

Asian Foods

Many healthful foods come from Asia, where traditional cultures have experimented with whole-food ingredients for thousands of years. As both whole foods and ethnic foods (which are most often whole foods) become more available, we will see an increasing array of popular Asian foods. Many other Asian foods are covered in the "Soy Foods," "Pasta," and "Condiments" sections of this chapter. Amasake, mochi, and seitan, however, are each unique, fitting into no other food category.

Amasake   Used as a beverage or as a cooking or table sweetener, amasake is a traditional unrefined cultured Japanese food. Amasake is made by inoculating a mixture of water and rice with koji. Koji, made of *Aspergillus oryzae* bacteria and rice, is prepared under controlled temperatures and moisture for a few days, until the bacteria have thoroughly invaded and digested the rice. As a bacterial culture starter, koji acts in a similar manner as the cultures used to make yogurt, except that in the case of koji, the bacteria are used to break down whole grains, making them more readily digestible and sweeter.

Amasake is thus naturally sweet, with a milder flavor than honey or maple syrup. Much of the naturally occurring sugar in amasake is maltose. This sugar is absorbed slowly into the body, contributing to sustained energy. Amasake is sold as a "shake" and is sometimes flavored with almond or other natural ingredients.

Mochi   A traditional Japanese energy food, mochi is made by steaming, pounding, and drying glutinous sweet brown rice. A favorite warming food among Japanese farmers on cold winter days, mochi comes in thick, fat cakes that must be cooked to be eaten. Mochi has a chewy, elastic texture and a delicious nutty grain flavor. It is best cut into squares and popped into an oven or a toaster oven for 10 minutes at 450°F. The squares pop up like biscuits and can be cut open and filled with nut butter or jam. Bigger squares can be used for sandwiches. Mochi is unlike any other food, and is wonderful. It comes plain, flavored with cinnamon, or mixed with mugwort, a spinachlike Japanese plant.

Seitan   Also known as "wheat meat," seitan is wheat gluten that has been extracted from whole-wheat flour with water. Seitan is a versatile meat substitute that is popular throughout Asia. Easy to make, it is available packaged in the refrigerated sections of natural food stores, though it rarely makes it into a conventional supermarket. Seitan is usually lightly seasoned and can be used in stir-fries, in stews, or as meatballs in pasta sauce. It has a satisfying flavor and a chewy, meatlike texture. Seitan is high in protein (about 18 percent) but contains none of the saturated fats or cholesterol found in meats.

Soups

Campbell's slogan is "Soup is good food." They're right, too. A well-made soup can be highly nutritious, easy to digest, and delicious. But commercial soups today are quite different from what Grandmother used to make. For starters, most brands of soup are loaded with salt, so they are very high in sodium—as much as 1,200 milligrams per can. That's outrageous. Commercial soups also often contain refined sweeteners, including dextrose, sugar, and corn syrup. It is completely unnecessary to add sugar to soup. In addition, many soups contain hydrogenated vegetable oils. Though soups usually contain only small amounts of these oils, they are highly processed and contribute to the body's production of cholesterol. So who needs them? Soups may also pick up small amounts of lead from cans with lead-soldered seams, although more and more soup cans are being made without seams.

Dry powdered soup mixes are usually filled with more salt, refined sugars, and chemical additives, including preservatives, MSG, and thickeners. When you buy soup, start with the label and avoid refined sweeteners, hydrogenated oils, and other unnecessary additives. Look for canned and dry soups made with natural ingredients such as vegetables, grains, beans, herbs, and spices. Read the nutrition panels on soups, and choose those brands that are lowest in sodium. A couple of soup brands use seamless cans or lead-free solder on the seams of their cans. This may be identified on the label.

Canned Fruits, Vegetables, and Beans

Canned goods, including fruits, vegetables, and beans, are subject to the usual parade of additives. Fruits may contain heavy syrups made of sugar and corn syrup. Dietetic fruits may contain sorbitol or saccharin or aspartame. Vegetables may contain preservatives. Beans and chili mixes may contain hydrogenated oils, or lard that has most likely been prepared with nitrites, which are carcinogenic.

Canned goods should never constitute a major part of the diet. They are alternatives when fresh foods are not available. When you buy canned goods, read the labels carefully. When possible, choose organically produced canned goods.

The least-mentioned problem with canned goods is that some cans have seams that are soldered tight with lead, trace amounts of which can get into the food. Lead is a toxic metal that causes mental retardation in children and irreversible brain damage. Though there are no studies that link soldered cans with brain damage, the toxicity of lead is widely acknowledged throughout the entire medical community. Dietary lead, in any amount, is a hazard. It is easy to detect a soldered can, because it has a full-length vertical groove. Welded cans, which are not held together with solder, have only a very thin vertical line. Seamless

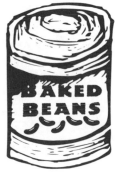

cans, which are becoming increasingly popular, have no vertical line or groove and are not held together with solder. Most companies are using welded or seamless cans.

Dinner Mixes

Many whole-food dinner mixes are available in natural food stores and some supermarkets. They range from falafel, which is a Middle Eastern dish made from garbanzo beans (chick-peas), to various grain pilafs and bean dishes. Whatever the product, the basic rules of label reading apply. Wherever a grain is listed, be sure that it is a whole grain. Do not assume that the grains in dinner mixes are whole. If they are, the label will say so, because this is an important selling point. Avoid any artificial colors, flavors, or preservatives as well as hydrogenated oils, thickening agents, sugar, and the many sources of added sodium (see "Salt").

Dinner mixes are convenient when you are traveling, camping, or in a hurry. However, you are always better off making meals from basic whole-food ingredients that you put together yourself. By doing so, you can be better assured of the quality and freshness of the meals you prepare. Some manufacturers of dinner mixes use organically produced ingredients, which are always preferred over conventionally produced ingredients.

Frozen Foods

Frozen foods, like all other foods, should conform to high standards of ingredient purity and nutrition without chemical additives, sugars, excessive salt, hydrogenated oils, and the many unnecessary or potentially harmful ingredients that have already been covered in this section.

Assuming that these bases are covered, the primary issues with frozen foods are those of packaging and handling. When you purchase frozen foods in your grocery store, look for a manufacturing date on the product you are choosing. Whenever dates appear, select the most recently produced product. Look for packaging that is completely intact, with-

out rips, tears, or punctures of any kind. Good supermarkets will display a thermometer in their freezer cases. The temperature in these cases should be 0°F (−18°C), or colder. This temperature assures maximum protection against spoilage or product deterioration. In the case of frozen fish fillets or other items that are visible through the packaging materials, avoid those products that show any freezer burn. This is an indication that the product has been stored at inconsistent temperatures. When you purchase frozen foods, bring them home and put them in your freezer as soon as possible. It is best not to run a bunch of errands after buying frozen foods (this is also true for dairy products, meat, and seafood). Instead, run other errands prior to shopping, whenever you can.

To thaw frozen foods, remove from your freezer only the amount required for immediate use.

Frozen foods should be thawed in the following ways:

- according to the manufacturer's instructions whenever given
- in a refrigerator at not more than 45°F
- under warm running water at not more than 70°F
- in an oven or microwave until the food is thoroughly cooked

Vinegars and Salad Dressings

The name *vinegar* comes from the French *vin aigre*, or "sour wine." Most vinegar today, however, is no longer a natural byproduct of wine but is a distilled alcoholic solution that is clarified and pasteurized, yielding a nonalcoholic, highly acidic liquid. **Distilled white vinegar** is nothing more than acetic acid and water. It is used widely in salad dressings and prepared foods, and has no nutritional value. Distilled vinegar is a fiber softener, a disinfectant, and an excellent cleaning agent, especially for glass. In a dilute solution with warm water, distilled vinegar is unsurpassed for removing wallpaper. It is not, however, much of a food.

Naturally fermented vinegars, by contrast, in-

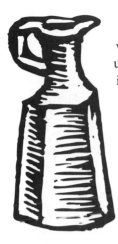

cluding apple cider vinegar and all varieties of wine vinegar, have unique flavors and colors characteristic of the raw materials from which they are made, and contain amino acids and other nutrients. **Herb vinegars** may be made with fermented vinegar, or they may be a combination of herbs and distilled vinegar. Read the label on the bottle to determine which is the case. Fermented vinegars have been used for thousands of years as flavorings in dressings and pickles. Naturally fermented vinegars are also highly regarded as traditional folk remedies. A small amount of vinegar drunk in warm water is said to be good for the digestion.

Among the various vinegars available, brown rice vinegar, balsamic vinegar, and umeboshi vinegar are the most flavorful. **Brown rice vinegar** has a light honey color, and a sweet flavor. It is used in Asian cookery but is equally wonderful in salad dressings and marinades. **Balsamic vinegar** receives its unique dark color and complex, sweet flavor from a mixture of wines and musts, and from years of aging in wood barrels. Balsamic vinegar has found its way into nouvelle cuisine and some of the world's poshest restaurants simply because it tastes wonderful. It is excellent in dressings and marinades. **Umeboshi vinegar,** made from the puckery-tart Japanese umeboshi plum, is salty, with a slight citrus flavor. It is an excellent substitute for vinegar in dressings and is so concentrated that a little goes a long way. In Japanese folk healing, umeboshi vinegar is used to treat colds, flu, weakness, and lassitude.

Mirin   A sweet rice wine, mirin is used in cooking, as a flavor enhancer, and in dressings and marinades. Mirin adds a light, sweet glaze to cooked foods and brings out the flavor of grains, fish, vegetables, and salads. Mirin has a 12 to 14 percent alcohol content that evaporates when it is cooked. The ingredients of high-quality mirin are brown rice,

koji (the same culture used in miso), and water. Read mirin labels, as some lesser brands are adulterated with corn syrup.

Salad dressings traditionally contain oil, vinegar, and various flavorings and seasonings. Today, however, salad dressing labels read like a college chemistry text, with long lists of gums, thickeners, artificial colors and flavors, preservatives, refined sugars, excessive sodium, hydrogenated oils, MSG, modified food starch, and a rogue's gallery of other additives.

A salad dressing should comply with the same quality standards as any other whole food. The ingredients, from unrefined oils to fermented vinegars, should be additive free. Look on the nutrition panel to make sure that the salad dressing you select is not unduly high in sodium (most are).

There are currently several brands of high-quality salad dressings on the market made from superior ingredients. You usually pay an absurd premium, however, to have someone else mix your salad dressing and bottle it for you. There is no question that your best strategy with salad dressings is to make your own. A little olive oil, some balsamic vinegar, a dash of mirin, and some dried herbs will result in a far better dressing than you will find on a supermarket shelf.

Condiments

Condiments add flavor, eye appeal, and an extra culinary dimension to foods of all kinds, from salads to sandwiches, casseroles to roasts. Following is a list of condiments that describe some of the things to look for when buying these products.

- **Capers**   The flower buds of a Mediterranean bush, capers are usually pickled in vinegar, water, and salt. They are used in salads, with lox, in vegetable platters, and in a variety of Mediterranean dishes. Capers do not usually contain any undesirable additives.
- **Garlic in Oil**   A definite convenience, bottled chopped garlic in oil is found in the refrigerated section of your grocery store and

is used whenever chopped garlic is required (which is all the time, by some accounts). Many people do not keep this product refrigerated, however, which is a serious mistake. The Food and Drug Administration has reported several cases of botulism poisoning attributable to the consumption of unrefrigerated chopped garlic in oil. So play it smart. Keep your garlic in oil cold to prevent the growth of harmful bacteria.

- **Hot Sauces**   Pure hot sauce is a simple unadulterated product consisting of hot chili peppers, vinegar, and salt. Hot sauce needs no chemical additives, keeps well without refrigeration (because of the antibacterial nature of vinegar), and adds a great deal of heat and zest to whatever you put it on. Start slowly with hot sauce, as brands vary in strength, and you can easily burn your mouth with an unfamiliar version if you use too much. A dash of hot sauce is wonderful in soups, stews, stir-fries, and just about every other food except dessert.

- **Ketchup**   One of the few foods that cannot be made legally with chemical additives, ketchup usually contains high amounts of salt and refined sugar or corn syrup. You can find natural brands with reduced sodium or no salt, sweetened with honey.

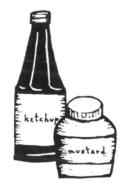

- **Mayonnaise**   Though artificial colors or flavors are not legally allowed in mayonnaise, preservatives are. Mayonnaise is made of oil, lemon juice or vinegar, and eggs. Many commercial brands include sugar and emulsifiers. Several natural brands, made without sugar or other additives, are available. Avoid "salad spread" and other mayo look-alike products, which are riddled with chemical additives.

- **Mustard**   Ideally, mustard should be ground mustard seed, a little vinegar, and some salt.

But today you'll find oil, gums, flour, and preservatives in many brands of mustard. One of the most popular brands of mustard in the United States is made primarily of turmeric and vinegar. Turmeric is a natural yellow spice that is cheaper than real mustard seed. It may be natural, but it has no place in mustard! Look for real mustards (read the labels) without additives.

- **Olives**   The fruit of an evergreen tree indigenous to Asia Minor and cultivated in the Mediterranean region, olives are widely used throughout the world. Green olives are picked when fully grown but unripe, whereas black olives are picked when ripe and are richer in oil. Both are treated with lye (mostly potassium carbonate) to remove bitterness. They are then packed in brine, a solution of water and salt. Olives need no additives, but some packers use preservatives anyway. Olives are usually available canned or bottled. Canned olives usually have a tinny taste and are not as tasty as those that are bottled. In addition, canned olives usually contain ferrous gluconate (iron) as a fixative. This nutrient helps canned olives keep their color. Some bottled olives are cured in brine and then packed in olive oil. Usually these are the highest-grade black olives, with the best flavor.

- **Pickles**   What is a pickle? It is any vegetable that is cured in either brine or vinegar. In Japan, pickles include radishes, sea vegetables, bitter carrots, and other root vegetables. In the United 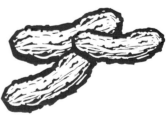 States, most pickles are cured cucumbers. Pickles do not need additives, but some contain refined sugar or corn syrup. Pickles of all kinds are a wonderful addition to almost any meal. Pickled cucumbers are a standard accompaniment to sandwiches and vegetable platters.

- **Relishes** From sweet chopped pickle to corn and spices, relishes usually are made with sugar or corn syrup, with few or no other additives. An increasing assortment of naturally sweetened relishes have entered the market in the past few years, so you now have a choice of a healthier alternative in this category. Relishes go with all sandwiches, from hot dogs to tofu burgers. They are traditionally eaten with meats and wild game.

- **Umeboshi** Used as long as four thousand years ago, the Japanese umeboshi plum is salted, pickled, and aged for several years. It has a sour, salty flavor and is used in salad dressings, dips, and spreads. It is also cooked with grains, beans, and vegetable dishes. Umeboshi plums come whole (with the pit inside), pitted, or in paste. In any form, they contain only umeboshi plum, salt, and shiso leaf, an herb that contains a naturally occurring preservative, perillaldehyde.

20

BEVERAGES

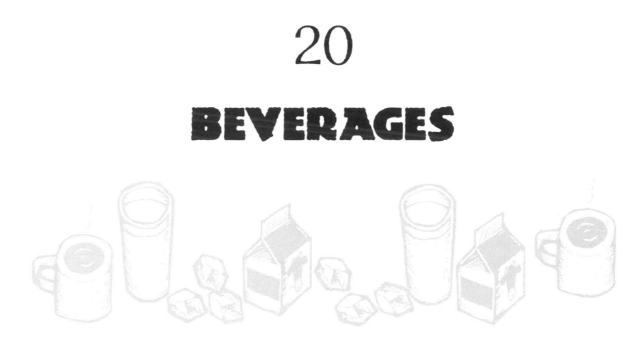

JUICES

Fruit and vegetable juices are popular, healthful beverages. Juices, the blood of fruits and vegetables, contain most of the nutrients in those foods. They are concentrated foods, and fruit juices in particular are high in natural sugars but low in calories. Juices are most healthful when drunk fresh, immediately after they are extracted. If juices sit, even for half an hour, they undergo oxidation and begin to lose nutrients. To obtain fresh juices as desired, your best strategy is to buy a juicer and keep a supply of fresh seasonal fruits and vegetables on hand. No orange juice from a package compares with fresh-squeezed orange juice. No carrot juice is as sweet and refreshing as when it comes right out of the spout of a juicer. Those who have discovered the secret of home juicing regard a vegetable juicer as an essential kitchen appliance.

We live in a fast-paced world, however. It isn't always possible to make juice every time you want it. In natural food stores and supermarkets you will be confronted by an array of bottled, boxed, and canned juices, with various label claims. Your mis-

sion, should you decide to accept it, is to figure out exactly what you're looking at, and to be aware that labels may often give pleasant impressions in place of real information.

Fresh Juices

The best-tasting, most nutritious juices you can buy are fresh. Though fresh juices are not widely available in the colder regions of the United States, they are popular in California and other warm areas. Fresh juices, blends, and smoothies (blended juices with banana, berries, and other puréed fruits) are a treat. Fresh juices are typically kept refrigerated in the dairy sections of most stores. Some are made with organically grown fruits, which is a real bonus. Fresh juices are not usually prepared with preservatives or other chemical additives. The one notable exception to this is apple cider, which is popular in New England and the Pacific Northwest, two major apple-growing territories. Apple cider is frequently preserved to extend its short shelf life.

The most popular fresh-squeezed juice is orange juice. Read orange juice labels carefully, however.

Look for orange juice that is not pasteurized and has a label that reads "100% fresh squeezed orange juice." Pasteurization destroys the nutrients and flavor in juices. Keep in mind that a juice with a label that touts "great fresh flavor" may not be fresh. Its manufacturer may simply be likening its taste to that of a fresh product. If a juice is fresh, its label should state that fact, explicitly.

Bottled, Boxed, and Canned Juices

Nonrefrigerated juices come in glass and plastic bottles, boxes (aseptic "brick" packages), and cans. These juices are pasteurized to halt enzymatic action and fermentation, and are vacuum packed for a long shelf life. Your best option, when you can find it, is 100 percent pure, organic juice from whole fruit. There are many packaged organic juices on the market today, though relatively few are available at conventional supermarkets.

Besides juice from whole fruit, there is a plethora of juices from concentrate. Concentrates are juices that have had much of the water evaporated out of them. Because concentrates are easier to store and transport than whole juices, they are preferred by a majority of manufacturers. When the product is ready to be made, water is added to the concentrate, and the juice is ostensibly restored to its original condition. Of course, this reconstituted product is quite different from the unpasteurized, fresh, whole, nutrient-rich original product. According to federal standards of identity for juices, producers are supposed to identify juice made from concentrate. The main thing to watch out for in juices made from concentrate is added sugar. A product label should read "no added sugar" if it is made from concentrate. Otherwise, it will most likely be sweetened. Extra concentrate, containing natural sugars, can also be added to a juice to perk up its sweet index.

Juice blends are increasingly popular. Apple juice is frequently used as a base to which other fruit juices or concentrates such as apricot, strawberry, peach, and other berries may be added. When you buy a juice blend, be sure to read the label carefully. Juice blends can contain added sugar, emulsifiers, and stabilizers. There is a lot of room for trickery with these products.

"Juice Drinks" and Other Scams

Watch out for juice drinks, fruit punches, fruit nectars, and other insults to nature, like Kool-Aid and Hi-C. For starters, these products are not 100 percent juice. They can contain 10 percent juice, or even less, or even none at all, regardless of how natural their labels may make them appear. Second, they can contain a full range of unidentified sweeteners, artificial colors, flavors, preservatives, emulsifiers, stabilizers, gums, and added sodium. There is no reason to buy these products.

The Fruit Juice Hall of Shame Award goes to Beech Nut, which in 1988 was found guilty of selling sugared water instead of apple juice for infants.

TEA

The most widely drunk hot beverage in the world, tea is made from the leaves of an evergreen bush or tree from the family Theaceae, known as *Thea sinensis, Camellia thea,* or *Camellia sinensis.* The tea plant is indigenous to India, China, and Japan and today is cultivated in warm, wet climates throughout Asia, Indonesia, and South America. Tea leaves are picked by hand during periods of active plant growth, called flushes, with the leaves at the tip of the plant being the most aromatic, desirable, and expensive. After picking, the leaves are dried, rolled, and heated. Black teas are fermented before heating, whereas green teas are not. Black teas typically have a strong, woody flavor compared with green teas, which tend to be more astringent. This is because the astringent flavor in tea is imparted by tannins, which are reduced during the fermentation of black tea varieties. Otherwise, the flavors of teas depend on each variety's unique combination of aromatic oils, tannins, and caffeine.

The caffeine content of teas varies widely. Contrary to some popular wisdom, tea is consistently lower in caffeine than coffee. Some mild teas may yield as little as 30 or 40 milligrams of caffeine per cup, whereas stronger varieties can yield 70 to 80 milligrams. See "About Caffeine" in the "Coffee" section. Following are a few of the world's most popular teas:

Assam   Over two million acres of tea are cultivated in the state of Assam in northeastern India, which is bordered by Burma, China, and Bhutan. Assam tea is the traditional Irish Breakfast Tea, and is pungent and heavy-bodied.

Ceylon   Now called Sri Lanka, Ceylon is an island south of the Indian mainland famous for its many teas, all of which are called Ceylons. The better Ceylon teas are full-bodied and brisk, with a clean, fresh aroma.

Darjeeling   The Himalayan resort area of Darjeeling in Northeast India yields one of the world's most highly prized teas. Darjeeling tea produces a red-gold color in the cup, with a delicate but hearty flavor and a sweet aroma.

Earl Grey   This scented tea blend is made with Ceylon and Keemun teas, to which bergamot oil is added. Bergamot oil is extracted from the rind of the Italian bergamot orange and is used in perfumes and colognes. Earl Grey tea is a strictly English concoction and has a lovely flavor and aroma.

Formosa Oolong   From the Chinese island of Formosa (Taiwan) come Oolong teas, which yield an amber cup and a penetrating, sweet flavor. The finer Oolongs have a flavor reminiscent of ripe peaches. Formosa Oolong is known as the "champagne of teas."

Keemun   The classic English Breakfast Tea comes from Keemun, a growing district in northern China. Sometimes referred to as the "Burgundy of teas," Keemun possesses a full, concentrated flavor and a toasty aroma.

Lapsang Souchong   From the island of Taiwan, Lapsang Souchong is treated with wood smoke as it dries. The result is a tangy, smoky-flavored tea with a woody aroma.

When purchasing tea, look for varieties that are identified by place of origin (Keemun, Darjeeling, etc.). Avoid generic teas. They are generic because they are inferior in flavor and aroma. Choose high-quality loose teas over bagged teas whenever possible. Store tea in a cool, dry, sealed container, but never frozen or refrigerated.

To brew tea, use a glass, porcelain, or earthenware pot. Place 1 teaspoon of tea leaves into the pot for each cup of water. Bring cold water to a rolling boil, pour it over the tea, cover the pot, and let the tea steep for 3 to 5 minutes. Do not judge tea by its color; the tannins in tea bleed into water quickly, but the full flavor takes longer. When the tea is fully brewed, strain it and drink.

Herbal Teas

Used as refreshing beverages and for medicinal purposes, herbal teas, also known as infusions, have been drunk throughout the world for thousands of years. Many natural food stores offer selections of bagged herbal teas, loose herbs, and mixed herbal blends. All herbs used for beverage purposes have some sort of medicinal value. Peppermint is an aid to digestion, and chamomile is a gentle relaxant. Eucalyptus is a decongestant, and senna is a very powerful laxative. If you are buying loose herbs or herbal blends that are not bagged and boxed name-beverage brands, be sure you know what you are buying. The guidelines for preparation and storage of herbal teas are the same as those for regular tea.

Following is a small list of herbs that can be drunk as infusions and that have been traditionally used for their purportedly medicinal values. This information is not intended to be a substitute for the advice of a trained health specialist. If you have a health problem, you should consult a physician. This information gives you a look at the many traditional medicinal uses of common herbs. Herbs have well-documented medicinal values and are used extensively in modern pharmacology.

Some herbal teas contain powerful alkaloids, which should be consumed sparingly. Consult a good herbal reference if you are going to experiment extensively with herbal teas not mentioned here.

Alfalfa *(Medicago sativa)*: A digestant that aids in urinary problems. It is high in minerals.

Burdock Root *(Articum lappa)*: A blood purifier used for skin eruptions and inflammations, bladder and kidney disorders, and colds.

Catnip *(Nepeta cataria)*: A relaxant and sedative for aches, pains, and nervousness.

Chamomile *(Anthemis nobelis, Matricaria chamomilla)*: A gentle relaxant, this herb soothes the stomach and alleviates colic, stomach cramps, and insomnia

Coltsfoot *(Tussilago farfara)*. Useful in treating coughs, colds, bronchitis, asthma, shortness of breath, and hoarseness.

Comfrey leaf and root *(Symphytum officinale)*: Used for skin problems of any kind, wounds, burns, broken bones, fractures, torn muscles or ligaments, coughs, colds, respiratory difficulties, intestinal mucus, diarrhea, and digestive troubles.

Dandelion *(Taraxacum officinale)*: Used for liver problems, edema, gallstones, and jaundice. Also a detoxifier.

Elder *(Sambucus nigra)*: A diuretic used for constipation, edema, and kidney problems.

Fennel *(Foeniculum vulgare)*: Used for colic, intestinal gas, and stomach cramps and as a diuretic.

Ginger *(Zingiber officinale)*: Stimulates appetite and promotes perspiration. Used for colds, flu, coughs, indigestion, and motion sickness.

Ginseng *(Panax quinquefolius)*: Good for just about everything, including general immunity, energy, stamina, endurance, and mental alertness.

Parsley *(Petroselinum crispum)*: A diuretic used for gallstones, intestinal gas, swollen glands, bad breath, kidney trouble, and anemia.

Peppermint *(Mentha piperita)*: Used for poor digestion, diarrhea, bowel problems, colds, flu, nausea, abdominal distress, intestinal gas, and vomiting.

Sarsaparilla *(Smilax officinalis)*: A blood purifier used for all skin eruptions, colds, intestinal gas, and fevers.

Senna *(Cassia acutifolia)*: A supreme cathartic useful in treating constipation. Senna is powerful. Use it sparingly!

Valerian *(Valeriana officinalis)*: Used for pain, nervousness, insomnia, spasms, cramps, fatigue, and neuralgia.

Yarrow *(Achillea millefolium)*: A blood purifier that induces perspiration and stimulates appetite. Used for fevers, intestinal gas, liver and gallbladder problems, and urinary disorders.

COFFEES

The history of coffee is embellished with colorful tales. Legend has it that a goatherd first discovered the stimulating effects of coffee when he observed his goats nibbling on the berries of a tropical evergreen shrub. After doing so, the goats became unusually frisky and rambunctious. When the goatherd tried eating some of the berries, he too became invigorated, and coffee was "discovered." Known in the ninth century

A.D. in Ethiopia as a food, crushed coffee was molded into balls of fat and eaten by African nomads. An invigorating wine made from coffee husks was perhaps the first coffee beverage. Eventually someone opened up some coffee berries, took out the inner "beans," and roasted and brewed them, and the beverage coffee as we know it was born. Coffee was subsequently introduced to Arabia in the fifteenth century. Today Arabia is the world's primary coffee production area.

The two primary types of coffee beans are arabica and robusta. Arabica beans are widely considered superior in every respect and are the beans chosen by those who appreciate fine regional coffees. Robust beans are used commercially in canned and vacuum-sealed blends, and in instant coffee. The primary coffee-growing areas today include Arabia and Africa, Indonesia and the Pacific Rim, and South and Central America. Coffee beans are harvested by hand, so to an extent the "Juan Valdez" commercials you see on television are at least partially authentic. The coffee berries must be picked before they are overripe. Each berry contains a bean that is removed, dried, sorted by hand according to size and condition, graded, and bagged. Coffee beans are roasted as close to use as possible, producing what we know as beverage coffee. The roasting of coffee, along with the variety of the bean, determines the flavor of the cup. Full, dark roasts yield a stronger, more flavorful cup, whereas a lighter roast yields a more delicate brew. Following are a few of the world's most popular coffees:

Colombian Supremo   The term "supremo" refers to large, uniform beans culled from high-grade stock. This coffee is Colombia's finest, with a smooth, sweet, nutty flavor, medium body, and delicate acidity.

Ethiopian Harrar   A unique coffee with a wild, spicy flavor, Ethiopian Harrar is excellent as a single brew or blended. It has medium body and medium to high acidity.

Ethiopian Yrgacheffe   Perhaps the finest of all Ethiopian coffees, Yrgacheffe has a complex, mellow flavor and a sweet aroma. Ethiopian Yrgacheffe has medium body and medium to high acidity.

Hawaiian Kona   Not to be confused with "Kona style," real Kona is a royal brew. Delicate and flavorful, Hawaiian Kona has a magnificent aroma, medium body, and medium acidity.

Jamaica Blue Mountain   From the high slopes of the Blue Mountains in central Jamaica, this exceptional and costly coffee is bold and clear, a perfect blend of full body and high acidity. Beware of imitations, of which there are many.

Kenya AA   The delineation "AA" indicates beans that are free of defects. This coffee is richly aromatic, with a bold, satiny flavor. Kenya AA yields an utterly distinctive cup, with heavy body and high acidity.

Mexican Oaxacan   The mountainous Oaxaca region of Mexico produces a wonderful coffee with a lush, complex flavor of chocolate and spice. Oaxacan coffee has a fine aroma, medium body, and medium acidity.

Mocha-Java   Arguably the most highly prized coffee blend, authentic Mocha-java is half Mocha Mattari from Yemen and half Javanese beans. The result is a complex cup with a sweet, mellow chocolate flavor and a fragrant, spicy aroma. Mocha-Java has a heavy body and medium to low acidity.

Sumatra Mandheling   This exceptional coffee has a sweet, velvety, nutty flavor and a fine finish. Sumatra Mandheling is one of the world's greatest coffees, with a very heavy body and low to medium acidity.

Organic Coffee

Coffee is a crop that is liberally sprayed with pesticides, because it grows in hot, sunny areas where there are many insects. Some coffee growers, however, particularly in Central and South America, are now growing certified organic coffees. The first thing you will notice about organic coffees is that they have slightly less of a bite to them. Perhaps this is due to the absence of pesticides? Who can say? But the taste difference is detectable. You will pay somewhat more for organically grown beans, but the difference is worth it.

Decaffeinated Coffee

The most common method for decaffeinating coffee is direct solvent extraction. Green beans are steamed until they soften and are then flushed with the toxic solvent methylene chloride, which soaks through the beans. The solvent is extracted from the beans along with most of the caffeine. The beans are steamed again, then dried. Another method of decaffeinating coffee is by the misnamed "European water process," also called indirect solvent extraction. By this method green beans are soaked in hot water to draw out the caffeine. This soaking also removes much of the flavor. The water and beans are then separated, and methylene chloride is added to the water to absorb the caffeine. The solvent is removed from the water. The water, which still contains many of the flavor components of the coffee, is added back to the beans, reflavorizing them. The beans are then dried.

In both the above processes, residues of methylene chloride remain in the coffee. No one knows the exact health consequences of drinking coffee containing traces of a chlorinated hydrocarbon solvent. However, the Food and Drug Administration has been concerned for two decades over the use of solvents in decaffeination.

The two safe methods of decaffeination are the Swiss Water Process and the carbon dioxide (CO_2) method. In the Swiss Water Process, green beans are soaked in water for several hours, until 97 percent of the caffeine is removed, along with many of the flavor components. The water is passed through a carbon block filter, which removes the caffeine but not the flavors. The water is then added back to the beans, and the beans are dried.

By the CO_2 method, the green beans are moist-ened with water and put into a vessel that is then filled with pressurized CO_2, the natural atmospheric gas that we exhale. By circulation through the coffee, the CO_2 draws the caffeine out of the coffee bean. In a separate vessel the caffeine precipitates from the CO_2, which is then pumped again into the coffee-containing vessel for a new cycle. When the required residual caffeine level is reached (99.9 percent caffeine free), the CO_2 circulation is cut short and the coffee is discharged into a dryer, where it is gently dried to about the original moisture content. After that the coffee is ready for roasting.

In both the Swiss Water Process and the carbon dioxide method, the coffee has been in contact only with the natural substances of water and carbon dioxide. The resulting decaffeinated coffee is solvent free and contains all the valuable flavor and aroma components of coffee.

When purchasing coffee, choose whole organic beans whenever you can. Look for beans with a clearly identified place of origin and a recent roast date. As with tea, generic coffees tend to be inferior varieties. Some coffee stores roast and sell whole-bean coffees the same day. This gives you the freshest, most flavorful, and aromatic coffee possible. The beans should be whole and intact, not chipped, dented, withered, gnarled, or cracked. Store your coffee in a sealed container either in the refrigerator or freezer for maximum freshness.

Coffee Filters

For those who brew their own coffee and use paper filters, there are now unbleached filters, which have a natural light brown color. Why should you care? Because the paper bleaching process leaves residues of dioxin in paper, and dioxin is the most carcinogenic chemical known. If you go to the trouble of brewing your own coffee and using paper filters, make sure to use an unbleached brand. Unbleached filters are labeled as such and are brownish in color, not bright white. You can also obtain reusable cloth filters and gold filters. The latter are expensive but will last for many years.

About Caffeine

Caffeine is the stimulant compound found in coffee and in black and green teas. It stimulates the central nervous system and also acts as a diuretic.

- A cup of coffee contains 100 to 150 milligrams of caffeine, whereas a cup of black tea contains 60 to 70 milligrams.

- As an over-the-counter drug, caffeine is approved as both a stimulant and a diuretic. The effective dose of caffeine as a drug is about 200 milligrams. Caffeine is also approved as a food additive in cola drinks.

- Doses of caffeine larger than 250 milligrams may cause insomnia or nervousness. This varies according to individual body weight and metabolism.

- The estimated fatal dose of caffeine is 10 grams (10,000 milligrams), or the equivalent of 100 cups of coffee, or 167 cups of black tea. It is obviously highly unlikely that one would die from a caffeine overdose as a result of drinking coffee or tea.

- Caffeine prolongs gastric secretion time. This can cause stomach acids to eat away at the stomach wall.

- Large doses of caffeine can cause cardiac irregularities, including irregular heartbeat and decreased cardiac output. During pregnancy, caffeine crosses the placenta. In animal studies, high caffeine intake increased the incidence of spontaneous abortion, premature births, and birth defects.

- Caffeine may interact with other prescription and nonprescription drugs in unpredictable or undesirable ways.

To sum it up, caffeinated beverages should be drunk judiciously. Keep your intake of these beverages moderate to avoid any undesirable side effects. Two cups of coffee or four cups of tea daily are well within the range of safe consumption.

GRAIN BEVERAGES

With a nutty flavor and an aroma somewhat similar to that of coffee, grain beverages do not contain the caffeine and acids found in coffee. They are made from various combinations of roasted grains, barley, chicory, and dandelion root and are sometimes flavored with cinnamon or some other aromatic spice. To the person who wants to drink less coffee, grain beverages offer a hot, flavorful drink that won't keep you awake at night staring at the ceiling.

NATURAL SODAS

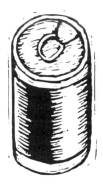

If you thirst for a good root beer, or if ginger ale does the trick for you, you will be pleased to find a growing selection of natural sodas in your local natural food store and in many supermarkets. Natural sodas are made with real fruits, herbs, natural flavors, and natural sweeteners, and without artificial colors, flavors, or preservatives. At first you may be surprised to see a clear root beer, because root beer has always appeared brown. If root beer is made from concentrated natural flavors instead of roots and barks that contain natural dyes and pigments, there is no reason for it to be dark unless it has been artificially colored.

The sweeteners used in natural sodas vary. Many sodas labeled "natural" are in fact sweetened with fructose, which is commercially refined from corn syrup solids. The "purist" natural soda brands sweeten their beverages with fruit concentrates and honey. From a nutritional standpoint, the difference is that fruit concentrates and honey contain some nutrients as they occur in nature, whereas fructose is nutritionally devoid.

ALCOHOLIC BEVERAGES

Throughout the course of history, humans have consumed a broad range of intoxicants of all kinds, from hallucinogenic mushrooms to mind-altering flowers, barks, cactus, and plant extracts. In fact, there is no known culture whose indigenous people do not use at least one, if not many, intoxicating substances. These substances are associated with various gods and spirit forces and have been influential in the formation of religions, shamanic rituals, and celebrations of all kinds.

A Social Intoxicant

Among the many intoxicants widely used today are alcoholic beverages, made either by the fermentation or the distillation of grains, fruits, and herbs. These beverages are believed to have been discovered by accident when primitive peoples drank the water from soaked fermented grains or fruits. Unexpectedly going into an altered state was something that often happened to the people of primitive cultures as they experimented with new and strange foods, as well as with various methods of food preparation, handling, and storage. The discovery of the potent intoxicating effects of fermented grain and fruit beverages led to ingenious methods by which beers and wines were made regularly as important beverages of many cultures. Methods of distillation eventually followed, producing thousands of different whiskies, brandies, and liquors, all of which are more highly concentrated and potent than fermented alcoholic beverages.

The worldwide use of alcoholic beverages makes alcohol the most widely used, and therefore the most influential, of all intoxicants. Alcoholic product manufacturing is a multibillion-dollar enterprise, and alcoholic beverages have played an enormous role in celebrations and festivities throughout the world as well as in the destruction of tribal cultures and urban and rural poor populations. The abuse of alcohol is the single largest substance abuse problem worldwide. Approximately 10 percent of all people who drink alcohol will become alcoholics.

Alcohol and Health

Despite this, there is very little evidence that the consumption of moderate amounts of alcohol can cause

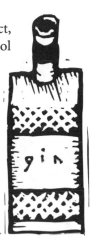

any harm, except during pregnancy. In fact, regular intake of a small amount of alcohol may be of benefit to health. In the Framingham Heart Study of five thousand men, those who consumed moderate amounts of alcohol actually lived longer, with less incidence of cardiovascular disease, than those who drank either heavily or not at all. Furthermore, beers and wines are known to contain numerous nutrients and enzymes that are prophylactic and beneficial to digestion. Specific herbal wines and liqueurs are important in the pharmacology of numerous cultures. Pure distilled grain alcohol is the primary solvent used in the extraction of medicinal herbs into liquid. It is therefore

The French Paradox

In a land blessed with Brie, pâté, and brilliant chefs, it is no wonder that the French have some of the highest per capita intakes of saturated fat on earth. What is a wonder, however, is the fact that the rate of heart disease in France is 2.5 times lower than it is in the United States. This situation, first identified in the 1980s, came to be known as the French Paradox. Why are the French able to consume a diet that would send scores of Americans to their graves and at the same time have such low rates of heart disease? The culprit, it turns out, is red wine.

Some of the chemicals in wine, called flavonoids, lower the levels of harmful cholesterol and prevent blood from clogging in the arteries. Flavonoids originate in the skins of wine grapes, which are only used in making red wine. Though white wine and grape juice have some preventive effect against heart disease, red wine has considerably more. Note that only a glass or two a day is recommended to achieve the best benefits.

In 1996 dark beer was added to the list of beverages with proven heart benefits. Turns out Guinness really *is* good for you! But then, the Irish knew that all along.

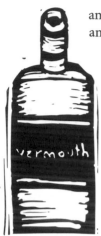

an important part of each herbal extract and of herbal pharmacology as a whole. Alcohol, as both a beverage and medicinal agent, is well established throughout the human race.

It is important to distinguish between the moderate intake of alcoholic beverages and alcoholism. Moderate and responsible use of alcohol is a socially acceptable practice enjoyed among the people of most cultures worldwide. The chronic and abusive consumption of alcohol, however, is a factor in diseases of the heart, brain, liver, kidneys, and gastrointestinal tract and is a major contributor to accidental death and injury. Here are a few health facts about alcohol:

- Alcohol is a sedative-hypnotic drug, a potent nervous system depressant that acts as a narcotic in the brain, putting nerve cells "to sleep."
- Alcohol is both a diuretic and an anesthetic.
- The overconsumption of alcohol can produce coma and death.
- Alcohol has 7 calories per gram.
- Alcohol can cause reduced motor control, slurred speech, blurred vision, numbness, erratic behavior, temporary amnesia, loss of reason, liver damage, kidney damage, brain damage, ulceration of the gastrointestinal tract, impaired digestion, fatigue, and lethargy.
- Alcohol can contribute to cardiovascular disease, including arteriosclerosis, heart attack, and stroke.
- Alcohol consumption during pregnancy can cause miscarriage, low infant birth weight, stillbirths, and fetal abnormalities. Fetal alcohol syndrome is a growing problem among poor, pregnant, alcohol-dependent women in the United States.
- Alcohol is an addictive drug. An estimated 10 million American adults abuse alcohol and are alcohol dependent.

- Alcoholic intoxication has caused more traffic fatalities than the combined death tolls of the Korean and Vietnam Wars.

To sum up, drink alcoholic beverages judiciously. Keep your intake moderate to avoid any undesirable side effects.

Beer

Made from fermented grains instead of being distilled, beer is one of the oldest of all alcoholic beverages and was widely consumed in ancient Egypt. According to the strict standards of the Bavarian beer purity law, beer is made only from water, malted barley, hops, and yeast, with no adjuncts of any kind. This law was initiated by Bavarian brewers at a time when some European brewmasters were using sugar in their brewing process.

Breweries today use an astonishing variety of ingredients, many of them chemical. Some commercial breweries, like Anheuser-Busch (Budweiser, Michelob, Busch) and Latrobe Brewing (Rolling Rock) add rice to their beer. Many other breweries add foam stabilizers, clarifying enzymes, natural and artificial flavors, antioxidants, and artificial colors to their products.

This "test tube beer" is a far cry from what the Bavarians had in mind. By federal law, beer must contain over 0.5 percent alcohol. Most beers range from 3 percent to 8 percent alcohol, although this information is rarely given on a label. There is no upper limit to the amount of alcohol allowed in beer according to federal standards, though many states have set limits.

There are several different types of beer:

Ale Traditionally a pale, strongly hopped malt beverage, today *ale* refers to any beer made with fast-acting yeast at room temperature.

Lager The word *lager* means "storage place" in German, and a lager beer is one that has been made with slow-acting yeast at a cellar temperature, usually between 45 and 55 degrees, then stored and aged for several weeks or months.

Bock   This is a dark, heavy lager beer.

Porter   A strong ale brewed with roasted malt for flavor and color, porter is nutty and aromatic.

Stout   Darker, maltier, and more heavily hopped than a porter, stout is definitely the Babe Ruth of beers for flavor and punch.

The question naturally arises: how do you know what you are buying? Full disclosure is your only real assurance. Many fine breweries, especially the new microbreweries, proudly display their full ingredients right on the label and are equally clear that they use no additives or adjuncts of any kind. Brands like Sierra Nevada, Samuel Adams, Anchor Steam, and Catamount have taken the lead in full-disclosure labeling, which is not legally required. In other words, a beer can contain a myriad of chemical additives, none of which need appear on the label. Some breweries argue that required full-disclosure labeling would force them to reveal secret recipes. This position is weak. Even if you know the ingredients of another company's beer, you don't know the proportions and methods used. It is one thing to know a beer's basic ingredients and quite another to reproduce the product.

Ideally you should look for an organic beer, produced entirely with ingredients that have not been exposed to agrichemicals. There are a few organic beers on the market today, but they are rare and hard to find.

Nonalcoholic Beer

Some consumers want a beer with little or no alcohol, simply for the refreshment. To this group breweries have responded with many brands of near beers, cereal beverages, and nonalcoholic beers. To qualify as a nonalcoholic beverage, a beer must contain less than 0.5 percent alcohol. If the product contains no detectable alcohol whatsoever, then it can be labeled "alcohol free."

Nonalcoholic beers can be made in two ways. One method is to brew a real beer and then vacuum-extract the alcohol. This allows for a full-bodied brew. The other method is to brew a beer and stop the brewing process before the beer contains more than 0.5 percent alcohol. Products made by this method tend to have less flavor. As with alcoholic beer, look for nonalcoholic beers with full-disclosure labeling.

Wine

Ever since the discovery of the intoxicating effects of the fermented juice of fruits and berries, wines have been important beverages throughout the world. From the high houses of wine production in southern France to regional makers of rice wines throughout Asia, skilled winemakers are prominent and celebrated in the societies in which they work. Wine is the primary beverage of traditional festivals of all kinds, particularly in Europe, the most well-developed area of wine production. Wine has played a major role in religion, especially Catholicism, whose tradition asserts that wine transmutes into the blood of Christ during Holy Communion. Not only does Catholicism give broad avenue for the consumption of wines throughout the year, but some of the world's most respected vintages have come from remarkable monk winemasters in monasteries throughout Europe.

By strict definition according to European tradition, wine is fermented grape juice. In regional wines throughout the world, however, other fruits, grains, berries, and herbs are used. Wine as referred to here is made with grapes. If you are a wine lover, though, you might want to investigate the wines of other cultures, such as the rice sake of Japan. If you are highly experimental you may wish to taste the *balché* of the Mayans in the Yucatán, which is made in a hollowed log with mashed roots, water, and spit, and which induces copious hallucinations of animals. But we will not cover exotic wines here.

Wines may be natural, fortified, or sparkling. Natural wines are still, without any carbonation, or bubbles. They are made from crushed grapes harvested at full ripeness. In some cases, as with late-harvest Riesling wines, the grapes are harvested when they are overripe and covered with mold. Natural wines generally have an alcohol content of 7 to 15 percent.

Fortified wines include port, sherry, and Madeira. These are still wines to which brandy and other distilled liquors have been added. Fortified wines are potent. Their alcohol content ranges from 16 percent to 35 percent.

Sparkling wines are wines with bubbles, the finest example of which is champagne. Sparkling wines undergo secondary fermentation when they are bottled, as the live yeasts in them continue to eat the natural sugars in the wine. Their alcohol content ranges from 7 percent to 15 percent. However, because of their carbonation, sparkling wines deliver their alcohol to the bloodstream faster than still wines.

Wine varies in flavor and aroma according to the variety of grape, the region in which it is grown, and the methods by which the wine is produced. It may be dry or sweet; red, white, or rosé in color. The drier the wine, the more the grape sugars have been eaten by enzymes in the fermentation process, reducing the residual sugar in the finished product. Red wines are made by crushing and fermenting the whole grape. Whites are made by fermenting only the juice of the crush. Rosé is made by fermenting the entire crushed grape for a short period of time, then separating out the skins and fermenting only the juice. The temporary fermentation of the skins, which contain various red pigments, leaves a blush-colored wine.

Wine, like beer, can be a chemical stew, made with an awesome array of clarifiers, stabilizers, preservatives, pH control agents, tannins, enzymes, and polyvinyl compounds. So much for the popular toast "to your health." Sulfur dioxide and potassium metabisulfite, two sulfite preservatives, are considered by many wine makers to be essential ingredients in the winemaking process. This inclusion of sulfites, however, poses a serious risk to sensitive consumers. In genetic experiments using yeasts, viruses, live cells, and bacteria, sulfites proved mu-

tagenic and caused chromosomal abnormalities. There is concern that sulfites in wine may do the same thing inside our bodies. Allergic sensitivity to sulfites is common. Asthmatics in particular are susceptible to sulfites in foods and can suffer attacks of wheezing, tightness in the chest, and difficulty breathing. A serious allergic reaction to sulfites in foods can render a person unconscious. Even if sulfites are not actually added to a wine, they most likely are in it, because sulfites occur naturally in aged wooden wine casks and are imparted to wine during the aging process. The Food and Drug Administration enacted legislation that mandated sulfite labeling on all wines by January 1988 if they contain more than 10 parts per million of sulfites. Almost all wines contain sulfites. A few wineries have managed to extract sulfites from wine after aging, producing 99.9 percent sulfite-free wines. We will most likely see more sulfite-free wines in the future, but the wines may nonetheless be processed with other additives.

Some organic wines are available today. Certainly the wineries producing organic wines are few at present, but we will see an increase in organically produced wines over the next few years as the urgency of removing pesticides from our food chain becomes more widely appreciated. The French organic certification program Nature et Progrés has already certified a few dozen European wines, apparently with more soon on the way. Several California vineyards are also producing organic varietal wines. The organic wine market is beginning to open.

In choosing wines, look for those that are organically produced whenever possible. Full disclosure labeling is not required on wines, and wineries just don't do it. You can find out about the possible additives in a wine by contacting the winery directly. Choose varietal wines, those named after the specific grapes with which they were made, such as chardonnay, riesling, sauvignon blanc, merlot, and zinfandel. The winery of origin makes a huge difference. Take the advice of some good books on wineries and particular vintages. Wine guides can be very helpful in directing you to good wine experiences. A poorly made varietal can turn you away from that grape, whereas a well-made wine is a true pleasure.

Nonalcoholic Wine

Nonalcoholic wines are subjected to pressure or heat after they are made, thus reducing the alcohol to less than 0.5 percent. They retain the full flavor and aroma of wine without producing intoxication. There are currently several brands of still and sparkling nonalcoholic wines on the market.

Part 2

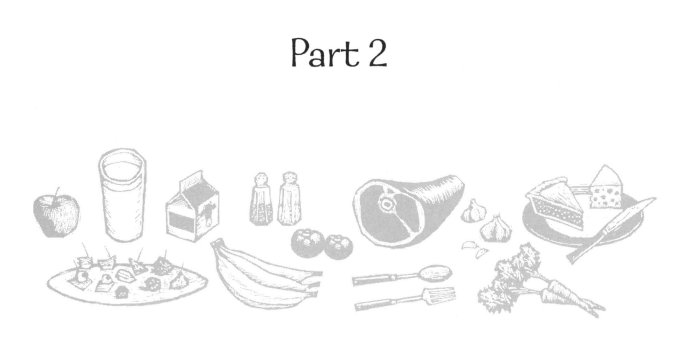

RECIPES

APPETIZERS

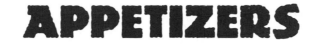

Cheddar Spread

Real cheddar cheese, which is aged naturally and without artificial colors, is the perfect partner for the sweet tartness of apple cider. These flavors conjure up the time of year when red and gold maple leaves begin to dazzle us with their glorious colors. Serve as a spread with apple wedges and rye bread or crackers, or place on bread and toast under the broiler for a grilled cheese sandwich unlike any you've ever had. Leftover spread can be used on turkey sandwiches.

Makes about 3 cups

2 cups (½ pound) grated sharp cheddar cheese
3 ounces fromage blanc or 2 to 3 tablespoons
   plain low-fat yogurt
½ cup apple cider
1 tablespoon prepared mustard
2 teaspoons caraway seeds

1. Combine all the ingredients and beat until smooth. Chill. (For a creamier texture, purée in a blender or food processor.)

2. Remove from the refrigerator ½ hour before serving.

Dill and Orange Miso Spread

Try this with grated carrot and watercress in pita bread, with sprouts on rice cakes, or with raw vegetables. It is also good as a sauce for udon or soba noodles or sautéed vegetables (try red bell pepper strips and broccoli for color). Store in refrigerator for up to 5 days.

Makes about 1 ½ cups

1 cup tahini
¼ cup white miso
3 tablespoons chopped fresh dill
2 tablespoons fresh orange juice

1. Place all the ingredients in a medium saucepan over low heat. Stir well to blend.

2. Simmer gently for 3 minutes, adding water to the desired consistency (more for sauce and less for spread).

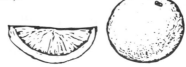

Tofu Spread

This spread can be served on bread or rice cakes, with sprouts, olives, tomatoes, avocados, greens, or any of your sandwich favorites. Serve on crackers for a snack or an hors d'oeuvre with a tiny dollop of mustard and paprika on top. This is a completely cholesterol-free spread.

Makes about 3 cups

1 pound firm tofu
²/₃ cup chopped lightly toasted walnuts*
2 tablespoons fresh minced dill
2 tablespoons low-sodium tamari
¹/₂ cup soy mayonnaise
¹/₃ cup chopped onion
¹/₄ teaspoon celery seed
3 tablespoons chopped dill pickle or sugar-free pickle relish

1. Cut the tofu into pieces that will fit on a steamer rack, and steam over boiling water for 4 minutes.

2. Wrap the tofu in a clean kitchen towel or cheesecloth and press to drain the excess moisture. Crumble the tofu and place, along with the remaining ingredients, in a blender or food processor and blend until smooth.

* To toast walnuts, place in a preheated 350°F oven for 8 to 10 minutes, or until lightly browned.

Toasted Nut Medley

Makes 3 cups

1 cup almonds
1 cup pumpkin seeds
2 teaspoons tamari
¹/₂ cup currants
¹/₂ cup dried apples, cut into small dice

1. Toast the almonds in a preheated 350°F oven for 7 minutes. Toast the pumpkin seeds in a dry cast-iron pan until they puff up. Sprinkle the hot nuts with tamari.

2. In a bowl, mix together the nuts, currants, and dried apples.

Spicy Popcorn

To 4 cups freshly popped popcorn, add 2 teaspoons curry powder. A great party pleaser.

Pistachio Popcorn

Makes 8 cups of popcorn

1 cup popcorn
1 cup shelled pistachios
¹/₂ cup pecan halves
2 tablespoons unsalted butter or canola oil
¹/₂ teaspoon curry powder
¹/₄ to ¹/₂ teaspoon sea salt
¹/₂ cup maple syrup

1. Air-pop the popcorn and place it in a large bowl along with the pistachios.

2. To toast the pecans, place on a baking sheet and toast in a preheated 350°F oven for 7 to 10 minutes. Be sure not to scorch them. Chop coarsely and add to the popcorn and pistachios.

3. In a small, heavy skillet or saucepan, heat the butter or oil over medium heat. Add the curry powder and salt, and sauté for a few seconds. Add the maple syrup and cook for 3 to 5 minutes. The syrup should boil and be uniformly bubbly.

4. Pour the hot syrup mixture over the popcorn and nut meats, and stir well to coat. Let cool completely before storing in an airtight container.

5. To serve, break into clusters.

Note: Brown rice syrup, honey, or barley malt may be substituted for the maple syrup.

Yogurt Cheese

This is a great way to use low-fat yogurt. Yogurt cheese can be used instead of much higher-fat dairy products (such as cream cheese and sour cream) for dips, dressings, and spreads. Yogurt cheese is also good as a breakfast spread with unsweetened fruit preserves.

Makes about 1 1/2 cups

32 ounces plain low-fat yogurt

1. Line a fine-mesh colander with a double-thick piece of cheesecloth.

2. Place 32 ounces of low-fat yogurt on top of the cheesecloth and place the colander over a bowl (the bowl must be as large as the colander, because the yogurt will be dripping liquid).

3. Place in the refrigerator and allow the yogurt to drip for 6 hours. At the end of this time, what's left in the cheesecloth will be thick, luscious, low-fat yogurt cheese.

Cool and Creamy Cucumber Salad

Reminiscent of lazy days in Greece, this salad is smooth and cooling

Makes 4 salad servings

1 1/2 cups of low-fat **Yogurt Cheese (see above)**
3 cucumbers, peeled, seeded, and diced fine
1 garlic clove, minced
1 tablespoon extra-virgin olive oil
2 tablespoons fresh lemon juice
Sea salt and white pepper to taste

Mix all the ingredients well and allow to sit in the refrigerator for 2 hours.

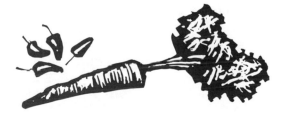

Crudités with Curry Dip

Here's a way to entertain without serving calorie-laden hors d'oeuvres. Use your imagination to cut vegetables into interesting shapes and arrange them in a vibrant, colorful display. The effect will be so dazzling that no one will miss the less healthful fare that is usually served at parties.

Makes about 1 1/2 cups

1 1/2 **cups low-fat Yogurt Cheese (at left)**
2 tablespoons mayonnaise
2 teaspoons curry powder
1/8 teaspoon freshly ground white pepper

1. Blend together the yogurt cheese, mayonnaise, curry powder, and white pepper. Allow to chill for 2 hours.

2. Serve with raw or slightly steamed vegetables, such as summer squash, red pepper, green beans, broccoli, carrots, celery, or cauliflower.

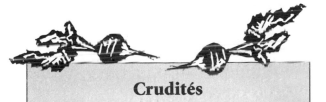

Crudités

For a healthful and colorful party platter, here are a few crudité (raw vegetable) ideas.

- Carrot sticks and celery (of course). After cutting up the carrot sticks, store in water with just a touch of lemon juice.

- Steam or blanch snow peas and cauliflower and broccoli florets.

- Raw mushrooms. To clean mushrooms, use a dish towel or a mushroom brush. Don't rinse with water, as this will make the mushrooms soggy and black.

- Strips of colored peppers such as red and yellow—be sure to core and seed.

Serve any of the above with a dip for a beautiful, low-fat hors d'oeuvre.

Low-Fat Jade Dip

Makes about 2 ½ cups

1 cup fresh watercress
1 cup fresh parsley sprigs
1 cup Yogurt Cheese (see page 161)
1 garlic clove, minced
2 tablespoons scallions, minced
1 tablespoon shoyu
2 teaspoons cider vinegar
1 tablespoon prepared mustard

1. Wash the watercress and parsley well. Remove heavy stems and measure loosely packed cups.

2. Mince the watercress and parsley finely with a knife or in a blender or food processor. Add 2 tablespoons of the Yogurt Cheese to facilitate chopping in the food processor.

3. Add the garlic, scallions, shoyu, vinegar, mustard, and remaining yogurt cheese to the watercress-parsley mixture and blend well. Refrigerate for at least 2 hours.

Variation:

1 cup cooked fresh spinach, drained well
½ cup fresh parsley, minced
½ cup fresh watercress, minced
¼ cup fresh basil, minced
2 tablespoons scallions, minced
1 tablespoon shoyu
2 teaspoons cider vinegar
1 tablespoon prepared mustard
1 cup Yogurt Cheese

Blend all the ingredients. Refrigerate for at least 2 hours.

Once Again: Hummus

Hummus has become a familiar part of our repertoire; it's easy to make and has lots of uses. Serve it as a dip with corn chips or vegetables, or put it in pita bread with sprouts and tomatoes for a sandwich. When hummus is served with a grain product, such as whole-wheat pita bread, it forms a complete protein. As with many other recipes for beans, it makes sense to cook extra beans and freeze them to use another time. The extra chick-peas (garbanzos) that you freeze can be used later in green salads, in a marinated chick-pea salad, and as an addition to soups and stews. Or you can sauté some garlic and red bell pepper strips in olive oil, add some chick-peas, heat through, and pour over noodles for a quick pasta dish.

Makes about 2 ½ cups

1 cup dried chick-peas, or 2½ cups cooked chick-peas plus ½ cup bean liquid
Bay leaf
3 garlic cloves, peeled
¼ cup tahini
2 tablespoons extra-virgin olive oil
Juice of 1 lemon
1 teaspoon sea salt
Lettuce leaves, or whole-wheat pita bread, sprouts, lettuce, and tomatoes or olives
Paprika

1. Place the dried chick-peas in a large bowl and cover with 3 times their volume of water. Soak 8 hours or overnight.

2. Drain and rinse the beans. Place in a medium saucepan with water to cover by 2 inches. Bring to a boil. Lower the heat and simmer for 15 minutes. Remove any foam that rises to the surface. Add the bay leaf. Simmer for 1 hour longer.

3. Drain the beans, saving ½ cup of the cooking liquid. Place the beans in a blender or food processor with the garlic. Purée until the beans begin to break down.

4. Add ¼ to ½ cup of the reserved liquid (depending upon the desired consistency), the tahini, olive oil, lemon juice, and salt. Continue to purée until all the ingredients are well blended and the mixture has a smooth consistency. Chill for at least 2 hours.

5. Serve the hummus on a bed of lettuce or in pita bread with sprouts, lettuce, tomatoes, or olives. Garnish with a sprinkle of paprika.

Mexican Tempeh Dip

Snappy southwestern flavors are matched with tempeh for a zesty dip to serve as an hors d'oeuvre with tortillas, chips, or crackers or as a sandwich filling.

Makes about 2 cups

8 ounces tempeh, cubed
3 tablespoons corn oil
¼ cup water
2 garlic cloves, crushed
2 teaspoons chili powder
2 teaspoons ground cumin
2 teaspoons tamari
1 cup salsa

1. Steam the tempeh over boiling water for 15 minutes.

2. Remove the cubes from the steamer and place in a blender or food processor. Add remaining ingredients except salsa and purée for 15 to 20 seconds. The texture will be slightly chunky.

3. Pour into a bowl and stir in the salsa. Chill well before serving.

Goat Cheese Spread

Makes about ½ cup

½ cup fresh goat cheese (chèvre)
1 tablespoon extra-virgin olive oil
5 Calamata olives, pitted and minced
1 teaspoon fresh thyme, minced
Freshly ground pepper to taste

Mix all the ingredients together and refrigerate. Serve on crackers or French bread.

Tempeh

Tempeh, a cake of cooked fermented soybeans, is one of the world's most nutritious foods. It is an excellent source of protein, fiber, iron, B vitamins (except B_{12}), and minerals.

This food is very low in sodium and saturated fat and contains no cholesterol. It's delicious marinated and then stir-fried or steamed, and in casseroles, pasta sauces, or sandwiches.

Made from soybeans, tempeh has a mild flavor. It is precooked and vacuum-packed for crunchiness and longevity (dark spots on tempeh are a normal, harmless result of tempeh fermentation).

Tempeh may be the best plant source of protein, roughly equaling the percentage of *usable* protein in beef and chicken. The enzymes produced in tempeh during fermentation make it a highly digestible food that can actually improve digestive health

Pan-fried Tempeh Heat about ¼ inch of light vegetable oil in a skillet until hot but not smoking. Slide sliced tempeh into the oil and sauté until a deep golden brown, about 10 minutes on each side. Drain on paper towels and serve as a snack with dips or in sandwiches.

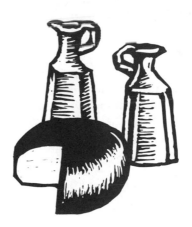

SOUPS

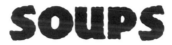

Lentil Soup

This is an easy recipe to make; any leftover soup can be frozen. Serve this soup with a piece of whole-wheat toast and you'll have a complete-protein meal.

Makes 6 to 8 servings

2 cups brown lentils

8 to 10 cups broth or water

2 tablespoons extra-virgin olive oil

4 garlic cloves, minced

1 large onion, chopped

2 celery stalks, chopped

2 carrots, scrubbed and chopped

2 tomatoes, peeled (see page 166), seeded, and chopped

3 tablespoons chopped fresh basil, or 1 tablespoon dried basil

Sea salt and freshly ground white pepper to taste

2 to 4 tablespoons balsamic vinegar

½ cup chopped fresh parsley

1. Wash and pick over the lentils and bring to a boil in the broth or water in a large soup pot. Lower heat and simmer for 10 minutes.

2. Meanwhile, heat the olive oil in a large skillet. Sauté the garlic, onion, celery, and carrots for 5 minutes over medium heat. Add the tomatoes and basil and sauté another 5 minutes.

3. Add the vegetable mixture to the lentils and simmer for 20 to 30 minutes, or until the lentils are tender but not mushy. Add the salt and pepper to taste. For a creamy soup, purée in a blender or food processor. Just before serving, add the balsamic vinegar to taste, and the parsley. Serve immediately.

Cream of Cauliflower Soup with Cardamom

This soup is elegant and easy to prepare. It works well in summer as a chilled soup, or as a steaming and filling dish for a winter's night.

Makes 6 servings

2 tablespoons extra-virgin olive oil

1 large garlic clove, minced

1 jalapeño chili, cored, seeded, and minced

2 medium onions, diced
½ teaspoon ground cardamom
⅛ teaspoon ground mace
1 large cauliflower (about 2 pounds), cored and chopped
4 cups vegetable stock or water
1 cup low-fat milk or soy milk
1 teaspoon sea salt
¼ teaspoon freshly ground white pepper
Chopped fresh chives for garnish (optional)

1. Heat the oil in a large saucepan or soup pot. Add the garlic, jalapeño, onions, cardamom, and mace. Sauté until the onions are soft, about 5 minutes. Add the cauliflower and stock or water. Bring to a boil, cover, and simmer for about 30 minutes.

2. Pour the soup through a sieve, reserving both liquid and vegetables. Purée the vegetables in a blender or food processor until smooth. Return to the soup pot and add the milk or soy milk and enough of the soup liquid to make a not-too-thick, not-too-thin soup. Season with salt and pepper. Gently reheat. Garnish with chives if you like (if you grow your own chives, add some chive blossoms as a garnish).

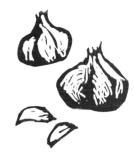

Vegetable Stock

Using a vegetable stock instead of water will give any soup more flavor and add to its nutritive value. Do not use lifeless old vegetables or your stock will taste—well, lifeless and old.

Before using vegetable scraps it's best to wash and chop them. Organic vegetables are the best place to start. You can sauté the vegetables in oil, a bit of water, or butter. This will concentrate their flavor. Once the vegetables are tender, add seasonings, such as whole garlic cloves or peppercorns, and twice as much water as vegetables. Bring the stock to a boil and immediately reduce to a simmer. It is important that the stock simmer gently, as boiling the vegetables creates a harsh flavor.

Strain the stock and discard the vegetables after about 45 minutes. Stock can be frozen in small containers for future use. Vegetable stock can replace water in soups and sauces and can be used to cook grains, beans, and vegetables. Served warm, it makes a delicious broth all by itself.

Making stock in a pressure cooker takes about the same amount of time as just thinking about it. Sauté the vegetables in a small amount of olive oil. Add water, lock the lid in place, and bring to high pressure. Cook for 10 minutes, run the pan under cold water, to release the pressure, and you have almost-instant vegetable stock.

Following is a list of some of the vegetables that can be used to make stock; the flavor of the soup itself will influence the choice of flavors you use in the stock.

Carrots, scrubbed
Parsnips, scrubbed
Onions, peeled
Parsley sprigs
Leeks, cleaned very well
Celery
Summer squash
Winter squash, peeled
Mushrooms (the trick here is to not use mushrooms with tightly closed caps: mushrooms with a bit of vintage work better)
Potato skins
Dried herbs
Thyme
Marjoram
Bay leaves
Basil
Spices
Curry spices (for curried soup)
Peppercorns

Cornwall Tomato Cobb Soup

The essence of vine-ripened tomatoes is all that's needed to make this cold soup a perfect refresher on a late summer day.

Makes 6 servings

5 ripe tomatoes, peeled (see below) and seeded
1 medium onion, grated
Sea salt and freshly ground white pepper to taste

Topping

½ cup plain low-fat yogurt
3 tablespoons canola mayonnaise
2 teaspoons curry powder
Parsley sprigs for garnish

1. Rough chop the tomatoes, or place them in a large mixing bowl and break up with your fingers to a coarse consistency. Add the onion, salt, and pepper and chill for at least 3 hours.

2. To make the topping, mix together the yogurt, mayonnaise, and curry powder. Pour the soup into individual serving bowls and place a dollop of topping on each serving. Place a small piece of parsley in the middle of each dollop and serve.

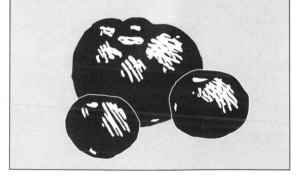

To peel tomatoes, bring a large pot of water to a rolling boil. Add the tomatoes and cook for about 10 to 30 seconds, until the skins begin to crack and burst; the riper the tomato, the shorter the time. Run under cold water, and the skins will slip off easily.

Minestrone Soup

This light and colorful soup is suitable for both warm and cold weather.

Makes 8 servings

¼ pound (about 1 cup) dried white navy beans
2 tablespoons extra-virgin olive oil
4 garlic cloves, minced
3 leeks, white part only, cleaned and sliced
3 carrots, scrubbed and cut into thin slices
2 cups sliced cabbage (Savoy if possible)
3 small new potatoes (about ¾ pound), scrubbed and cut into large dice
1 tablespoon minced fresh oregano
½ teaspoon dried thyme
¼ teaspoon red pepper flakes
8 cups vegetable stock or water
1 bay leaf
½ pound green beans, cut on the diagonal
Sea salt and freshly ground pepper to taste
1 bunch red chard or collard greens, sliced into strips
3 tablespoons chopped fresh parsley
Freshly grated Romano cheese (optional)
Lemon slices

1. Wash and pick over the white navy beans. Soak the beans in triple their volume of water for 8 hours or overnight. Rinse and drain.

2. Heat the olive oil in a stockpot. Add the garlic and leeks. Sauté over medium heat for 5 minutes, or until translucent.

3. Add the carrots, cabbage, potatoes, oregano, thyme, and red pepper flakes. Sauté over medium heat for 10 minutes, stirring frequently to prevent sticking. You may need to add a ½ cup of stock or water to prevent sticking.

4 Add the remaining stock or water, the navy beans, and bay leaf. Bring to a boil, reduce heat, cover, and simmer for about 40 minutes, or until the beans are just tender.

5. Add the green beans. Bring to a boil, reduce heat, and season with salt and pepper. Simmer for 15 minutes. Remove the bay leaf.

6. Add the chard or collard greens and simmer until wilted, about 5 minutes.

7. Place in serving bowls and sprinkle with parsley and Romano cheese, if desired. Serve with a slice of lemon.

Hearty Miso Soup

Reheat gently so that the beneficial enzymes of the miso are not destroyed.

Makes 8 servings

1 tablespoon sesame oil

2 small carrots, scrubbed and cut into thin matchsticks

2 small parsnips, scrubbed and cut into thin matchsticks

1 medium onion, thinly sliced

8 cups water

$^1/_2$ pound extra-firm tofu, cut into $^1/_2$-inch cubes

5 tablespoons dark miso

1 bunch watercress, stemmed

1. Heat the oil in a soup pot over medium heat. Add the carrots, parsnips, and onion and sauté for 10 minutes, stirring frequently.

2. Add the water and simmer for 10 minutes. Add the tofu and simmer 5 minutes longer. Turn off heat. Remove 1 cup of the soup liquid and allow to cool for a minute. Dissolve the miso in this liquid and return to the soup pot, making sure the soup is not boiling. Stir to blend. Add the watercress and allow to wilt. Serve.

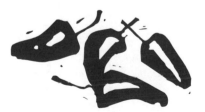

Moroccan Tomato Soup

There is no reason to buy canned tomato soup when you can make this soup in such a short time. Honey and cinnamon are often combined in Moroccan foods and in foods of the Middle East.

Makes 4 servings

2 tablespoons extra-virgin olive oil

1 large onion, chopped

1 teaspoon sea salt

3 tablespoons honey

$^1/_2$ teaspoon ground cinnamon

2 pounds tomatoes, peeled (see page 166), seeded, and puréed, or 1 28-ounce can puréed tomatoes

2 tablespoons tomato paste

5 cups water

$^1/_4$ cup minced fresh dill

2 tablespoons balsamic vinegar

Fromage blanc or plain low-fat yogurt

1. Heat the olive oil in a large soup pot and sauté the onion and sea salt over medium heat until the onion is translucent, about 5 minutes.

2. Add the honey and cinnamon. Sauté, stirring until the onion is glazed, about 4 minutes.

3. Add the puréed tomatoes, tomato paste, water, and 3 tablespoons of the dill. Stir well to blend. Bring to a rapid boil and cook, uncovered, until the contents are reduced by half, about 30 minutes, stirring occasionally.

4. Remove the soup from heat and add the balsamic vinegar. Purée the mixture in a blender or food processor (you may have to do this in batches). Return to the soup kettle and reheat gently.

5. Ladle the soup into individual serving bowls. Place a dollop of fromage blanc or low-fat yogurt in each bowl, and sprinkle the remaining tablespoon dill over the top. Serve immediately.

Oriental Noodle Soup

This simple and satisfying noodle soup is the essence of Oriental cuisine: subtle, yet hearty and full of nutrition. It is extremely low in fat (only a teaspoon of oil is used). Its soothing appeal is a healthful answer to heavier "comfort foods."

Makes 2 generous main-course servings,
or 4 to 6 first-course servings.

6 to 8 cups water
6 to 8 dried shiitake mushrooms
1 8-ounce package dried soba noodles
1 carrot, scrubbed and cut into matchsticks
3 scallions, white and pale green parts only,
    cut thinly or on the diagonal
1/2 pound firm tofu, cut into 1 1/2-inch dice
3 tablespoons shoyu
3 tablespoons mirin
1 tablespoon minced fresh ginger
2 garlic cloves, minced
1 teaspoon sesame oil

1. In a large saucepan, heat 6 to 8 cups water (depending on how thick you want your soup) to boiling. Place the shiitakes in a medium bowl and pour the boiling water over them. Let steep for 2 hours or as long as overnight.

2. Cook the noodles according to the package instructions,* but undercook them slightly, as they will be reheated in the broth. Drain and rinse well. Set aside.

3. Steam the carrots until they are brightly colored and just tender. Rinse with cold water and set aside.

4. Drain the mushrooms, reserving the liquid. Place the liquid in a soup pot. Remove and discard the stems from the mushrooms. Chop the mushroom caps and add to the saucepan.

5. To the mixture add the scallions (reserving 1 tablespoon), tofu, shoyu, mirin, ginger, and garlic. Simmer gently for 15 minutes.

6. Add the cooked noodles and steamed carrots to the saucepan. Simmer a few more minutes, until the noodles and carrots are heated through. Remove from the heat and add the sesame oil. Serve in warmed bowls, garnished with the reserved scallions.

* **See instructions for cooking Japanese noodles, page 180.**

Mushroom-Barley Soup

This soup can be frozen, so make extra. If you do freeze it, don't add the miso until you're ready to serve the soup. The white miso adds sweetness and body.

Makes 8 servings

3 1/2 cups plus 4 cups water
Pinch of sea salt
1 cup whole barley
1 ounce dried black Chinese or porcini mushrooms
3 tablespoons extra-virgin olive oil or butter
2 garlic cloves, minced
2 medium onions, diced
3 celery stalks, diced
1 large carrot, scrubbed and diced
3/4 pound fresh mushrooms, cut into 1/4-inch slices
1 teaspoon dried thyme
1/2 teaspoon dried sage
1/2 cup dry red wine
4 cups vegetable stock or water
1 bay leaf
3 to 5 tablespoons white miso dissolved in 1 cup water
Fresh minced dill for garnish

1. In a medium saucepan, bring the 3 1/2 cups water and the salt to a boil. Rinse the barley well and add to the boiling water. Bring the water back to a boil, reduce to a simmer, and cook for 45 to 60 minutes, or until all the water is absorbed.

2. Pour the 4 cups boiling water over the mushrooms in a large bowl. Let steep while the barley is cooking.

3. Heat the olive oil or butter in a large skillet. Add the garlic, onions, celery, and carrot and sauté over medium heat for 10 minutes, or until the celery and onions are soft. Add the fresh mushrooms, thyme, and sage and sauté for 5 more minutes. The mushrooms will release their liquid.

4. Turn the heat to high and add the red wine. Boil to reduce the liquid to a thick consistency, stirring constantly.

5. Strain the mushroom liquid from the dried mushrooms. Reserve the liquid and discard the mushrooms.

6. When most of the liquid has evaporated from the celery-onion mixture, add the vegetable stock or water, bay leaf, cooked barley, and reserved mushroom liquid. Bring the soup to a boil, reduce the heat, and simmer for at least 30 minutes.

7. Turn the heat off and allow the soup to cool to lukewarm. Add the miso-water mixture to the soup and stir. Gently ladle the soup into individual serving bowls and serve garnished with fresh dill.

Ambrosial Melon Soup

This is summer itself. Make this cooling and delightful soup in the morning to enjoy on a warm and balmy night.

Makes 4 servings

1 cantaloupe, peeled, seeded, and cubed
2 peaches, peeled, pitted, and cubed
1 cup fresh orange juice
1 tablespoon fresh lemon juice
½ teaspoon ground cloves
Mint sprigs and blueberries or raspberries for garnish

1. Place the fruits, juices, and cloves in a medium saucepan. Bring the mixture to a simmer and cook for 1 minute.

2. Purée in a blender or food processor. Chill for at least 2 hours

3. Garnish with a sprig of mint and a few blueberries or raspberries.

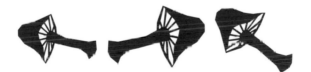

SALADS

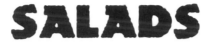

Quinoa Fiesta Salad

This light, zippy dish is a colorful introduction to the delightful versatility of quinoa. The pecans help make the recipe a complete-protein meal.

Makes 4 to 6 side-dish servings

2 cups water
1 cup quinoa
Pinch of sea salt

Dressing

1 garlic clove, minced
¼ cup canola oil
1 teaspoon ground cumin
2 teaspoons honey
1 tablespoon fresh lemon juice
2 teaspoons rice, raspberry, or champagne vinegar
1 red bell pepper, cored, seeded, and cut into small dice
1 carrot, scrubbed, cut into small dice, and steamed for 4 to 5 minutes
6 scallions, white and pale green parts only, minced

½ cup cooked corn (optional)
2 tablespoons minced fresh cilantro or parsley
½ teaspoon sea salt
½ cup lightly toasted pecans,* chopped
½ cup currants

1. Bring the water to boil in a 2- to 3-quart saucepan. Rinse the quinoa several times in cold water. Add the quinoa and salt to the saucepan, reduce to a simmer, and cook for about 20 minutes, or until all the water is absorbed. Fluff with a fork, replace the cover, and let sit off heat for 5 minutes. Place the quinoa in a large mixing bowl to cool.

2. To make the dressing, in a small skillet, sauté the garlic in the canola oil for 2 minutes. Add the cumin and sauté another minute. Add the honey, stir to melt, remove from heat, and allow to cool. Add the lemon juice and vinegar. Mix well and pour onto the quinoa along with all the vegetables, cilantro, sea salt, pecans, and currants. Mix gently but thoroughly, and serve, or place in the refrigerator to chill. Serve on a bed of greens.

* **To toast the pecans, place in a preheated 350°F oven for 8 to 10 minutes, or until lightly browned.**

170

Southwestern Black Bean Salad

Cooking with whole foods opens the door to many ethnic cuisines: the original whole-foods diet. It is an adventure to play with the world of spices and seasonings that cultures from around the globe have enjoyed as part of their culinary heritage. Often, the imaginative use of unusual seasonings creates dishes that have no need for salt or fat as a flavor source. In this recipe the taste buds are treated to the combination of spicy and cool that makes Southwestern food so much fun.

Makes 6 to 8 side-dish servings

2 cups dried black turtle beans
1 bay leaf

Dressing

3 tablespoons minced fresh cilantro, chopped
2 tablespoons corn oil
Juice of ½ lime
Juice of ½ orange
1 teaspoon grated orange zest
1 teaspoon sea salt
1 teaspoon ground cumin
¼ teaspoon paprika
1 teaspoon sherry or rice vinegar
2 garlic cloves, minced

½ red onion, diced
2 red bell peppers, roasted, cored, seeded, and diced
3 tomatillos, husked and diced
2 ears fresh corn, cooked and kernels cut off, or 1½ cups frozen corn

1. Sort through the beans and remove any stones or debris. Rinse, cover with 3 times their volume of water, and let soak 8 hours or overnight.

2. Drain and rinse the beans. Cover by 3 inches with fresh water in a large soup pot. Add the bay leaf and bring to a boil. Reduce to a simmer and cook until the beans are just tender, about 45 minutes to an hour (do not overcook; the beans should retain their shape). Discard the bay leaf.

3. Combine the dressing ingredients and mix well.

4. When the beans are done, drain well. Place in a large mixing bowl along with the vegetables and dressing (the dressing will penetrate the beans better while they are warm). Mix gently, adjust the seasonings, and marinate for 2 to 3 hours in the refrigerator.

Tabouli

This version of tabouli (and there are many) leaves the bulgur slightly crunchy, a texture that complements the abundant mint and parsley in this recipe. Make some tabouli in the morning and come home to a light and refreshing meal.

Makes 6 side-dish servings

1½ cups bulgur
2 cups boiling water

Dressing

½ cup fresh lemon juice
⅓ cup extra-virgin olive oil
2 to 3 garlic cloves
1 tablespoon tomato paste
1½ teaspoons sea salt

6 scallions, minced
2 plum tomatoes, cut into small dice
1 cup minced fresh mint
2 cups minced fresh parsley
1 cup lightly toasted sesame seeds*
Salad greens
Black olives and sliced tomatoes for garnish

1. Place the bulgur in a medium saucepan with a tight-fitting lid. Add the boiling water, cover, and let sit for 45 minutes.

2. While the bulgur is soaking, place the dressing ingredients in a blender or food processor and blend until smooth.

3. Line a colander with cheesecloth and place the bulgur in the colander. Wrap the cheesecloth around the bulgur and twist until the excess water is strained out. Place the bulgur in a large bowl.

4. Add the vegetables, herbs, sesame seeds, and dressing to the bulgur. Mix well and chill for at least 2 to 3 hours. Serve on a bed of greens with olives and tomato slices.

* **To toast sesame seeds, stir in a dry skillet over medium heat until lightly browned.**

Tofu Udon Salad

This is a snap to make, and it slips easily into lunch boxes or brown bags for a filling and nutritious lunch. Daikon, thought by people in Asia to have many health benefits, brings a lot of crunch and pizzazz to this recipe.

Makes 4 main-course servings, or 6 side-dish servings

$\frac{1}{2}$ **pound extra-firm tofu**
1 large carrot, scrubbed and cut into julienne
1 8-ounce package udon noodles
1 tablespoon Asian (toasted) sesame oil
$\frac{1}{4}$ **cup sesame seeds**
1 small daikon, scrubbed and cut into julienne, or 4 thinly sliced small radishes
1 bunch scallions, white and pale green parts only, cut thinly on the diagonal

Marinade for Tofu

1 tablespoon Asian (toasted) sesame oil
1 tablespoon tamari

Dressing

1 tablespoon Asian (toasted) sesame oil
1 tablespoon tamari
1 tablespoon brown rice vinegar
2 teaspoons prepared mustard

1. Preheat the oven to 425°F.

2. Place the tofu between 2 flat plates. Place a heavy object on the top and let the tofu drain for about $\frac{1}{2}$ hour.

3. Steam the carrot over boiling water for 5 minutes, or until just tender. Run it under cold water to set the color. Drain and set aside.

4. Place the marinade ingredients in a medium glass jar with a lid. Cut the tofu into $\frac{1}{2}$-inch cubes and place in the jar with the marinade. Shake well to coat and let marinate for 15 minutes.

5. Place the tofu cubes on a flat baking sheet and bake for 10 minutes, shaking the pan periodically to prevent the tofu from sticking. Remove the tofu from the oven and lower the oven temperature to 350°F.

6. Cook the udon noodles according to the package directions. Rinse and drain well. In a large bowl, toss the noodles with the toasted sesame oil.

7. Place the sesame seeds on a baking sheet and toast for 5 minutes, shaking the pan to prevent scorching.

8. Add the tofu, sesame seeds, carrot, daikon, and scallions to the udon noodles.

9. Place all the dressing ingredients in a glass jar with a lid and shake well. Pour over the noodle mixture and mix well. Serve at room temperature or chilled.

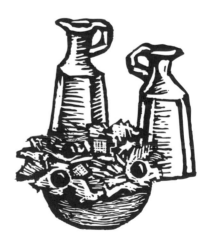

Jícama-Orange Salad

This is a light and refreshing salad that goes well with grilled foods of all sorts.

Makes 4 side-dish servings

1 large jícama, peeled
3 oranges, peeled
1 bunch red radishes
3 tablespoons minced fresh cilantro
1 tablespoon extra-virgin olive oil
1 tablespoon fresh lime juice
Big pinch of cayenne pepper or red pepper flakes

1. Cut the jícama into thin wedges or ½-inch cubes.

2. Cut the oranges into ⅓-inch thick slices and then into quarters.

3. If the radishes are small, cut them in half for an interesting shape contrast. If not, slice them into rounds.

4. Toss the jícama, orange pieces, radishes, and cilantro with the olive oil, lime juice, and pinch of cayenne. Refrigerate for at least an hour.

Jícama

Jícama (hē-cuh-mah) is a vegetable "talent" deserving wider recognition. Its light, crunchy texture and sweet, juicy taste make it welcome during warm weather. Jícama is turniplike in shape and has a brown outer skin and fibrous white underskin that should be peeled away from the white interior. Once cut it will not discolor, and it will also retain its crunch. At only 50 calories per cup, jícama offers a surprising amount of flavor, making it a great low-calorie hors d'oeuvre or snack.

Jícama is good cut into strips or "chips" and served with a touch of lime juice and either cayenne or salt. It's great raw in salads of all sorts, and relishes also benefit from its delicate crispness. Jícama is an excellent alternative to water chestnuts in both cold and hot dishes, since it's much less expensive and holds its shape and crunch better.

Whole jícama or large pieces will keep 1 to 2 weeks in the refrigerator. Store small pieces in cold water to retain freshness and moisture.

Green Bean Salad with Red Onion and Caper Vinaigrette

Makes 4 to 6 first-course or side-dish servings

1 pound green beans, trimmed
1 tablespoon capers, drained
½ red onion, minced
2 tablespoons fresh chopped parsley

Dressing

4 tablespoons extra-virgin olive oil
2 tablespoons balsamic vinegar
1 garlic clove, minced
½ teaspoon sea salt
¼ teaspoon ground black pepper

1. Bring a large pot of water to boil and add the beans. When the water returns to a boil, drain the beans and run them under cold water to set the color. Drain.

2. Place the beans in a bowl with the capers, onion, and parsley. Shake the dressing ingredients together in a glass jar. Pour over the beans, toss to coat beans with dressing, and serve at room temperature or chilled.

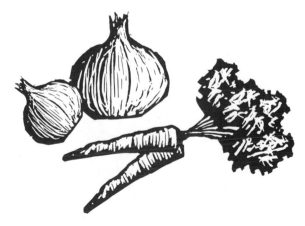

Red Lentil Salad

Plan a bit ahead for this salad. Soaking the lentils for 48 hours to sprout them increases their digestibility and keeps them separate and beautiful for this delicious salad.

Makes 6 to 8 servings

2 cups red lentils
8 cups water
2 plum tomatoes, diced
1 small red onion, diced
¼ cup fresh parsley, chopped
2 tablespoons fresh mint, chopped
2 garlic cloves, minced

Dressing

3 tablespoons extra-virgin olive oil
2 tablespoons balsamic vinegar
1 tablespoon fresh lemon juice
2 teaspoons prepared mustard
1 teaspoon sea salt

1. Wash the lentils and soak them in plenty of water for 48 hours, changing the water twice a day. When you're ready to make the salad, drain and rinse the lentils.

2. Bring 8 cups water to a rolling boil. Add the soaked lentils and return to a boil. Cook for 1 minute. Drain immediately and rinse well with cold water to cool. Drain again.

3. While the lentils are draining, prepare the salad vegetables and place them in a large bowl.

4. Combine the dressing ingredients in a small jar and shake well.

5. Add the drained lentils to the bowl with the vegetables and pour the dressing over the salad. Toss gently to combine. Allow to sit at room temperature for 30 minutes, if possible, to enhance the flavor of the lentils.

Veal and Orange Salad

The delicate pink color of humanely raised veal along with the bright green beans and vibrant orange segments makes this dish perfect for a spring or summer day. Leftovers make great sandwiches on sourdough bread.

Makes 4 to 6 servings

3 tablespoons extra-virgin olive oil
2 garlic cloves, crushed
½ pound free-range veal cutlets, pounded thin
⅓ cup dry white wine
1½ teaspoons minced fresh rosemary
¼ cup fresh orange juice
3 tablespoons wine vinegar
1 tablespoon grated orange zest
Sea salt and freshly ground pepper to taste
1 pound green beans
2 cups salad greens
1 orange, peeled and separated into segments

1. Heat a heavy skillet, pour in 1 tablespoon of the oil, swirl to coat the pan, and add the crushed garlic. Add the veal and sauté over medium heat for about 2 minutes on each side. Remove the cutlets (leave the juices in the pan) and cut into thin strips about 1½ inches long.

2. Remove the garlic from the pan and add the wine and rosemary. Turn the heat up to high and reduce the liquid to 3 tablespoons.

3. Combine the reduced liquid with the remaining oil, orange juice, vinegar, zest, and salt and pepper to make a dressing.

4. Steam the beans over boiling water until bright green and crisp-tender, about 5 to 8 minutes.

5. Marinate the meat and green beans in half of the dressing for at least 1 hour in the refrigerator.

6. Create a mound of greens on a platter or on individual plates. Arrange the beans and veal on top. Garnish with the orange segments and pour the remaining dressing over the salad.

Warm Arame Salad

If you have never tried sea vegetables, this recipe is the place to start. It is subtle and faintly reminiscent of the sea. Make a simple and very healthy dinner by combining this dish with brown rice and steamed broccoli.

Makes 4 servings

1 2-ounce package (approximately 3 cups) dried arame
Juice of ½ lemon
3 tablespoons low-sodium tamari
3 tablespoons mirin
1 carrot, scrubbed and cut into matchsticks
⅓ cup sesame seeds
3 scallions, white and pale green parts only, cut thinly on the diagonal

1. Soak the arame in water to cover for 10 minutes.
2. Rinse and drain the arame. Place in a medium saucepan with the lemon juice, tamari, and mirin. Add water to cover by one half. Simmer uncovered until all the water is absorbed, stirring occasionally to prevent scorching.
3. Add the carrot to the arame mixture after it has been simmering for 15 minutes.
4. While the arame is simmering, toast the sesame seeds by stirring them in a dry skillet over medium heat until lightly browned. Place in a blender or food processor and grind to a coarse powder (do not grind too long or the seeds will become nut butter).
5. Place the cooked arame in a large mixing bowl. Add the sesame seed mixture and scallions. Mix well. Serve warm or at room temperature.

Rice, Arame, and Asparagus Salad

This salad is best if made while the rice is still warm.

Makes 4 to 6 servings

2 cups arame
1 bunch asparagus, woody stems removed,* cut into thin slices on the diagonal (tips left intact)
2 carrots, scrubbed and cut into thin matchsticks
¼ cup sesame seeds
4 cups cooked brown rice

Dressing

3 tablespoons sesame oil
2 tablespoons rice vinegar
2 tablespoons lemon juice
2 tablespoons tamari

1. Soak the arame for 10 minutes. Drain and rinse. Chop into 1-inch pieces and set aside.
2. Steam the asparagus for 3 to 4 minutes, until tender but still bright green. Run under cold water and drain.
3. Using the same hot water, steam the carrots for 3 minutes. Run under cold water and set aside.
4. Toast the sesame seeds in a dry skillet or in a 350°F oven until they are lightly browned. Remove from the pan and place in a bowl to cool.
5. Place the brown rice, arame, asparagus, carrots, and sesame seeds in a large bowl and mix gently but well. Combine the dressing ingredients in a small jar and shake to blend well. Pour the dressing over the salad and toss gently. Serve immediately at room temperature, or chilled, on a bed of red leaf lettuce and radicchio.

* **If desired, peel the lower 4 inches of the asparagus stalks.**

Indian Rice Salad

When cooking brown rice, make some extra and use it in this amazingly simple dish. It's great for lunch (the complex carbohydrates in the brown rice will give you energy all afternoon) and is an inexpensive way to transform brown rice into something quite exotic. This salad turns out best when it is put together while the grain is still warm. Taking some time to cut the vegetables into striking shapes adds finesse to this dish.

Makes 6 side-dish servings

4 cups cooked brown rice
4 scallions, white and pale green parts, cut thinly on the diagonal
2 celery stalks, cut very thinly on a sharp diagonal
1/4 cup fresh cilantro, chopped
1/2 cup raisins
1/2 cup dried apricots, cut into julienne
3/4 cup toasted cashews* (optional), chopped coarsely
1/3 cup extra-virgin olive oil
1 tablespoon curry powder
1 teaspoon ground cumin
1/2 teaspoon ground nutmeg
1/2 teaspoon ground cardamom
1 teaspoon dried thyme
1 tablespoon tamari
Juice of 1/2 lemon
1 tablespoon maple syrup

1. Place the rice, scallions, celery, cilantro, raisins, apricots, and cashews (if using) in a large bowl and mix well.

2. In a small skillet, gently warm the oil. Add the spices and thyme and sauté over low heat for 1 minute. Pour over the rice mixture along with the tamari, lemon juice, and maple syrup. Stir well and allow to marinate in the refrigerator for at least 1 hour.

* **To toast cashews, place in a preheated 350°F oven for 8 to 10 minutes, or until lightly browned.**

Carrot Salad

Even people who have never before liked carrot salad love this one. It is light and lively, with the flavors of ginger and orange juice blending perfectly with the natural sweetness of the carrots.

Makes 6 first-course servings

1 2-inch piece fresh ginger, peeled
1/2 cup sunflower seeds
8 medium carrots, scrubbed and grated
1 cup currants
1/2 cup plain low-fat yogurt
1/4 cup fresh mint
2 tablespoons fresh parsley
1/2 teaspoon ground cumin
1/2 teaspoon ground cinnamon
1/3 cup fresh orange juice

1. Grate the ginger and squeeze the pulp to produce 1 tablespoon of juice.

2. Toast the sunflower seeds by stirring them in a dry skillet over medium heat until they are lightly browned. Remove seeds from pan and cool.

3. Mix all of the ingredients together in a medium bowl and refrigerate overnight.

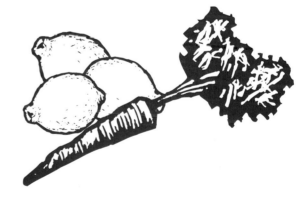

PASTA

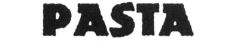

Quick Pasta-Veggie Medley

Makes 4 to 6 servings

Water
1 stalk broccoli, florets and stems
1 zucchini
1 carrot
8-ounces whole-wheat udon noodles or other
    whole-grain pasta
1 cup cooked chick-peas
1 to 2 tablespoons extra-virgin olive oil
1 medium tomato, diced
Parmesan cheese to taste
Freshly ground pepper

1. Bring a large pot of water to a boil. Do not add salt to the water if using udon noodles because they are already salted.

2. While the water is coming to a boil, prepare the vegetables. Cut the stems off the broccoli and separate the florets. Peel the stems and cut the inner parts into thin matchsticks. Cut the zucchini and carrot into similarly sized matchsticks. Set aside.

3. When the water has come to a rolling boil, add the pasta and return the water to a boil. Cook the pasta according to package directions or until *al dente*, cooked through but not overcooked. Add the broccoli, carrot, zucchini, and chick-peas. Cook for 1 minute. Drain the pasta and vegetables in a colander. Place in a large bowl and toss with the olive oil and tomatoes.

4. Serve hot and pass the Parmesan cheese and pepper.

Pesto Pasta

This is the perfect summer meal: easy, colorful, and full of the flavors of fresh herbs and vegetables. Note the snazzy (and effortless!) way the vegetables are "cooked."

Makes 2 main-course servings or 4 to 6 side-dish servings

1 8-ounce package soba noodles
2 carrots, scrubbed and cut into julienne

1 medium zucchini, cut into julienne
1 cup Pesto (see page 212)

1. Cook the noodles according to package directions or see "Japanese Noodles," page 180. Place the vegetables in the bottom of a colander. When the noodles are done, pour the noodles *and* cooking water into the colander over the carrots and zucchini. This blanches the vegetables just enough to make them tender.

2. Drain the noodles and vegetables well and place in a large bowl. Pour the pesto over the noodle mixture, mix well, and chill.

Angel Hair Pasta

Makes 6 servings

1 pound angel hair pasta
4 tablespoons extra-virgin olive oil
1 bunch watercress, stemmed
1 cup chopped fresh Italian parsley
25 calamata olives, pitted and cut into thirds
1 cup (8 ounces) sheep's milk feta cheese
Juice of $\frac{1}{2}$ lemon
Grated zest of 2 lemons
$\frac{1}{2}$ cup thinly sliced red onions, cut into $\frac{3}{4}$-inch pieces
Sea salt to taste
Black olives, lemon slices, and watercress sprigs for garnish (optional)

1. Cook pasta *al dente* or according to package directions. Drain.

2. Toss with 2 tablespoons of the oil.

3. Let cool 5 minutes and toss with the remaining 2 tablespoons of the oil and the watercress, parsley, olives, feta cheese, lemon juice and zest, onion, and salt. Serve warm, garnished with lemon slices, watercress, and additional black olives if desired.

Cooking Whole-Wheat Pasta

Whole-wheat pasta, like many other whole-grain products, has a different taste and texture from those of its refined counterparts. Many people spend a bit of time and experimentation acquainting themselves with these differences, and after some initial resistance, come to love the richness and fullness of flavor that whole-grain products offer.

Whole-grain pastas are denser than white-flour products, but this can be an advantage, as it provides a wonderful background for other flavors. To cook whole-wheat pasta bring a *large* pot of water to a *rolling* boil. Add the pasta and a pinch of sea salt, and cook according to the time on the package, usually about 12 minutes, always keeping the water at a high boil. When the pasta is done (test by removing a piece from the water and cutting it in half; it should be the same color throughout), pour it into a colander and rinse with cold water. Drain the pasta well and place it in a medium bowl. Toss with a bit of olive oil and return to the cooking pot. Warm over medium heat, stirring to prevent the pasta from sticking to the bottom of the pot. You'll have all the benefits of a whole-grain food and great taste to boot.

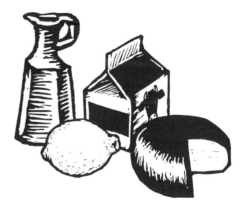

Leek and Fennel Pasta e Fagioli

Pasta e fagioli (pasta fazool) was originally a bean soup with pasta; here it refers to a pasta dish with a sauce of vegetables and white beans. It is interesting to note that every ethnic cuisine has, at its root, dishes that combine grains and beans to make a complete-protein meal. These meals are typically high in fiber and low in fat. The wisdom of indigenous peoples in combining foods for health and survival is something we would do well to adopt.

Fennel is used extensively in Italy, where it is sautéed, roasted, baked, and served raw as an appetizer. Its aniselike flavor perks up the taste buds without a lot of fat or calories. In this recipe it's a wonderful contrast in texture to the pasta and beans. This meal can be dressed up for company or enjoyed as the centerpiece of a relaxed family meal.

Makes 6 main-course servings

1½ cups whole-wheat pasta shells

2 medium carrots, scrubbed and cut into ¼-inch diagonal slices

1 large fennel bulb, stalks and core removed, roughly chopped

3 tablespoons extra-virgin olive oil

3 garlic cloves, minced

3 leeks, white part only, cut into ½-inch slices, rinsed, and drained well

1 teaspoon sea salt

1 tablespoon dried basil

2 teaspoons dried oregano

⅛ teaspoon red pepper flakes

¼ teaspoon fennel seeds

6 fresh plum tomatoes and ½ cup tomato juice, or 1 14-ounce can of plum tomatoes with juice

Juice of ½ lemon

1½ cups cooked (½ cup uncooked) small white beans

Fresh pepper to taste

Grated Pecorino Romano or Parmesan cheese (optional)

Chopped fresh parsley

1. Bring a large pot of water to a boil. Add a pinch of sea salt and the pasta shells. Cook for 12 minutes. Drain and rinse.

2. Heat the olive oil in a large soup pot over medium heat. Add the garlic, leeks, and ½ teaspoon of the salt. Sauté, stirring often, for 5 minutes.

3. Add the carrots, fennel, basil, oregano, red pepper flakes, and fennel seeds and continue to sauté, stirring often, for 10 minutes.

4. In a blender or food processor, purée the tomatoes and tomato juice to a coarse consistency. Add to the leek mixture along with the lemon juice and cooked beans. Stir well, bring the mixture to a boil, immediately reduce the heat to a simmer, and cook for an additional 10 minutes, stirring often.

5. Add the pepper and the rest of the salt. Place the noodles on serving plates and spoon a large serving of leek-fennel mixture over the pasta. Sprinkle with grated cheese (if using) and chopped parsley. Serve immediately.

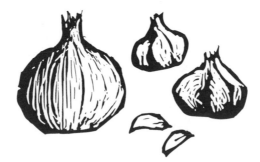

Japanese Noodles

Udon, soba, ramen, and *somen*—with the possible exception of ramen, they're not exactly household words. Japanese pastas should attract the attention of anyone interested in healthier fast meals. They're light in texture and boast a subtlety of flavor unusual in whole-grain pastas. These advantages over most Western whole-grain pastas are the result of both the type of flours and the meticulous methods used to make Japanese noodles.

In the West, pasta is made from hard winter wheat and is produced by forcing dough through a noodle machine and then drying the pasta quickly under heat. In contrast, Japanese pasta is made from light spring wheat, the thin sheets of dough are knife-cut into noodles, and they are allowed to dry very slowly.

Soba The slightly sweet taste and firm, smooth texture of soba comes from the buckwheat flour that distinguishes it from other Japanese pastas, which are made primarily from wheat flour. Soba noodles are the stuff of hearty meals, lending themselves to a wide range of warm and cold dishes. Soba readily absorbs and retains all sorts of flavors while keeping its distinct character.

Buckwheat is not related to wheat and is not even a true cereal grain. It's virtually fat-free, has a high protein content, and is abundant in B vitamins, fiber, vitamin E, and rutin. It has traditionally been considered a "blood-building" food, and in the East buckwheat is thought to cleanse and soothe the digestive system.

Soba is made with either 100 percent buckwheat flour or a 40 to 60 percent mix of buckwheat and wheat. There are also *jinenjo* sobas containing wild mountain yam flour, which lends an orange tint and subtle flavor, and *mugwort* soba, made with the spinachlike mugwort plant (it's great with pesto sauce).

Udon and Somen Udon and somen are made from whole-wheat flour. Udon is thicker and heartier than somen and is traditionally eaten in cooler weather, usually in a hot miso broth with steamed vegetables. *Genmai* udon, a variety made with about 25 percent rice flour, is slightly lighter than regular udon.

Somen is usually served cold with shoyu and garnished with scallions, sliced nori, and grated ginger. Thanks to its light texture and rapid absorption of flavors in dressings, many prefer somen to udon or to Western whole-grain pastas for salads.

Cooking Udon and Soba The key to the enjoyment of udon and soba is proper cooking. When done right, these noodles stay firm and separate, allowing you to cook extra for future meals. There are two basic methods of cooking Japanese noodles: a traditional "shock" method, or simple boiling. While straight boiling is fine, the shock method produces the finest texture.

"Shocking" Noodles Bring 3 to 4 quarts of water to a full, rolling boil, and add the noodles a little at a time to keep the water temperature high. Stir the noodles well at first to keep them from sticking to the pot and to each other. When the water returns to a full boil, add a cup of cold water. For soba noodles, repeat this step twice more; for udon, three times more. The noodles are done when they are the same color inside and out, or are *al dente*. If noodles are to be incorporated into another dish, it is best to undercook them a bit, since the second heating will finish them off. Drain them in a colander and rinse well with cold water. This method produces a "springy" noodle that can be cooked in a stir-fry with other ingredients and can be enjoyed in soups, with sauces, or in cold pasta salads

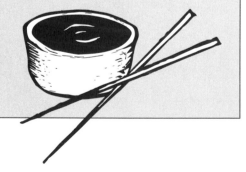

VEGETARIAN ENTREES

Hints of the Himalayas Lentil-Rice Casserole

Exotic spices, red lentils, and basmati rice team up in this Indian-accented casserole. Good hot or cold, a dollop of plain yogurt finishes off this dish perfectly. Serve with sliced cucumbers for extra crispness, and dark green steamed broccoli for a contrast in color. The combination of a grain (rice) and a bean (lentils) makes this a complete-protein entree.

Makes 6 main-course servings, or 8 side-dish servings

4 cups water
2 cups brown basmati rice
1 cup red lentils, soaked 4 to 8 hours in plenty of water
2 onions, diced
2 teaspoons fresh ginger
3 large garlic cloves, minced
1 teaspoon ground turmeric
1 teaspoon ground cumin
¼ teaspoon ground cardamom

2 to 3 tablespoons ghee (clarified butter), unsalted butter, or safflower oil
1 large carrot, scrubbed and cut in large dice
2 large tomatoes, chopped
½ cup red seedless raisins or sultana raisins
½ teaspoon sea salt or vegetable seasoning salt
Freshly ground pepper to taste
1½ cups plain low-fat yogurt, plus extra for garnish
½ cup lightly toasted cashews or sesame seeds (optional)
Fresh parsley or cilantro for garnish

1. Bring the water to a boil in a large saucepan. Add the rice, cover pot, reduce heat, and simmer for 45 minutes, or until all the liquid is absorbed. Preheat the oven to 325°F.

2. Place the soaked lentils in a medium bowl. Pour boiling water over the lentils to cover. Let sit for 1 minute. Drain and repeat this step. This process will cook the soaked lentils without causing them to lose their color or become mushy.

3. In a medium skillet, sauté the onion, ginger, garlic, and spices* in 2 tablespoons of the ghee,

butter, or oil over medium heat for 5 minutes, stirring often. Add the carrot and tomatoes and continue sautéing for 7 more minutes

4. In another small skillet, heat about 1 teaspoon of butter or oil and sauté the raisins briefly. Add to the onion-tomato mixture, season with salt and pepper, and cook 3 minutes more over low heat.

5. When the rice is cooked, rinse it and pour it into a large bowl. Add the yogurt and lentils and mix well until the mixture is creamy.

6. Grease a 3-quart casserole dish. Either alternate layers of vegetables and rice-lentil mixture, or fold the vegetables into the rice-lentil mixture and then place in the casserole dish. Bake covered for 30 minutes.

* **If you prefer a spicier version, add ¼ teaspoon cayenne pepper along with the spices.**

Two-Bean Vegetarian Chili

Use precooked beans for a chili on the table quick, quick, quick.

Makes 6 to 8 servings

2 tablespoons extra-virgin olive oil
1 large Spanish onion, chopped
3 cloves garlic, minced
1 each red, yellow, and green bell peppers, blanched, peeled, and chopped
1 tablespoon ground cumin
2 tablespoons chili powder
2¼ cups cooked white beans, drained
2¼ cups cooked red kidney beans or black turtle beans, drained
1 2-pound can plum tomatoes, chopped, with liquid
1 tablespoon balsamic vinegar
Sea salt, pepper, and Tabasco sauce or cayenne pepper to taste
Chopped black olives, scallions, and grated cheese

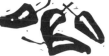

1. In a 5- to 6-quart soup pot, heat the olive oil and sauté the onion, garlic, and peppers for 10 minutes over medium heat. Add the cumin and chili powder and cook another 5 minutes.

2. Add the cooked beans, chopped plum tomatoes and their liquid, and balsamic vinegar. Cook covered for 15 minutes.

3. Add the salt, pepper, and Tabasco sauce to taste and cook covered another 15 minutes. Serve piping hot garnished with chopped olives, scallions, and grated cheese.

Note: Other beans may be substituted for those suggested.

Sweet and Sour Tofu and Vegetables

Making your own stir-fries will show you how simple it is to create better-than-restaurant fare at a fraction of the cost. Once you get the knack of it, it's a dramatic and fun way to prepare food. Stir-fries are also a good way to use up bits and pieces of leftover vegetables. This recipe is colorful and festive, and takes little time to prepare.

Makes 4 generous servings

Sweet and Sour Sauce

2 garlic cloves, minced
2 tablespoons grated fresh ginger
3 tablespoons shoyu
3 tablespoons fresh lemon juice
2 teaspoons rice vinegar
2 tablespoons honey
¼ teaspoon red pepper flakes
1 tablespoon arrowroot
1 tablespoon canola oil

½ package (8 ounces) firm tofu, cut into ½-inch dice
2 tablespoons peanut oil
1 medium zucchini, cut into matchsticks
1 yellow summer squash, cut into matchsticks

1 red bell pepper, cored, seeded, and cut into
matchsticks

1 green or yellow bell pepper, cored, seeded,
and cut into matchsticks

1 bunch scallions, sliced thinly on the diagonal

Cooked brown rice or soba noodles

3 tablespoons toasted sesame seeds*

1. Mix together all the ingredients for the sweet and sour sauce. Drain the tofu by placing it between two flat plates with a heavy object on the top plate for at least ½ hour. Place the drained tofu in the sauce and marinate for at least 15 minutes.

2. Heat 1 tablespoon of the peanut oil in a wok or heavy skillet. Add the zucchini and yellow squash, and stir-fry over high heat for 3 minutes. Remove from the wok.

3. Reheat the wok. Add the remaining 1 tablespoon of the oil. Add the peppers and scallions. Stir-fry for 1 to 2 minutes. Remove the tofu from the sauce with a slotted spoon and add to the wok. Stir-fry for 2 minutes, stirring constantly to keep the ingredients from sticking.

4. Mix the sauce well to dissolve the arrowroot and add to the wok along with the zucchini mixture. Heat the vegetables through and allow the sauce to thicken. Serve immediately over brown rice or soba noodles and sprinkle with sesame seeds.

* **To toast sesame seeds, stir them in a dry skillet over medium heat until lightly browned.**

Polenta Pizza

This is whole-grain goodness from northern Italy, where it is traditional to combine corn and buckwheat to create the region's famous polenta. This is less complicated than a yeast-dough pizza crust, but the crust is still crispy and delicious.

Makes 4 servings

Crust

5½ cups water or broth

½ teaspoon sea salt

⅓ cup kasha (toasted buckwheat groats)

2 cups polenta or yellow corn grits

Olive oil

Topping

2 to 3 tablespoons extra-virgin olive oil

3 medium onions, thinly sliced

2 garlic cloves, minced

1 sprig fresh rosemary or thyme or 1 teaspoon
crumbled dried thyme

½ cup grated Parmesan cheese or 1 cup
crumbled fresh goat cheese

Fresh ground pepper to taste

1. Preheat the oven to 400°F.

2. Bring the water or broth to a boil in a heavy 2½-quart saucepan. Add the salt and whisk in the kasha. Cook for 5 minutes. Add the polenta and whisk constantly until the mixture thickens. Turn the heat to low, cover, and cook for 15 minutes, stirring occasionally.

3. Brush a pizza pan or pizza stone with olive oil and spread the polenta-kasha mixture evenly on the pan or stone. Set aside to cool and become firm.

4. While the crust is cooling, heat 2 tablespoons of the olive oil in a large skillet. Add the sliced onions and garlic and sauté over medium heat for 10 minutes. Add the rosemary or thyme and continue to cook over medium-low heat for 10 to 15 minutes, until the onions are soft, translucent, and slightly browned. They will be very sweet and delicious.

5. Spread the onion mixture on top of the firm polenta and top with cheese, grindings of pepper, and the remaining olive oil, if desired.

6. Bake 15 minutes in the preheated oven. Broil for the last 2 or 3 minutes to brown the top a bit.

◆ **Variations:**

• Add thin slices of red bell pepper to the onion mixture for the last 10 minutes of cooking.

• Use jack cheese instead of Parmesan.

• Use buckwheat flour instead of the kasha.

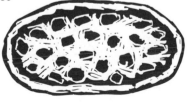

Tempeh with Sauerkraut, White Miso, and Mustard

Cabbage and sauerkraut are paired with miso and mustard for hearty fall and winter fare. Leftovers can be heated and served on onion rolls for sandwiches.

Makes 3 servings

1 pound tempeh
¼ cup canola oil
½ cup thinly sliced cabbage
1½ tablespoons white miso
1 tablespoon Dijon mustard
¼ cup sauerkraut with brine
1½ to 2 cups water
1 tablespoon arrowroot dissolved in 2 tablespoons water
Cooked noodles

1. Cut the tempeh into 1-inch cubes. Heat the oil in a large skillet and sauté the tempeh until golden brown. Carefully place the tempeh in a colander or sieve and rinse with water to get rid of excess oil. Drain the tempeh on paper towels.

2. Place the cabbage on the bottom of a large, heavy saucepan. Place the tempeh on top of the cabbage.

3. In a bowl, combine the miso and mustard with the sauerkraut and water. Cover the tempeh and cabbage with this mixture and bring to a boil. Reduce heat, cover, and simmer for 25 to 30 minutes.

4. Pour the dissolved arrowroot into the saucepan, stirring constantly until the mixture thickens. Serve over noodles.

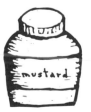

Mediterranean Stuffed Peppers

Either red or green bell peppers work in this recipe, the red being sweeter. This is a good dish to make for guests, as you can make it in advance up to the point of baking the peppers. A meal in itself, this dish is complemented by a simple salad of bitter greens with Barely Tangy Vinaigrette (see page 214). Make extra peppers—they're great for lunch the next day.

Makes 3 main-course servings, or 6 side-dish servings

2 tablespoons extra-virgin olive oil
1 large onion, minced
1 cup short-grain brown rice
1¾ cups water
6 medium red or green bell peppers
½ cup pine nuts
¼ cup freshly grated Pecorino Romano cheese
¼ cup fresh mint, minced
¼ cup fresh parsley, minced
¼ cup fresh lemon juice
¼ cup dry white wine
½ teaspoon ground cinnamon
Sea salt and freshly ground pepper to taste

1. In a 2- or 3-quart saucepan, heat the olive oil and sauté the onion over medium heat until tender, about 10 minutes. Add the rice and sauté, stirring often, for a few minutes. Add the water, bring to a boil, reduce heat, and simmer for 45 minutes, or until all the water is absorbed.

2. Bring a large pot of water to a boil. Meanwhile, cut off the tops of the peppers with care, as they will be used later. Gently remove the cores and seeds to create an empty cavity. Blanch the peppers in the boiling water for 5 minutes. Remove from the water and place upside down on paper towels to drain.

3. Roast the pine nuts on a baking sheet in a preheated 350°F oven for about 5 minutes, shaking the pan often. Remove and set aside, leaving the oven on for the peppers.

4. When the rice is done, toss it with the pine nuts, cheese, herbs, lemon juice, wine, cinnamon, salt, and pepper in a large bowl. Mix well and adjust the seasonings. Stuff the peppers with the rice mixture, put the tops back on the peppers, and place them in a baking dish just large enough to hold them upright. Bake for 25 to 30 minutes, or until the rice is heated through. Serve immediately.

Tostadas

If the only tostadas you've ever had have been fast-food or frozen versions, then the taste and texture of these will be a pleasant surprise. Their texture is soft without being mushy, and the taste is a delicious blend of healthful ingredients.

Tostadas are a good meal to put together when you need to use up leftovers. Many kinds of beans can be used in place of the pinto beans in the recipe. Leftover millet or couscous can be substituted for the rice. Add small pieces of steamed vegetables, such as broccoli and zucchini, for extra nutrition and color.

Corn tortillas made from whole corn bring an authentic flavor (and a good dose of fiber) to this dish.

Makes 6 to 8 servings

3 garlic cloves, minced
1 teaspoon sea salt
2 tablespoons canola oil
2 carrots, scrubbed well and minced
1 large onion, diced
2 teaspoons ground cumin
1 tablespoon dried marjoram
$^{1}/_{2}$ to 1 teaspoon chili powder
1 tablespoon dried basil
1$^{1}/_{2}$ cups cooked pinto beans, plus $^{1}/_{2}$ cup bean liquid
2 tablespoons white miso
$^{1}/_{2}$ cup water
6 to 8 corn tortillas
1$^{1}/_{2}$ cups cooked rice
1 cup ($^{1}/_{4}$ pound) grated jack or sharp cheddar cheese (optional)
Salsa or other hot sauce (optional)
Shredded lettuce, guacamole, or scallions (optional)

1. In a mortar and pestle or in a small bowl with a fork, mash the garlic with the sea salt.

2. Heat the oil in a large skillet. Add the garlic-salt mixture, carrots, and onion and sauté until tender, about 12 minutes (if the vegetables begin to stick to the bottom of the pan, add a very small amount of water). Add the cumin, marjoram, chili powder, basil, and beans and simmer, stirring frequently, for 10 minutes. As the mixture becomes dry, add a small portion of the reserved bean liquid.

3. Dissolve the miso well in $^{1}/_{2}$ cup water. Turn heat to a low simmer and add the miso-water mixture, stir, and gently heat through.

4. Mash the beans with a potato masher or the back of a spoon. For a creamier consistency, place in a blender or food processor and purée to a coarse consistency.

5. Warm the corn tortillas in a cast-iron pan or in the oven. Spread some of the bean mixture on each tortilla. Place the rice over the beans and sprinkle a small amount of the grated cheese over the rice. (Don't spread the toppings too thick or it will be difficult to manage the finished tostadas.)

6. Place the tortillas under a broiler until the cheese is bubbly. Invite people to place their own toppings, such as salsa, lettuce, guacamole, or scallions, on the tortillas.

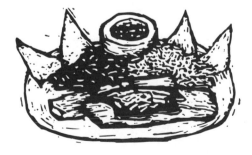

FISH & SHELLFISH

Savory Swordfish with Braised Red Peppers and Leeks

This is a simple dish to make, but it will taste as if you've spent hours on it. The slightly sweet, slightly smoky flavor of braised red peppers is a perfect match for succulent marinated swordfish. You can cook this on the grill or under the boiler. Serve with a grain to soak up the marinade.

Makes 4 generous servings

1½ pounds swordfish (about 2 medium steaks)

2 red bell peppers, cored, seeded, and cut into thin strips

3 medium leeks, white part only, sliced thin and washed well

Marinade

3 tablespoons extra-virgin olive oil

2 tablespoons low-sodium shoyu

2 tablespoons fresh lemon juice

2 tablespoons mirin

2 garlic cloves, minced

2 quarter-sized pieces fresh ginger, peeled and minced

1. Wash and pat the swordfish dry. Combine the marinade ingredients and place the swordfish and marinade in a glass or ceramic dish. Marinate 1 hour in the refrigerator, turning several times.

2. Light a charcoal fire in an open grill 45 minutes before cooking, or preheat the broiler 15 minutes before cooking.

3. Remove the fish from the marinade and set aside. Pour the marinade into a large skillet and heat. Add the leeks and red pepper and sauté for 15 minutes, or until tender.

4. After the vegetables have sautéed for 5 minutes, place the swordfish over white coals or under the boiler, 4 to 6 inches from heat. Cook 4 to 5 minutes on each side, or until the flesh is opaque throughout and flakes easily.

5. Place the swordfish on serving plates and top with the braised red peppers and leeks.

Fish Teriyaki

The teriyaki sauce in this recipe can also be used with chicken or tofu. If you are using wooden skewers, be sure to soak them in water first to prevent them from scorching.

Makes 4 servings

Teriyaki Sauce

¼ cup tamari
¼ cup dry sherry
1 tablespoon maple syrup
1 tablespoon sesame oil
1 tablespoon grated fresh ginger
2 garlic cloves, put through a press

2 pounds salmon or tuna steaks
Oil
Lemon wedges

1. Combine the ingredients for the sauce
2. Place the fish in a glass or ceramic dish, pour the marinade over, and marinate in the refrigerator for 2 hours.
3. Light a hardwood fire in an open grill or preheat the broiler.
4. Remove the fish from the marinade and transfer to a plate.
5. Grill the fish over white coals (or under the broiler), basting with marinade, for 3 to 4 minutes. Turn and grill, basting again, for another 3 to 4 minutes. Do not overcook.
6. Any leftover marinade can be reheated and served with the fish. Garnish with lemon wedges.

Sesame Tuna on a Bed of Wilted Greens

Thinly sliced marinated tuna rests atop a bed of greens, creating a subtle combination of tastes and textures. Because strips of tuna are used, it is also a less costly way to enjoy this fabulous fish. Serve any leftovers in a whole-wheat sourdough roll for the ultimate in tuna sandwiches.

Makes 4 to 6 servings

Marinade

2 tablespoons white miso
Juice of ½ lemon
Juice of ½ orange
3 tablespoons sesame oil
2 tablespoons extra-virgin olive oil
1 heaping tablespoon minced fresh ginger
2 garlic cloves, minced

2 pounds fresh tuna, sliced into ½-inch strips
⅓ cup sesame seeds
3 tablespoons minced fresh parsley

Dressing

3 tablespoons extra-virgin olive oil
1 tablespoon balsamic vinegar
2 teaspoons grainy mustard
¼ teaspoon sea salt
⅛ teaspoon ground pepper

6 cups assorted greens such as spinach, radicchio, chicory, and arugula

1. Place all the marinade ingredients in a glass jar with a lid. Shake well. One hour before eating, place the tuna strips in a ceramic or glass dish, cover with the marinade, and place in the refrigerator. Turn several times to recoat.
2. Light a charcoal fire in an open grill about 45 minutes before cooking tuna, or preheat a broiler 15 minutes before cooking.
3. Toast the sesame seeds by stirring them in a dry skillet over medium heat until lightly browned. Grind the sesame seeds in a blender or food processor to make a coarse powder. (Do not overgrind.) Place on a flat plate and mix in the parsley.
4. Remove the tuna from the marinade and place 4 to 6 inches from heat in the broiler or on the grill. Cook for 2 minutes on each side, or until the flesh is white except for a hint of pink in the middle.

5. Place the dressing ingredients in a small saucepan and warm over low heat. Toss the greens with the dressing until the greens become slightly wilted and softened. Place on individual serving plates.

6. When the tuna is done, roll it in the sesame-parsley mixture. Arrange the tuna pieces on the beds of greens and serve immediately.

Bouillabaisse

Our version of bouillabaisse is a richly flavorful and easy way to incorporate seafood into a meal. The orange peel and honey are typical ingredients from the south of France. This dish can be made in advance up to the point of adding the fish, then be refrigerated or frozen. In fact, it is best left to "settle" a day or so ahead of when you plan to serve it. The white fish can be any variety of firm, white-fleshed fish: scrod, pollack, hake, and cusk are all good, relatively inexpensive choices. The mussels, clams, and shrimp are optional. Serve with French bread and a salad.

Makes 6 first-course servings or 4 main-course servings

1 ounce dried black mushrooms
1½ cups boiling water
3 tablespoons extra-virgin olive oil
3 garlic cloves, minced
2 large onions, diced
2 red bell peppers, cored, seeded, and diced
1 tablespoon dried basil
1 tablespoon honey
1 tablespoon dried orange peel
3 tablespoons tomato paste
4 large tomatoes, peeled (see page 166), seeded, and diced, plus 1 cup tomato juice, or 1 pound canned tomatoes with juice
1 cup dry white wine
1 cup fish stock or bottled clam juice
2 cups water
1½ pounds firm white-fleshed fish such as monkfish, scrod, hake, or cusk
1 pound shrimp, mussels, or clams in the shell (optional)

Sea salt and freshly ground pepper to taste
3 tablespoons chopped fresh parsley
3 tablespoons chopped fresh basil

1. Rinse the mushrooms well to remove the grit. Soak the mushrooms in boiling water in a medium bowl for 20 minutes. Strain and reserve the liquid. Chop the mushrooms and set them aside.

2. Heat the oil in a large soup pot over medium heat. Add the garlic and onions. Sauté over medium heat until they are translucent, about 10 minutes.

3. Add the chopped mushrooms, peppers, dried basil, honey, and orange peel to the onion-garlic mixture. Sauté for 10 minutes, stirring frequently.

4. Add the tomato paste, blend well, and sauté for 2 minutes, stirring. Add the tomatoes and juice or canned tomatoes and liquid. Simmer for 5 minutes. Add the wine, fish stock, or clam juice, water, and reserved mushroom liquid. Bring to a boil, reduce heat, and simmer, uncovered, for 30 minutes.

5. Bring the broth to a high simmer. Add the fish and shellfish if using and cook for 5 minutes, or until the fish is opaque. Season to taste. Place in bowls and garnish with parsley and basil.

Simple and Savory Winter Fish Stew

This is a Mediterranean-style fish stew using lots of tomatoes and garlic. The base of the stew can be made in advance and either refrigerated or frozen. Look for cut-up pieces of tuna, salmon, and swordfish, which are often available in seafood departments at very good prices. Serve with whole-wheat bread sticks and a green salad.

Makes 8 servings

1 28-ounce can plum tomatoes plus juice
2 tablespoons extra-virgin olive oil
2 onions, chopped
5 garlic cloves, minced
2 cups dry white wine*
3 tablespoons chopped fresh mixed basil, oregano, and thyme

4 cups water

2 cups fish stock or clam juice

$1/4$ to $1/2$ pound whole-wheat pasta shells

A few threads of saffron

2 pounds halibut, tuna, salmon, or shrimp, or a combination of white-fleshed fish such as scrod or cusk, cut into bite-sized cubes

Sea salt and freshly ground pepper

1. Drain and chop the tomatoes, reserving the juice, and set aside.

2. In a large soup pot, heat the olive oil and gently sauté the onions and garlic until translucent, about 5 minutes.

3. Add the wine, tomatoes, tomato juice, and herbs and continue sautéing for another 5 minutes.

4. Add the water and stock or clam juice and bring to a boil. Add the pasta and saffron and gently simmer for 5 to 8 minutes.

5. Add the fish and gently simmer, covered, for 10 minutes. Season with salt and pepper to taste and serve.

* **Once the wine boils, most of its alcohol content evaporates.**

Curried Shrimp with Pineapple

Curry, ginger, garlic, and pineapple combine in this easy "flash-in-the-pan" recipe to create an unusual and exotic meal. Brown rice is the perfect bed for this dish.

Makes 4 servings

$1^1/4$ pounds shrimp, shelled and deveined

1 teaspoon sea salt

Juice of 1 lime

1 tablespoon butter

2 tablespoons canola oil

3 small onions, coarsely chopped

3 garlic cloves, minced

2 quarter-sized pieces fresh ginger, peeled and minced

1 to 2 tablespoons curry powder to taste

3 large tomatoes, chopped, plus 1 cup tomato juice, or 1 14-ounce can tomatoes plus juice

1 cup fresh or frozen peas

$1^1/2$ cups canned cubed pineapple plus $1/4$ cup juice

1. Sprinkle the shrimp with the salt and lime juice and set aside.

2. Heat the butter and canola oil in large skillet. Add the onions, garlic, and ginger. Cook over medium heat, stirring often, until the onions are translucent, about 5 minutes.

3. Add the curry powder, stir well, and continue to sauté the mixture for 3 more minutes, stirring frequently.

4. Add the tomatoes and juice, peas, and pineapple juice. Stir, cover, and let simmer for 15 minutes, stirring occasionally.

5. Uncover the skillet and add the pineapple and shrimp. Stir well and cook over medium heat for 3 to 5 minutes, or until the shrimp turns pink. Serve immediately.

Baked Scrod with Tomato-Basil Sauce

This recipe couldn't be simpler or more delicious. Serve with a grain and a green salad for a complete meal.

Makes 4 servings

2 tablespoons olive oil

2 pounds scrod, cut into 4 serving pieces

Sauce

2 cups chopped fresh basil

3 large garlic cloves, chopped

$1/2$ teaspoon sea salt

$1/4$ teaspoon ground pepper

$1/8$ teaspoon cayenne pepper

2 tablespoons extra-virgin olive oil

2 tablespoons red wine vinegar

2 cups minced plum tomatoes

1. Preheat the oven to 400°F.

2. Sprinkle the olive oil over the bottom of an ovenproof casserole large enough to hold the fish. Place the fish on top of the oil.

3. Place the basil, garlic, salt, pepper, cayenne, olive oil, and vinegar in a blender or food processor. Purée for 10 seconds. Add the tomatoes and blend until the tomatoes are chopped but not puréed.

4. Spoon the sauce over the fish, cover, and bake for 15 to 20 minutes, or until the flesh is opaque and flakes easily.

Caribbean Seafood Marinade

The foods of the Caribbean are an exotic blend of flavors from all over the world. In this recipe, Central American mangoes combine with Asian ginger and tamari to create an exotic and mouthwatering marinade. This marinade works well with the full flavor of either tuna or shark. Small, kebab-sized pieces of fish can also be marinated and sautéed instead of cooked on the grill.

Makes 4 generous servings

Marinade

2 garlic cloves, minced
1 tablespoon peeled and minced fresh ginger
1/4 cup minced fresh cilantro
2 tablespoons tamari
1/4 cup fresh lime juice
1/3 cup extra-virgin olive oil
1 tablespoon prepared mustard
2 mangoes, peeled and sliced
2 pounds tuna or shark steaks

1. Place all the marinade ingredients in a large glass jar with a lid and shake well. Place the mangoes in a blender or food processor and purée to a coarse consistency; some tiny chunks of mango should remain. Mix the mango purée with the marinade in a glass or ceramic dish just large enough to hold the fish.

2. Place the fish in the marinade and turn several times to coat. Cover the fish with the marinade and place in the refrigerator for 45 minutes. Do not marinate longer or the fish will begin to "cook" in the acidic ingredients of the marinade.

3. If grilling, light a hardwood fire 45 minutes before serving. If broiling, preheat the broiler 15 minutes before cooking the fish.

4. Remove the fish from the marinade and place the marinade in a small saucepan. Gently warm over low heat. (If sautéing fish, add the fish along with the marinade to a large skillet and cook until done, about 10 minutes.)

5. Place the fish over white coals or under the broiler. Cook approximately 5 minutes on each side, or until the fish is opaque throughout and flakes easily with a fork.

6. Place the fish on plates or a serving platter. Spoon a bit of the warmed marinade over the fish and serve immediately.

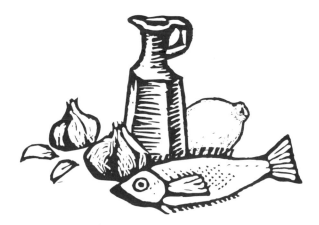

MEATS & POULTRY

Lamb Stew

This recipe shows off the remarkable flavor of naturally raised lamb. Serve with wild rice and homemade applesauce. This recipe freezes well.

Makes 6 servings

2 pounds leg of lamb, naturally raised
1 cup whole-wheat pastry flour
$^1/_4$ teaspoon ground pepper
$^1/_4$ teaspoon sea salt
$^1/_8$ teaspoon ground allspice
5 tablespoons extra-virgin olive oil
10 small boiling onions, peeled and left whole
5 whole cloves
5 garlic cloves, smashed and peeled
2 large carrots, scrubbed and cut into $1^1/_2$-inch chunks
2 tomatoes, peeled (see page 166), seeded, and chopped coarsely
2 fresh rosemary sprigs
6 small Yellow Finn, Yukon Gold, or red potatoes, halved
$1^1/_2$ cups dry red wine

$^1/_2$ cup water or broth (optional)

1. Cut the lamb into 1-inch pieces.
2. In a brown paper bag, combine the flour, pepper, salt, and allspice. Dredge the meat in this mixture by shaking 10 pieces of it at a time in the paper bag with the flour. Set aside each batch and repeat.
3. Preheat the oven to 350°F.
4. Heat 4 tablespoons of the oil in a large Dutch oven. Brown the meat evenly in 2 to 3 batches, removing each batch to a plate lined with paper towels.
5. Stud 5 of the onions with a clove. In the Dutch oven, sauté the clove-studded onions, garlic, and carrot chunks for 5 minutes. Add the tomatoes and rosemary sprigs and continue to cook for another 5 minutes. Add the potatoes, wine, water or broth (if using), and meat. Bring to a boil, reduce heat, cover, and cook on top of the stove for 15 minutes over medium-high heat. Place the Dutch oven on the lower rack in the preheated oven and cook the food for 30 minutes, or until the meat is tender, the potatoes are cooked, and a sauce has formed. (If water or stock is used, the sauce will be thinner.)
6. Test the meat for doneness and correct the seasoning.

Rib Roast of Beef with Parsnips and Potatoes

A succulent standing rib roast is a classic part of a holiday meal and makes any meal feel festive. This recipe is almost a meal in itself with the addition of root vegetables and yellow potatoes.

Makes 6 servings

1 head garlic, cloves separated and peeled
1 naturally raised beef rib roast (6 pounds with bones or 3 pounds boneless)
2 bay leaves
Salt and pepper to taste
3 carrots, scrubbed and diced into ¼-inch pieces
3 parsnips, scrubbed and diced into ¼-inch pieces
8 Yellow Finn, Yukon Gold, or red potatoes, quartered

1. Preheat the oven to 450°F.

2. Purée the garlic in a blender or food processor. Rub the purée over the surface of the roast.

3. Place the roast on a rack in a roasting pan filled with ¼ inch of water (if bone is in, place the bone side down in the pan). Place the bay leaves in the water.

4. Place the roast in the oven and reduce the heat to 325°F. Roast for 18 to 20 minutes per pound for a medium-rare roast (see Note). After 30 minutes of roasting, season with salt and pepper.

5. For the last 45 minutes of roasting time, add the vegetables and potatoes to the roasting pan, coating well with juices.

6. Allow the roast to rest at least 15 minutes before serving. Remove the vegetables to a separate warming plate and discard the bay leaves.

Note: Roasting times vary, so use a meat thermometer and remove the roast from the oven when the thermometer reads 150° to 160°F for medium rare to medium. Make a slit halfway through the roast to test for doneness, then push the roast together and roast for a while longer if necessary until the meat is the desired doneness.

Fajitas

Fajitas are a good way to make a little bit of meat go a long way. Here sirloin shares the stage with vegetables. Serve with fresh tortillas and guacamole.

Makes 6 servings

2 pounds naturally raised beef sirloin

Marinade

⅓ cup fresh lime juice
⅓ cup fresh lemon juice
¼ cup low-sodium shoyu
1 cup vegetable stock
2 serrano or jalapeño chilies, sliced (with seeds)
¼ teaspoon sea salt
1 teaspoon paprika or ground achiote
3 garlic cloves, smashed

3 tablespoons canola, safflower, or olive oil
1 medium green bell pepper, cored, seeded, and cut into strips ½ inch wide
1 medium onion, sliced into crescents ½ inch wide
2 medium tomatoes, cut into wedges
Fresh tortillas
Guacamole (optional)
Salsa (optional)

1. Cut the steak into thin strips about ⅛ inch thick and 2 inches long (putting the steak in the freezer until it is very cold, but not frozen solid, makes it easier to cut). Place it in a glass or ceramic container just large enough to hold the meat. Combine the marinade ingredients and pour over the meat. Cover and marinate in the refrigerator for 2 hours.

2. Heat a cast-iron skillet to very hot. Add 1 tablespoon of the oil and sauté the green peppers and onion over high heat for 3 minutes. Add the tomato wedges and cook 1 minute more. Remove the vegetables to a platter.

3. Remove the meat from the marinade with a slotted spoon and place on a plate.

Chili Peppers

The appearance of chili peppers in more and more produce departments attests to their popularity in enhancing many dishes with their hot spiciness. When combined correctly with complementary and balancing seasonings, chili peppers can add just the right excitement to a wide variety of ethnically inspired foods.

Handling Chili Peppers Because of the volatile oils in chilies, it is recommended that you handle them with care. Always wash your hands, knife, and cutting board well after cutting chilies. Be sure not to rub your eyes while chili pepper juice is on your hands. Should you get some of this hot stuff on your skin, apply a bit of flour to draw out the heat, then wash the area with soapy water.

To Check Hotness Slice off the top of the chili pepper and rub the cut surface with your finger. Delicately touch your finger to your tongue. If it does not seem too hot, cut off a little piece and taste. Adjust the amount of chili used in the recipe to personal taste.

Nutritional Value All chili peppers are a rich source of vitamins A and C, having more of both than oranges, lemons, or grapefruits.

The Anaheim Chili This chili is approximately 6 inches long and 1½ inches wide, and is relatively flat. It has a mildly hot flavor. A medium green or red color when fresh, it ripens to a dark red.

When fresh, the Anaheim is often roasted and peeled to make *chiles rellenos,* and diced into soups, stews, or vegetable casseroles. Anaheims are also good roasted, peeled, cut into strips, and tossed with olive oil, garlic, and a touch of salt.

Dried Anaheims are ground and added to dishes as a seasoning or soaked and made into tasty sauces.

Cayenne Chilies Cayenne chilies are about 3 inches long and ⅜ inch wide.

They are widely available and can be used in place of jalapeño, serrano, and habañero chilies if necessary.

Poblano Chilies Poblanos have a wavy triangular shape, which varies in size; a typical poblano is 5 inches long and 5 inches wide at the top and center, tapering to a point. They are a shiny, very dark green and have a rich flavor that ranges from mild to medium hot.

Poblanos are delicious with cheese and corn, and are used in chilies rellenos. They are roasted and peeled before use and can therefore be prepared ahead of time and stored in the freezer.

Guero Chilies These chilies are pale yellow and average 4 to 5 inches in length and 1 inch in width. They are hot or very hot.

Gueros are used in salads after being toasted and skinned; they can be used in stews without skinning.

Habañero Chilies These lantern-shaped chilies are light green to bright orange with a smooth surface. They are extremely hot.

Habañeros can be used in sauces for beans and pork, and in tomato sauces.

Jalapeño Chilies These chilies are about 3 inches long and range in width from ¾ inch to 1½ inches. Jalapeños are bright green when fresh and scarlet when dried. They are hot to fiery in taste.

Fresh jalapeños are minced and added to salsas, soups, guacamole, vegetable dishes, egg dishes, and almost any dish that needs a bit of zip.

Serrano Chilies Serranos are about 1½ inches long and about ½ inch in diameter. They usually have pointed ends and are bright green in color. These little chilies pack a big punch; their flavor is very hot to fiery, and they are somewhat sharper in taste than jalapeños.

The serrano chili pepper is usually used in its fresh, green state, minced or sliced crosswise into thin rounds and added to salsas, sauces, and vegetable dishes or used as a garnish.

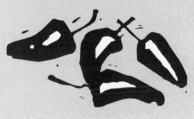

4. Add the remaining oil to the skillet and heat until very hot but not smoking. Add the meat and sauté over high heat for about 5 minutes, or until the meat is browned. Remove the meat from the skillet and place it on a platter with the vegetables.

5. Pour the marinade into the skillet and heat through. Pour over the vegetables and meat and serve sizzling hot. To serve, place meat and vegetables in warmed fresh tortillas and serve with guacamole and salsa if desired.

Grilled Indian Chicken

Serve with basmati rice, grilled red peppers, and a crisp green salad. Leftovers make a delicious salad with chopped celery, apple, and shredded lettuce.

Makes 4 servings

2 pounds boneless, skinless chicken breasts

Marinade

1 cup plain low-fat yogurt
1 teaspoon turmeric
1 teaspoon paprika
$1/4$ teaspoon ground cardamom
1 tablespoon fresh lemon juice
2 tablespoons fresh lime juice
2 tablespoons extra-virgin olive oil
1 tablespoon finely grated ginger
4 large garlic cloves, minced
$1/2$ teaspoon ground cumin
4 scallions, greens included, minced
$1/4$ teaspoon sea salt
White pepper to taste

Lemon or lime wedges for garnish

1. Cut skinless chicken breasts into 1-inch pieces. Place in a medium bowl.

2. In another bowl, combine the yogurt, turmeric, paprika, cardamom, lemon and lime juices, olive oil, ginger, garlic, cumin, scallions, salt, and pepper. Pour the marinade over the cubed chicken and mix well with your hands to coat the pieces

evenly. Marinate in the refrigerator for 2 hours.

3. Thread the chicken onto skewers and cook over a medium-hot fire for 5 to 7 minutes, turning frequently. Baste the chicken with leftover marinade after turning.

4. Serve with the lemon or lime wedges.

Variation: This recipe may also be made with 4 pounds of cut-up chicken pieces. If using chicken pieces, cut a few slits in the skin of each piece and place the pieces in a bowl that is large enough to accommodate them. If you prefer, skin the chicken pieces and prick the flesh to allow the marinade to penetrate. Marinate in refrigerator for 4 hours.

When using chicken pieces, cook bone-side down over a medium-hot fire for 15 minutes, covered. Baste the uncooked side with a little of the leftover marinade, turn, and cook about another 10 to 15 minutes. Serve with the lemon or lime wedges.

Whole Roasted Chicken

Makes 4 servings

1 $3^{1}/2$- to 4-pound roasting chicken
2 teaspoons tamari
1 bunch fresh rosemary or thyme
1 lemon, cut into quarters

1. Preheat the oven to 425°F.

2. Wash off the chicken, trim excess fat from the cavity area, and dry the exterior.

3. Rub the skin of the chicken with tamari and place it on a rack in a roasting pan that will accommodate the rack well.

4. Place the bunch of rosemary or thyme and the quartered lemon pieces inside the chicken cavity.

5. Place the pan in the oven and immediately turn the heat down to 350°F. Cook approximately 15 to 20 minutes per pound, or until the juices run clear from the leg when pierced.

6. Remove from the oven and let rest for 15 minutes before carving. The meat should be tender and juicy. Serve with whole-grain rice, quinoa, or roasted potatoes and a green salad.

Leftover Turkey Ideas

Variations on a turkey sandwich theme:
- Place cooked turkey on a bed of Country Corn Bread Stuffing (see page 217)
- Serve cooked turkey with Cranberry Chutney (see page 213) on sourdough bread
- Combine cooked turkey with leftover Fruits of the Fall Wild Rice (see page 200) for a turkey–wild rice salad

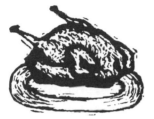

Turkey Noodle Soup

Many people have a ritual of making turkey soup the day after Thanksgiving. Try this easy recipe, which fits in well with a relaxed day around the house. The simmering stock will fill your home with its hearty fragrance.

Makes 8 to 10 servings

Stock

Carcass from a 12- to 16-pound turkey, skin and fat removed
3 celery stalks, cut into quarters
2 carrots, scrubbed and cut into quarters
1 unpeeled onion, cut into quarters

Turkey Talk

Naturally raised turkeys are especially moist and flavorful, but as with all turkeys, care should be taken to keep the bird moist and juicy until it reaches your table. Here are some tips and cooking instructions that will help ensure the most delectable turkey you've ever had.

Turkey Tips Plan on ³/₄ to 1 pound per person for turkeys weighing 12 pounds or less, and ¹/₂ to ³/₄ pound for turkeys weighing more than 12 pounds. If you want leftovers, plan on 1¹/₄ pounds of turkey per person. A nice touch is to send guests home with all the fixings for turkey sandwiches.

You should not partially roast a turkey one day and finish roasting it the next. Interrupted cooking enhances the chance of bacterial growth. For the same reason, do not stuff the bird until right before you're ready to put it in the oven. Remove stuffing after the bird has finished cooking.

Cooking Instructions

1. Preheat the oven to 425°F.
2. Rinse the completely defrosted (if frozen) turkey with warm water and pat dry. Stuff and truss.
3. Cut cheesecloth to a length that will cover the turkey and unfold to a single thickness.
4. Melt ¹/₂ cup (1 stick) butter or olive oil in a small saucepan and add ¹/₂ teaspoon each crumbled dried sage, thyme, marjoram, and rosemary.

Place the cheesecloth in the pan and completely saturate it

5. Place the turkey breast-side up on a rack in a shallow roasting pan. Add ¹/₄ inch water and 1 quartered onion to the roasting pan.
6. Place the turkey in the oven and turn the heat down to 325°F. After 10 minutes, drape the butter-soaked cheesecloth over the bird so that it is completely covered (don't forget the wings). After an hour, baste the turkey every 30 minutes or so to keep the cheesecloth moist. Remove the cheesecloth for the last 30 minutes of cooking time for a crisp skin.
7. Allow turkey to sit for at least 20 minutes before carving.

Cooking Times

Up to 10 pounds	20 minutes per pound
10–14 pounds	18 minutes per pound
14–16 pounds	15 minutes per pound

Add at least 30 minutes of cooking time for a stuffed bird.

The turkey is done when the drumsticks move slightly in their joints, or a meat thermometer inserted into the center of the thigh (take care not to touch the bone) reads 180° to 185°F.

2 garlic cloves, cut in half
1 bay leaf
10 peppercorns
2 parsley sprigs
10 to 12 cups water

1 8-ounce package udon noodles, broken in
  half and cooked*
3 carrots, scrubbed, cut into thin strips, and
  steamed until tender
Sea salt and freshly ground white pepper to
  taste

1. If the carcass is too large for the soup pot, break it into pieces and place it in the pot. Cover with water. Add the remaining stock ingredients. Bring to a boil and reduce to a simmer. (It is important not to cook the broth above a simmer after this point. If it is allowed to boil, it will become cloudy and greasy.) Skim off the fat and foam that come to the surface. Add additional cold water if necessary to keep the bones submerged in the liquid.

2. After 2 hours, remove the carcass and, when cool enough, pick off any pieces of meat that still remain. Reserve the meat and discard the carcass.

3. Strain the stock and discard the vegetables and seasonings. Place the strained stock in the refrigerator for several hours, or until the fat rises to the surface. Skim off the fat and discard.

4. Place the stock in a large soup pot. Add the turkey meat, noodles, carrots, and salt and white pepper. Simmer for 10 minutes and serve.

* **Cook noodles separately, to keep soup from getting cloudy and starchy.**

Ground Turkey Loaf

Ground turkey is becoming a familiar item in meat cases. It is extremely low in fat (only 5 to 6 percent), is lower in cholesterol than ground beef, and has a light taste and color that appeal to many people who do not (or cannot) eat red meat. Here you have the homey comfort of "meat" loaf with less fat and cholesterol than the traditional dish. Serve this with Creamy Mushroom Sauce (see page 212).

Makes 4 to 6 servings

1⅓ pounds ground naturally raised turkey
¼ cup minced onion
¾ cup bread crumbs
2 egg whites, or 1 whole egg
½ teaspoon ground white pepper
¼ cup minced celery
¼ cup low-fat milk or soy milk
1 teaspoon sea salt
1 minced garlic clove
3 tablespoons chopped fresh parsley

1. Preheat the oven to 350°F.

2. Mix all the ingredients well. Form into a loaf and pack into lightly oiled 8-by-4-inch baking pan. Bake for approximately 45 minutes, or until the loaf begins to pull away from the pan.

3. Remove from the oven and let sit for several minutes before cutting.

◆ **Variation:** This recipe can also be cooked in a pie plate to make "turkey pie."

Lemon Chicken

The rich flavor of free-range chicken makes this easy dish elegant. When you start with chicken that has such taste advantages, there is not much you need to do to make a meal special. Many people who have tasted free-range chicken say that it reminds them of what chicken tasted like before it became such an industrialized product.

Serve over basmati or wild rice or noodles and with stir-fried carrots for a balanced and colorful meal.

Makes 4 generous servings

1 teaspoon sea salt
¼ teaspoon ground pepper
½ cup unbleached all-purpose flour
2 pounds free-range chicken breasts, halved,
  skinned, boned, and pounded to a ¼-inch
  thickness

2 tablespoons butter
1 tablespoon canola oil
$\frac{1}{4}$ cup dry white wine
$\frac{1}{4}$ cup fresh lemon juice
1 tablespoon butter
2 tablespoons minced fresh parsley
1 lemon, thinly sliced

1. Mix the salt and pepper into the flour. Dredge the chicken pieces in the flour. Shake off the excess flour and set aside.

2. In a large skillet, melt the butter with the oil over medium heat. Sauté the chicken breasts until lightly browned, about 3 minutes per side. Remove from the pan and place on paper towels, turning once to absorb excess oil.

3. Combine the wine and lemon juice and pour into the skillet. Bring to a boil and scrape down any bits of chicken stuck to the sides of the pan. Add the chicken pieces and simmer in the liquid for 5 minutes. Remove to a heated platter.

4. Raise the heat to high, bring the liquid in the pan to a boil, and reduce the liquid to $\frac{1}{4}$ cup. Whisk in the butter and pour over the chicken. Garnish with parsley and lemon slices.

Chicken Almond Ding

Don't let the list of ingredients intimidate you; stir-frying is a quick and easy way to put together a meal. The tenderness of the chicken and the delectable sauce created in this recipe will make this meal a favorite one. Serve over brown rice.

Makes 6 servings

Marinade

3 tablespoons shoyu
3 tablespoons dry sherry or mirin
2 tablespoons Sucanat
3 garlic cloves, minced
2 tablespoons minced fresh ginger
1 tablespoon canola oil

$1\frac{1}{4}$ pounds chicken breast, skinned, boned, and cut into $\frac{1}{2}$-inch strips
3 tablespoons canola oil
3 cups broccoli florets
2 carrots, scrubbed and cut into julienne strips
$\frac{1}{4}$ pound mushrooms, cleaned and cut into $\frac{1}{4}$-inch slices
3 celery stalks, cut into $\frac{1}{4}$-inch diagonal slices
$\frac{1}{8}$ pound snow peas, trimmed
1 cup lightly toasted almonds*
2 tablespoons arrowroot dissolved in $\frac{1}{4}$ cup water
1 teaspoon Asian (toasted) sesame oil

1. In a medium glass or ceramic bowl, combine all the ingredients for the marinade. Add the chicken and let sit at room temperature for at least 15 minutes and up to an hour.

2. Meanwhile, heat a wok or large skillet. Add 1 tablespoon of the canola oil. Stir-fry the broccoli and carrots until they turn a bright color, 3 to 4 minutes. Remove and set aside.

3. Reheat the wok. Add 1 tablespoon of the canola oil. Stir-fry the mushrooms, celery, and snow peas for 2 to 3 minutes. Remove from the wok and set aside.

4. Reheat the wok. Add the remaining tablespoon of the canola oil. Remove the chicken from the marinade with a slotted spoon, add to the wok, and stir-fry until the chicken is opaque throughout, about 5 minutes. Add all the vegetables and the almonds, and stir to mix well. Re-dissolve the arrowroot well in the marinade mixture and pour into the wok. Stir and allow the mixture to thicken. Remove from the heat. Sprinkle with the toasted sesame oil. Serve immediately over brown rice.

* **To toast the almonds, place in a preheated 350°F oven for 8 to 10 minutes, or until lightly browned.**

Busy People's Stir-Fry

Marinate the meat before you go to bed, pick up the vegetables on your way home from work (it's particularly handy to get these vegetables already cut up at a salad bar) and once you set to work it will only be 20 minutes before the main course is ready.

Makes 6 servings

1¼ **pounds naturally raised beef flank steak**
¾ **cup teriyaki sauce (store-bought without preservatives, or make your own; see page 187)**
2 **tablespoons peanut oil**
½ **pound snow peas**
1 **pound cherry tomatoes, quartered**
½ **cup thinly sliced red onions**
¼ **cup chopped scallions**
1 **cup radish or mung bean sprouts**

1. Cut the flank steak lengthwise, with the grain of the meat, into 3 equal strips each approximately 1½ inches wide. Cut each strip across the grain into thin slices. Place in a glass or ceramic bowl. Pour the teriyaki sauce over and marinate overnight in the refrigerator.

2. Remove the meat from the marinade with a slotted spoon to a separate plate. Reserve the marinade. Heat a wok or skillet for 1 minute and add the oil. Swirl the oil in the hot wok to coat the sides. Add the meat and stir-fry for 3 minutes over high heat.

3. Add the snow peas, cherry tomatoes, red onions, and scallions and stir-fry for 1 minute. Add 2 tablespoons of the reserved marinade and heat through briefly. Add the sprouts and toss well to combine. Serve hot over Asian noodles or rice.

◆ **Variation:** Substitute blanched broccoli for the snow peas.

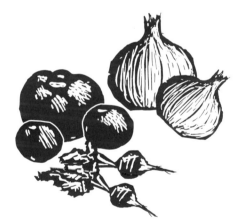

SIDE DISHES

Baked Barley

Barley takes well to baking, remaining firm and chewy. Baked barley can be enjoyed with seafood and chicken dishes, and leftovers can be turned into a hearty grain salad. Also try half barley and half brown rice, the "two immortal sons of heaven" of Vedic literature, in this recipe. Serve plain or with Creamy Mushroom Sauce (see page 212).

Makes 6 side dish servings

½ cup sunflower seeds
3 shallots, peeled and minced
1 onion, minced
1 leek, well-cleaned and thinly sliced
3 tablespoons butter or canola oil or
    combination
½ pound mushrooms, sliced
3 celery stalks, chopped
1 cup barley
1 teaspoon dried thyme
1 teaspoon dried rosemary
1 teaspoon dried marjoram
2 tablespoons tamari
3 cups boiling vegetable stock or water

1. Preheat the oven to 350°F. Toast the sunflower seeds in the oven for about 7 minutes, or until lightly browned; remove from the oven, leaving it at 350°F.

2. In a large skillet, sauté the shallots, onion, and leek in the butter or oil for 5 minutes over medium heat. Add the mushrooms, celery, sunflower seeds, barley, herbs, and tamari and continue sautéing for 5 more minutes, stirring frequently.

3. Add the vegetable stock or water to the barley mixture. Bring to a boil and transfer the mixture to a casserole dish. Bake, covered, for 1¼ hours.

◆ **Variation:** For a slightly sweet and fragrant variation, place the barley in a baking dish with boiling stock or water. Add 1 cinnamon stick, 2 whole cardamom pods, and a pinch of sea salt. Bake as above. Remove the cinnamon stick and cardamom pods before serving.

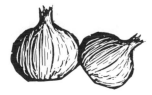

Fruits of the Fall Wild Rice

Apples, cider, sage, and wild rice: these are the tastes and textures of fall in New England. But this recipe transcends any season or place, blending the taste of wild rice with the sweet-tangy flavor of the apples and cider. Pecans bring just a touch of crunch, and the combination of wild rice and pecans makes this a complete-protein dish. Serve by itself with a green vegetable, or as an accompaniment to chicken, Cornish game hens, or game of any sort. This is a good dish for those new to wild rice or who find the flavor of wild rice too strong. See Variations for a scrumptious way to use this recipe with winter squash as a vegetarian entree.

Makes 6 side-dish servings

2³/₄ cups water
1 cup wild rice
3 tablespoons canola oil or butter
4 scallions, white and pale green parts only, roughly chopped
2 small, tart, firm apples, such as Macintosh, Granny Smith, or Cortland, cored and diced
1 cup pecans, lightly toasted and roughly chopped
¹/₄ teaspoon ground sage
¹/₄ teaspoon ground nutmeg
¹/₂ teaspoon sea salt
¹/₈ teaspoon freshly ground pepper
3 tablespoons apple cider or apple juice
Chopped scallions and chopped fresh parsley for garnish

1. Bring the water to a boil in a medium saucepan. Add the wild rice, return the water to a boil, and reduce to a simmer. Cook for 35 to 60 minutes. (The cooking time varies a great deal with wild rice. When done, it should be somewhat firm to the bite or *al dente*. Wild rice that is cooked too long will get mushy and lose a great deal of its flavor and appeal.)

2. Heat the oil or butter in a large skillet over medium heat. Add the scallions and sauté for 4 minutes. Add the apples, pecans, sage, nutmeg, salt, and pepper. Sauté for 5 minutes, stirring often. The apples should be soft but not mushy.

3. Add the cider or juice and sauté for 5 minutes. Add the cooked wild rice and continue sautéing for another 5 minutes. Sprinkle with scallions and parsley and serve.

◆ **Variations:**

• Bake 6 small, seeded acorn squash halves at 350°F for 45 minutes, cut-side down in a baking dish with ¹/₄ inch of water. Carefully remove the cooked flesh; place in a blender or food processor. Purée until the squash is smooth and creamy. Fill each acorn shell two-thirds full with the squash purée. Top each acorn squash with one-sixth of the wild rice mixture.

• Add cranberries to the apple-pecan mixture and sauté until the cranberries burst.

Saffron-scented Rice Pilaf with Parsley

Makes 8 servings

4 cups water or stock
$^1/_8$ teaspoon saffron, crushed
2 tablespoons extra-virgin olive oil or butter
1 shallot, minced
1 medium yellow onion, diced
2 cups long-grain brown rice
1 teaspoon sea salt
$^1/_2$ cup fresh parsley

1. Boil 1 cup of the water or broth and pour over the saffron. Set aside.

2. Heat the oil in a large saucepan. Sauté the shallot and onion over medium heat for about 5 minutes.

3. Add the rice and stir to coat all the grains. Cook over medium heat for about 5 minutes, stirring frequently.

4. Add the remaining 3 cups water or broth to the rice; add the saffron mixture and salt and bring to a boil. Reduce the heat to a simmer and cook, covered, for 45 to 60 minutes, or until all the water is absorbed.

5. Remove the cover, fluff the rice with a fork, fold in the parsley, and serve immediately.

Millet with Easy Curried Vegetables

Millet is a greatly underutilized grain, which goes well with the spicy flavor of curried vegetables. Millet is very easy to digest and lends a light nutty flavor to heartily flavored vegetable dishes.

Makes 8 servings

2 cups millet
2 tablespoons ghee (clarified butter) or light sesame oil
1 teaspoon whole cumin seeds
1 teaspoon brown mustard seeds
1 small onion, diced
$3^1/_2$ cups vegetable stock or water
$^1/_4$ teaspoon sea salt

1. Rinse the millet with water and set aside to drain.

2. Heat the ghee or oil in a $1^1/_2$- to 2-quart saucepan and add the cumin and mustard seeds. Sauté for 10 seconds, until the mixture is aromatic. Add the onion and sauté 5 minutes. Add the millet and sauté for another 5 minutes.

3. Bring the stock or water to a boil. Add the boiling liquid and the sea salt to the sautéed millet mixture. Reduce heat and simmer for 20 minutes, or until all the liquid is absorbed. Remove from heat and let rest for 10 minutes. Fluff with a fork and serve with Easy Curried Vegetables (see page 209).

Note: If you make this whole-grain millet dish ahead of time, reheat millet by steaming over boiling water.

Savory Grilled Polenta

This dish is great with grilled foods of all sorts, or as an accompaniment to bean dishes. The rich flavor of cornmeal that is *not* degerminated adds a wonderful nutty sweetness to this dish.

Makes 8 servings

5½ cups water
1 teaspoon sea salt
1½ cups polenta or yellow corn grits
Leaves from 4 or 5 sprigs of fresh thyme
¼ cup sun-dried tomatoes (dry pack), cut into
   ¼-inch pieces
Extra-virgin olive oil

1. Bring the water to a boil in a 2-quart saucepan. Add the salt. Gradually pour in the polenta, stirring constantly with a whisk. Add the thyme leaves and the sun-dried tomatoes. Continue to stir with a wooden spoon until the polenta begins to thicken. It will bubble and "heave." After about 20 minutes the polenta should be thick enough for the spoon to stand upright in it.

2. Pour the cooked polenta into an 8-by-8-inch Pyrex baking dish. Let cool completely. Placing the pan in the refrigerator speeds the cooling time.

3. When the polenta is completely cooled and firm, cut into 9 pieces. Brush the slabs with olive oil and grill for 5 minutes per side, to brown and heat through.

4. Serve with Tuscan Vegetable Stew (see page 203).

Note: If you do not have a grill, heat a large cast-iron skillet or pancake griddle. Add 2 to 3 tablespoons olive oil and fry the slabs until they are a bit crusty on both sides.

Quinoa, Corn, and Carrots

Makes 6 to 8 servings

2 cups water
1 cup quinoa
1 large carrot
1 ear corn
Pinch sea salt
Parsley for garnish
Butter (optional)
Freshly ground pepper

1. Wash the quinoa well and drain in a fine sieve. Set aside.

2. Bring the water to a boil in a small saucepan that has a tight-fitting lid.

3. Meanwhile, scrub and dice the carrot. Shuck the corn and cut the kernels off the cob.

4. When the water has come to a boil, add the salt, quinoa, carrot, and corn kernels and return to a boil. Reduce the heat, cover, and simmer for 15 to 20 minutes, until all the water is absorbed.

5. Serve hot, garnished with parsley, a dab of unsalted butter if desired, and lots of freshly ground pepper.

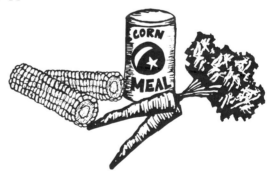

VEGETABLES

Tuscan Vegetable Stew

This recipe takes a bit of extra time to prepare but is well worth the effort. Make a large amount and have some on hand for the week. It can be served over Savory Grilled Polenta (see page 202) or any other grain, including brown rice, quinoa, and couscous. This recipe can also be frozen.

Makes 8 servings

1 medium eggplant, cut into ¹/₂-inch chunks
1 teaspoon sea salt
2 cups water
1 cup sun-dried tomatoes (dry pack)
2 red bell peppers, roasted, peeled, seeded, and chopped
4 tablespoons extra-virgin olive oil
1 large onion, chopped
5 garlic cloves, minced
3 6-inch zucchini, quartered lengthwise and cut into ¹/₂-inch chunks
3 tablespoons chopped fresh basil
3 tablespoons chopped fresh parsley

Sea salt and pepper to taste
2 tablespoons fresh lemon juice
Pecorino Romano cheese (optional)

1. Place the eggplant chunks in a non-aluminum colander or strainer, sprinkle with the salt, toss, and let drain for 30 to 60 minutes.

2. Bring 2 cups water to a boil. Place the sun-dried tomatoes in a Pyrex bowl and add the boiling water. Let soak for 10 minutes.

3. Roast the red peppers on a cookie sheet in a 400°F oven until their skins blacken and blister (about 30 minutes), turning them frequently. Place the blackened peppers in a paper bag to sweat for 10 minutes. Peel, seed, and chop the peppers.

4. Heat 1 tablespoon of the olive oil in a large skillet. Add the onion and garlic and sauté over medium heat for 10 minutes.

5. Drain the soaked tomatoes, reserving liquid. Chop roughly and add to the sautéing onion and garlic. Cook 5 minutes more. In blender or food processor, purée the onion-garlic-tomato mixture with the reserved soaking liquid and prepared, roasted red peppers. Set aside.

6. Wash and dry the skillet. Heat 1 more

203

tablespoon of the olive oil and quickly sauté the zucchini chunks for 5 minutes. They should be firm, slightly crunchy, and a bright green color. Remove from the pan to a plate.

7. Rinse the eggplant with water and gently squeeze out the excess moisture.

8. Heat the remaining 2 tablespoons of olive oil in the same skillet in which you sautéed the zucchini. Sauté the eggplant for 5 to 8 minutes to brown lightly.

9. Return the zucchini to the pan with the eggplant, add the onion-garlic-tomato–red pepper purée, basil, and parsley and bring to a gentle simmer. Cook for 10 minutes to allow the flavors to blend. Season with salt and pepper to taste and squeeze in the fresh lemon juice. Serve hot or at room temperature with grilled or pan-fried polenta slabs.

Note: If you are serving the sauce hot, a few gratings of Pecorino Romano cheese, that distinctive Italian sheep's milk cheese, is delicious.

Broccoli-Carrot Amandine

Makes 4 servings

1 bunch broccoli
3 carrots, scrubbed and cut diagonally into ¼-inch slices
1½ tablespoons butter
1 teaspoon low-sodium shoyu
2 teaspoons fresh lemon juice
½ cup whole almonds, lightly toasted* and roughly chopped

1. Cut the florets from the broccoli. Cut 2 inches off the bottom of the stalk. Peel the rest of the stalk and cut into thin slices on the diagonal.

2. Bring a large pot of water to a boil. Blanch the broccoli for 3 minutes. Remove with a slotted spoon. Add the carrots to the same water and blanch for 2 minutes. Remove.

3. In an 8- or 10-inch skillet, heat the butter. Add the broccoli and carrots and toss to coat with

butter. Place a cover on the skillet and steam the vegetables for 2 minutes.

4. Add shoyu, lemon juice, and almonds to the broccoli mixture. Sauté, stirring, for 1 minute and serve immediately.

* **To toast the almonds, place in a preheated 350°F oven for 8 to 10 minutes, or until lightly browned.**

Brussels Sprouts with Lemon-Mustard Sauce

Makes 4 servings

1 pound Brussels sprouts, prepared as described in box (opposite page)
¼ cup sesame seeds
1 tablespoon butter
2 tablespoon fresh lemon juice or mirin
2 teaspoons whole-grain mustard

1. Preheat the oven to 350°F.

2. Steam the sprouts over boiling water for about 8 minutes, or until they are tender but not soft.

3. While the sprouts are cooking, toast the sesame seeds in a dry pan, for about 5 minutes, shaking the pan frequently to keep them from scorching. Remove seeds from the pan and place in a bowl to cool.

4. Combine the Brussels sprouts, sesame seeds, butter, lemon juice, and mustard in a medium bowl and toss. Serve immediately.

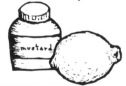

Herbs

If a recipe calls for fresh herbs, and they are not available to you, substitute with one-third the amount of dried herbs. Conversely, if a recipe calls for dried herbs and you have fresh herbs on hand, multiply the amount by three.

Brussels Sprouts

Brussels sprouts are a delectable vegetable that has had bad press. If cooked properly, they are sweet and slightly crunchy. Like broccoli and cauliflower, they are at their best in the fall after a frost or two.

Brussels sprouts are a good source of vitamins A and C, and of iron and potassium. They are part of the cruciferous family of vegetables, recommended by the American Cancer Society as having properties that may help to inhibit certain types of cancer. Other vegetables in this family are broccoli, cabbage, and cauliflower.

To prepare Brussels sprouts, slice off the woody part of the stem and remove the outer, coarser leaves. With a sharp paring knife, make an X in the remaining stem. Soak the Brussels sprouts in a large bowl of salted water for at least 30 minutes prior to cooking (this will get rid of bitterness and help with digestibility).

Confetti Cabbage

Napa or Chinese cabbage is mellower tasting than most other cabbages. Cooked as it is in this recipe it becomes very tender and mild, and is well complemented by an international cast of seasonings. Carrots and red peppers add color and extra nutrition.

Makes 4 servings

1 2-inch piece fresh ginger
1 2-pound (approximately) napa cabbage
2 tablespoons corn oil
1 small onion, cut into thin slices
1 large carrot, scrubbed and cut into julienne
    strips
1 large red or green bell pepper, cored, seeded,
    and cut into thin strips
1 tablespoon rice vinegar
$\frac{1}{2}$ teaspoon sea salt
Freshly ground white pepper
2 teaspoons honey
2 teaspoons whole-grain mustard

1. Peel and grate the ginger. Squeeze ginger pulp. You should get between 2 and 3 teaspoons of ginger juice; set aside.

2. Cut the base from the cabbage and separate the leaves. Rinse well and cut the thick stems from the leaves. Stack the leaves and cut them into thin strips.

3. Warm the oil in a large skillet. Add the cabbage, onion, carrot, and red pepper. Stir well, turn the heat to medium-high, and cook for 5 minutes.

4. Reduce the heat to medium and add the ginger juice, rice vinegar, sea salt, and pepper. Simmer, stirring often, for 5 minutes.

5. Add the honey and mustard and sauté, stirring, for 2 minutes. Serve immediately.

Spangled Spaghetti Squash

Spaghetti squash is a relative newcomer to the produce section, providing a different texture and taste than most winter squashes. Its flesh comes out in spaghettilike strands and has a delicate sweetness and mild crunch that complement many different seasonings. Spaghetti squash is a favorite with dieters, as a 3-ounce serving has only 20 calories. It contains a great deal of beta-carotene, which is recognized by both the National Cancer Institute and the American Cancer Society as an important dietary protection against certain types of cancer.

Here is an easy way to cook spaghetti squash: pierce the squash with a fork in several spots and bake in a preheated 350°F oven for about an hour, or until the outside is slightly soft to the touch. Once the squash is cooked, cut it in half and scoop out the seeds, or the squash will continue to cook and will become mushy. When the squash has cooled, use a fork to gently separate the strands of squash.

Makes 6 servings

1 spaghetti squash, about 3 pounds
2 tablespoons light sesame oil

1 tablespoon minced fresh ginger

2 garlic cloves, minced

6 plum tomatoes, peeled (see page 166), seeded, and roughly chopped, or 1 14-ounce can of tomatoes

$\frac{1}{2}$ teaspoon sea salt

$\frac{1}{4}$ teaspoon freshly ground white pepper

3 tablespoons minced fresh cilantro

1. Cook the spaghetti squash according to the above directions. Separate the strands of squash with a fork. Place the strands in a cheesecloth or a dish towel and squeeze to remove excess moisture. Set aside.

2. In a large skillet, warm the oil. Add the ginger and garlic, and sauté over low heat for 2 to 3 minutes, stirring often.

3. Add the spaghetti squash, tomatoes, salt, and pepper and mix well. Sauté for 5 minutes, crushing the tomatoes with the back of a wooden spoon so that they blend into the spaghetti squash.

4. Add the cilantro, mix well, sauté for 1 more minute, and serve. Any leftovers can be refrigerated and eaten as a salad the next day.

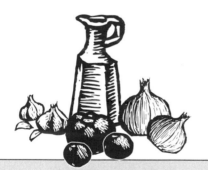

Sweet Potatoes

Sweet potatoes are loaded with beta-carotene and are delicious. Wash them in cold water and pat dry with a towel. Prick them with a fork a few times and bake in a preheated 400°F oven for about 30 to 35 minutes (they do not take as long as regular potatoes). You can eat them plain, or with a little butter, parsley, allspice, or salt and white pepper. Or try puréeing baked sweet potatoes with a little low-fat yogurt.

Greens with Garlic and Ginger

This recipe will make fans even of those who have never tried these remarkably nutritious vegetables. Serve leftovers in whole-wheat rolls for sandwiches.

Makes 4 servings

1$\frac{1}{2}$ pounds turnip greens, mustard greens, kale, or collard greens, roughly chopped

2 tablespoons light sesame oil, or 1 tablespoon canola oil and 1 tablespoon light sesame oil

3 garlic cloves, minced

1 tablespoon minced peeled fresh ginger

$\frac{1}{8}$ teaspoon red pepper flakes (optional)

$\frac{1}{4}$ cup water

1 tablespoon tamari

2 teaspoons maple syrup

Toasted sesame seeds* for garnish

1. Wash the greens very well (they tend to be sandy). If using kale or collard greens, steam them for 5 minutes prior to sautéing.

2. Heat the oil in a large skillet. Add the garlic, ginger, and red pepper flakes (if using). Cook over medium heat for 30 seconds, stirring often.

3. Add the greens and stir for 1 minute to blend. Add the water and continue to sauté, stirring, until the greens are completely wilted.

4. Combine the tamari and maple syrup. Add to the greens, stir, and sauté for 3 minutes. Remove the greens to a platter with a slotted spoon. Bring to a boil and reduce the liquid in the pan to a syrup; drizzle over the greens. Serve immediately, garnished with toasted sesame seeds.

◆ **Variation:** Add sliced radishes to the greens while they are sautéing.

* **To toast sesame seeds, stir in a dry pan over medium heat until lightly browned.**

Sautéed Spinach, Chard, or Beet Greens

Makes 4 servings

1 bunch fresh spinach, red or green chard, or
  beet greens
1 tablespoon extra-virgin olive oil or unsalted
  butter
1 garlic clove, minced
Water
Dash sea salt (optional)

1. Wash the greens well by plunging them into a large basin or bowl of cold water. Swish them around a bit to loosen any sand or dirt, which will sink to the bottom. Remove the leaves to a colander, drain the water and sand from the basin or bowl, and repeat. Remove the leaves to a colander.

2. Remove the stems from the greens and discard them or finely chop. Set aside. Chop the leaves coarsely and set aside.

3. Over medium heat, warm the olive oil or butter in a large, noncorrosive skillet that has a tight-fitting lid. Add the garlic and sauté 1 minute. Add the chopped stems if using, cover, and cook 2 minutes. Add the chopped leaves and toss to coat with the oil. If the pan seems dry, add 1 to 2 tablespoons water. Cover and cook for 5 minutes until the leaves are just wilted. They should still be bright green.

4. Sprinkle with a dash of salt if desired, stir gently to distribute, and serve hot or at room temperature.

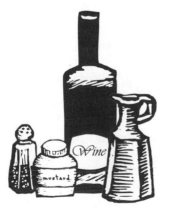

Colorful Coleslaw

Makes 8 to 10 servings

4 cups thinly shredded green cabbage
1½ cups thinly shredded red cabbage
1 cup carrot, finely grated
1 cup red bell pepper, minced
⅓ cup Vidalia or red onion, minced
2 tablespoons fresh dill, minced

Dressing No. 1: Tahini Dressing

4 tablespoons sesame tahini
4 tablespoons white wine or brown rice vinegar
2 tablespoons rice syrup
6 tablespoons water
½ teaspoon sea salt
2 teaspoons Dijon mustard
Freshly ground black pepper to taste

Dressing No. 2: Yogurt Cheese Dressing

2 cups Yogurt Cheese (see page 161)
2 tablespoons white wine or brown rice vinegar
3 tablespoons rice syrup
2 teaspoons Dijon mustard
½ teaspoon sea salt
Freshly ground black pepper to taste

1. Shred the cabbage and carrot for the salad using a sharp knife or food processor. Mince the red pepper, onion, and dill by hand. Place all prepared vegetables in a large bowl.

2. Whisk together the ingredients for the dressing of choice and pour over the salad vegetables, tossing gently but well. Your hands will work well. Serve immediately or refrigerate until ready to serve.

Winter Cooking Greens

When you crave something fresh and green in your winter diet, a crisp and verdant relief awaits you: "cooking greens" such as kale, chard, collards, and mustard greens. It is a handy coincidence that the flavors of these vegetables reach their height just as the fall vegetables have begun to fade and before spring brings new crops to fruition.

Nutrition Cooking greens are very high in beta-carotene and vitamin C and are full of potassium, calcium, fiber, and, in many instances, iron. Beta-carotene is the chemical precursor to vitamin A. The body stores beta-carotene and makes it into vitamin A on an as-needed basis. The National Cancer Institute recently stated that the risk of certain cancers (including lung cancer) can be decreased by as much as 40 percent when the diet is rich in beta-carotene.

Kale, mustard greens, and collards also belong to a family of vegetables called crucifers, which includes broccoli and cauliflower. Cruciferous vegetables contain certain compounds called indoles, which are believed to act as detoxifying agents that remove carcinogens from the body. The National Cancer Institute, the National Academy of Sciences, and the American Cancer Society all recommend plentiful amounts of cruciferous vegetables for their apparent ability to protect against cancer.

Culinary Uses Cooking greens are great down-home foods with strong personalities that complement foods with assertive flavors. Here are some basic suggestions and guidelines for preparing greens:

- 1 pound greens will serve 3 to 4 people as the vegetable portion of a meal.

- All greens should be well washed. Dip the amount you are going to use in a sink or bowl of cold water, and swish the greens around so that all sand and dirt falls to the bottom. For salads, spin or towel-dry well. Drying is unnecessary to prepare greens for braising, steaming, sautéing, or puréeing.

- Greens should be used within a few days of purchase. At home, wrap them in a damp towel, place them in a plastic bag with holes punched in it, and put them in the crisper drawer to keep them moist and vibrant.

- If the leaves are small, simply chop the green and use it stem and all. If the leaves are large, strip them from the stem first, because the stems will likely be tough.

Preparing Greens

- **Sauté** steamed greens in a small amount of olive oil with garlic, or try sautéing greens with ginger and tamari, roasted pine nuts and currants, hot peppers, or honey and mustard. Like spinach, sautéed kale is enhanced by a dash of nutmeg or caraway seeds.

- **Steam** chopped greens and add a squeeze of lemon juice before serving. Regardless of the cooking method, the "heartier" greens, such as kale and collards, should be steamed over boiling water first. Save the steaming water for soups or cooking grains. Following steaming, place the greens in a colander and squeeze out excess water.

- **Purée** combined greens (such as kale or mustard greens and green chard) to create a balanced flavor. Steam the greens first, squeeze out excess liquid, and purée in a blender or food processor. Serve plain or with a generous helping of freshly ground black pepper. Add the purée to grain and bean dishes, or to soups and casseroles for a rich, pungent flavor (puréed kale is traditionally added to many barley dishes in Scotland).

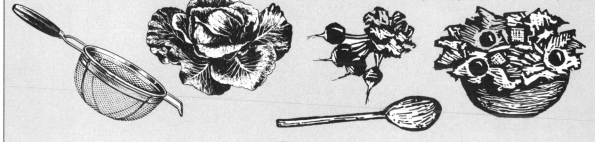

Broccoli-Udon Stir-Fry

The secret to great stir-fried noodles is to cook and chill them before adding them to the wok. Chilled noodles absorb less oil and have a better texture. Blanching the vegetables first keeps them crisp and colorful and makes the whole dish surprisingly light.

Makes 4 generous servings

1 8-ounce package udon noodles
1 small bunch broccoli
2 medium carrots, scrubbed and cut thinly on the diagonal
2 tablespoons peanut or canola oil
2 teaspoons light sesame oil
1 bunch scallions, minced
2 garlic cloves, minced
1 tablespoon minced fresh ginger
2 teaspoons umeboshi vinegar or rice vinegar
2 teaspoons mirin or fresh lemon juice
¼ cup toasted sesame seeds*

1. Cook the noodles according to the directions on the package (or see "Japanese Noodles," page 180). Rinse under cold water, drain well, and refrigerate.

2. Bring a large pot of salted water to a rolling boil. Cut the florets from the broccoli. Trim the bottom 2 inches of the stalk and discard. Peel the remaining stalk and cut thinly on the diagonal. Add the broccoli to the boiling water and blanch for 1 to 2 minutes, or until the broccoli turns bright green. With a slotted spoon, remove the broccoli from the water and run it under very cold water. Add the carrots to the boiling water and repeat the process. Drain the vegetables well and set aside. Use the water for stock or to cook grains.

3. Add 1 tablespoon of the peanut or canola oil and 1 teaspoon of the sesame oil to a hot wok or skillet. Immediately add the scallions, garlic, and ginger. Stir-fry for 30 seconds. Add the vegetables and continue to stir-fry for 3 to 4 minutes. Remove the mixture from the wok.

4. Reheat the wok. Add the remaining table-spoon of peanut or canola oil and the remaining teaspoon of sesame oil. Add the noodles and stir-fry for 2 minutes. Add the vegetables and mix well. Add the vinegar, mirin or lemon juice, and sesame seeds. Stir-fry for 1 to 2 minutes, or until all the ingredients are heated through; serve immediately.

◆ **Variation:** Add small cubes of marinated and baked tofu along with the vegetables.

* **To toast sesame seeds, stir in a dry skillet over medium heat until lightly browned.**

Easy Curried Vegetables

Make extra and place in pita sandwiches for brown bag lunches. Serve over millet (see page 201).

Makes 6 to 8 servings

6 small Yellow Finn or other potatoes
1 large yellow onion
1 to 2 tablespoons ghee (clarified butter),* unsalted butter, or canola oil
2 cups diced carrots
2 teaspoons curry powder or kuzu
½ teaspoon dry basil leaves, crushed
½ cup water or vegetable stock
2 cups plain low-fat yogurt
2 cups fresh or frozen peas
2 tablespoons arrowroot powder or kuzu dissolved in ¼ cup cold water
Sea salt to taste
Freshly ground black pepper
2 tablespoons chopped fresh cilantro for garnish

1. Peel the potatoes and cut into bite-sized pieces. Dice the onion.

2. Heat the ghee, unsalted butter, or canola oil in a large skillet. Add the onion and carrots and sauté over medium heat for 5 minutes. Add the potatoes, curry powder, and basil and sauté another 5 minutes.

3. Add the water, bring to a boil, and reduce heat

to low. Cover and cook for 10 to 15 minutes, until the potatoes are tender but not overcooked.

4. Stir in the yogurt and peas and heat through over low heat. When heated, add the dissolved arrowroot powder. Cook for a minute or two until thickened. Season to taste with salt and freshly ground black pepper. Serve hot, garnished with chopped cilantro. Or serve with toasted cashews over millet or in whole-wheat chapatis or pitas as a sandwich. Or serve with Millet with Easy Curried Vegetables (see page 201).

* **To clarify butter, melt it in a small pot over low heat, remove it from the heat, and let it stand until the milk solids have settled to the bottom. Carefully skim the clear butter from the top, and discard the solids.**

SAUCES & DRESSINGS

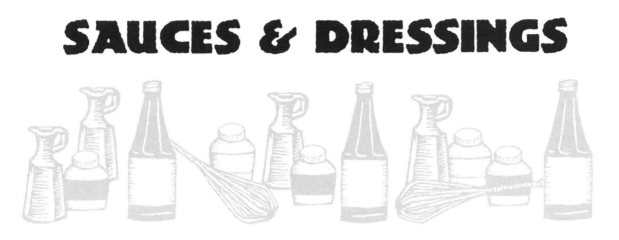

Miso-Tahini Sauce for Grains and Vegetables

This is a handy sauce, as it can dress up many different grains and vegetables. Steam some vegetables (like carrots and broccoli) and serve with miso-tahini sauce over whole-grain noodles for a filling and super-quick meal (soba or udon noodles are especially good). Remember to not let the miso come to a boil, as this will destroy its beneficial enzymes. The sauce will keep in the refrigerator for about a week.

Makes 1¼ cups

1 tablespoon sesame oil
4 scallions, white and pale green parts only, minced
½ cup tahini
1 tablespoon white miso
¾ cup water
½ teaspoon dried basil

1. Heat the oil in a medium saucepan. Add the scallions and sauté over medium heat until soft, about 5 minutes. Add the tahini and stir constantly until lightly toasted, about 3 to 5 minutes. Do not let the tahini burn. The tahini will have a light brown color and will give off a nutty aroma. Allow the mixture to cool for a few minutes.

2. Dissolve the miso well in the water and slowly pour into the tahini mixture, stirring constantly with a whisk.

3. Add the basil and allow the mixture to simmer for 5 minutes, stirring often, until thick and smooth.

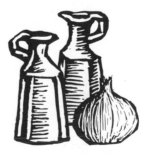

Creamy Mushroom Sauce

This easy-to-make sauce goes well with grain dishes and Ground Turkey Loaf (see page 196). If made with soy milk, it is cholesterol-free.

Makes about 3 cups

2 tablespoons canola oil
½ pound mushrooms, sliced
⅓ cup minced onion
1 garlic clove, minced
1 carrot, scrubbed well and cut into tiny dice
½ teaspoon dried thyme
2 scallions, thinly sliced
1 cup low-fat milk or soy milk
1 cup water or vegetable stock
2 tablespoons arrowroot
1 teaspoon tamari
Pinch of sea salt or vegetable seasoning salt
15 grinds fresh pepper

1. Warm the oil in a medium skillet.

2. Sauté the mushrooms over high heat for 4 minutes, or until they begin to "squeak." Lower the heat to medium and add the onion, garlic, and carrot; continue to sauté for another 4 minutes, or until the mushrooms are lightly browned and there is no liquid in the bottom of the pan.

3. Add the thyme and scallions and cook for 1 minute. Combine the milk or soy milk and water or stock. Add the arrowroot to the liquid and dissolve well. Pour the arrowroot mixture over the mushrooms and cook for 3 minutes, or until thickened. Season with the tamari, sea salt or vegetable seasoning salt, and pepper. Taste and adjust the seasoning.

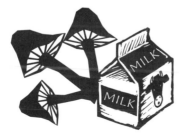

Pesto

Pesto is a summer favorite that makes use of the fresh basil available at this time of year. It is a rich indulgence, but a little goes a long way. Fresh cilantro or mint can be substituted for part of the basil.

Freezing pesto is a cinch and makes the warm and verdant days of August last all winter long. Once you've made the pesto, pour it into an ice cube tray. Once it is frozen, pop the pesto cubes into a plastic bag for later use on pasta, in soups and casseroles, over fish and chicken, and over grains.

Makes about 1½ cups

3 cups loosely packed fresh basil leaves
1 cup fresh parsley sprigs, stems removed
⅔ cup extra-virgin olive oil
¾ cup pine nuts, or ½ cup pine nuts and ¼ cup almonds
¼ cup freshly grated Parmesan cheese
¼ cup freshly grated Romano cheese
2 to 3 garlic cloves

1. Place the basil and parsley in a blender or food processor. Purée.

2. Add all other ingredients and process until the mixture is smooth and creamy.

Quick Cranberry Sauce

This recipe takes only minutes to make.

Makes 4 cups

1 12-ounce bag cranberries
½ cup apple cider
1 teaspoon minced orange zest
½ cup Sucanat

1. Place all the ingredients in a medium saucepan. Boil until the berries pop open (about 5 minutes).

2. Refrigerate for several hours before serving.

Cranberry Chutney

This chutney can be served on a smoked turkey sandwich, with grilled chicken, or as a relish for venison. It is a tangy accompaniment to plain grain dishes, especially wild rice dishes. Make extra to give as gifts.

Makes about 4 cups

¹/₃ cup molasses
¹/₃ cup barley malt syrup
¹/₃ cup white wine vinegar
1 teaspoon curry powder
1 teaspoon dry mustard
¹/₂ teaspoon each ground ginger, cloves, cinnamon, and allspice
1 12-ounce bag fresh cranberries
1¹/₂ cups fresh pineapple, coarsely chopped
¹/₂ cup raisins
1 cup toasted walnuts,* coarsely chopped

1. Place the molasses, barley malt, vinegar, and spices in a medium saucepan and bring to a boil. Reduce heat and simmer for 15 minutes.

2. Add the cranberries, pineapple, raisins, and walnuts and simmer for 30 minutes or until the cranberries have burst and are tender.

3. Refrigerate the mixture for several hours before serving.

* **To toast walnuts, bake in a preheated 350°F oven until lightly browned, 8 to 10 minutes.**

Cranberries

The bright color, high vitamin C content, and tangy taste of cranberries can be a tart addition to many dishes.

Buy cranberries in the fall and freeze them, whole and unwashed, for use throughout the year. It is easier to chop cranberries while they are frozen, so keep them this way until you are ready to use them.

Cranberries are low in calories (44 per cup) but usually need to be coaxed to an enjoyable flavor with a bit of sweetener.

Mellow Barbecue Sauce

Once you try this sauce, barbecues will never be the same. Use it to baste chicken, burgers, pork, and even tofu. Serve extra sauce on the side—this is so good it can be spread on bread or crackers.

Makes 1 cup (enough for 2 pounds of chicken, meat, or tofu)

2 tablespoons extra-virgin olive oil
1 large onion, diced
Pinch of sea salt
2 tablespoons tomato paste
1 tablespoon prepared mustard
1 teaspoon dry mustard
2 tablespoons blackstrap molasses
1 cup puréed tomatoes
1 tablespoon mirin
1 tablespoon sherry or balsamic vinegar
Pinch of cayenne pepper
Pinch of paprika

1. Heat the oil in a medium skillet. Add the onion and salt and sauté over medium heat for 5 minutes, or until the onion is translucent

2. Add the tomato paste, prepared mustard, dry mustard, and molasses. Sauté, stirring over medium heat for 4 to 5 minutes.

3. Add the tomatoes and bring to a boil. Lower heat and simmer for 15 minutes.

4. Remove the mixture from the heat and add the mirin and sherry or vinegar. Purée the sauce in a blender or food processor until slightly chunky in consistency.

5. Marinate whatever you are cooking in the barbecue sauce for at least 1 hour. Baste grilled foods the last 10 minutes of cooking time. Leftover sauce can be heated and served separately.

Hot tip! Mirin is great to use in all sorts of barbecue sauces and marinades. It adds a subtle sweetness and helps sauce stick to the food while grilling.

Egg-, Dairy-, and Vinegar-Free Curry Dressing

A zesty salad dressing for those who avoid mayonnaise or milk-based dressings because of milk allergies or a need to limit cholesterol. It has a variety of uses and can help toss a meal or side dish together in minutes.

Makes 1¼ cups, enough for 8 cups salad greens

1-inch piece fresh ginger
2 tablespoons extra-virgin olive oil
¼ cup grated onion
1 garlic clove, pressed
1 10-ounce package soft tofu, drained
2 tablespoons fresh lemon juice
1 teaspoon curry powder
1 teaspoon sea salt

1. Peel the ginger, grate it, and squeeze out the juice using a garlic press. Set aside.

2. Heat the olive oil in a small skillet over medium heat. Sauté the onion and garlic for 2 to 3 minutes; set aside.

3. In a blender or food processor, purée the tofu and lemon juice until creamy smooth.

4. Add the curry powder, salt, sautéed onion mixture, and ginger juice. Purée for 30 seconds.

5. Mix with the salad ingredients of your choice (see below) and refrigerate for 2 to 3 hours before serving.

- **Shrimp Salad**   Toss 2 cups cooked shrimp and 1 cup chopped celery with ½ cup dressing. Serve in avocado halves.
- **Pasta Salad**   Toss 3 cups cooked whole-grain pasta, 2 cups steamed sliced carrots, 2 cups steamed chopped broccoli, and 1 cup chopped red bell pepper with 1¼ cups dressing.
- **Sweet Potato Salad**   Steam 3 pounds whole unpeeled sweet potatoes over boiling water until the outer parts are soft and the centers are still firm, about 15 minutes (be sure not to overcook). Plunge into cold water to prevent overcooking once the potatoes are out of the pan. Peel, cube, and toss with 1¼ cups dressing. Garnish each serving with 1 teaspoon grated coconut and a sprinkle of ground cinnamon.

Barely Tangy Vinaigrette

This is a good, all-around vinaigrette which you can make up (doubling the recipe is a good idea) and use for all sorts of toss-together meals. This is where a really fine olive oil counts; its taste will make or break the results.

Use this dressing

- on green salads.
- in grain salads (toss with still-warm grains, along with a few slightly steamed vegetables, for a quick salad. You can add leftover pieces of chicken, fish, or tofu for extra protein, or toss with some toasted nuts).
- with warm beans along with some chopped onion, for a bean salad. Chopped celery, carrots, and other vegetables can be added.
- on potatoes as a healthier alternative to sour cream or butter.

Makes about ¾ cup

6 tablespoons extra-virgin olive oil
1 tablespoon balsamic vinegar
1 tablespoon orange juice
2 teaspoons whole-grain mustard
1 teaspoon maple syrup
1 garlic clove, minced
1 tablespoon minced fresh herbs (basil, dill, and marjoram work well)
Sea salt and freshly ground pepper to taste

1. Combine all the ingredients (a small glass jar is ideal for this) and mix well.

2. Store in the refrigerator up to 2 weeks.

Tofu Green Goddess Dressing

This creamy dressing has no cholesterol. It makes even the simplest salad something special and can liven up leftover grains.

Makes about 2 cups

½ pound silken tofu, crumbled
3 scallions, coarsely chopped
3 tablespoons olive oil
1 tablespoon prepared mustard
2 tablespoons fresh lemon juice
1 tablespoon rice vinegar
4 teaspoons white miso
3 tablespoons coarsely chopped fresh parsley
2 teaspoons rice syrup or honey
¼ to ⅓ cup water

1. Place all the ingredients except the water in a blender or food processor and purée. Slowly add ¼ cup of the water while the machine is running and blend until smooth (add more water if a thinner dressing is preferred).

2. Store up to 4 days in the refrigerator.

Yogurt Fruit Dressing

Yogurt's tanginess brings out the natural sweetness of many different fruits. Try kiwis in fruit salad—their bright emerald color does not fade, and they are exceptionally high in vitamin C. Peel them and then cut into half-moon shapes. Other good salad fruits are strawberries, bananas, grapes, and apple and pear slices. The combination of yogurt and fruit is great for breakfast, lunch, or as a low-calorie snack.

Makes enough for 6 fruit-salad servings

2 cups plain low-fat yogurt
1 teaspoon vanilla extract

2 tablespoons maple syrup
½ teaspoon ground cinnamon
Mint sprigs (optional)

1. Blend all the ingredients until smooth.

2. Serve over a selection of chilled fruit and garnish with mint, if you like.

Corn Relish

Makes 4 cups

4 ears sweet corn
1 small red onion, finely diced
1 red bell pepper, cored, seeded, and cut into small dice
4 tablespoons minced fresh cilantro
2 to 3 tablespoons fresh lime juice
1 tablespoon brown rice vinegar or other mild vinegar
1 tablespoon extra-virgin olive oil
¼ teaspoon sea salt

1. Bring a large pot of water to a boil. Add the corn and cook for 5 to 8 minutes, or until the kernels are bright yellow and just tender. When the corn is cool enough to handle, cut the kernels from the cob, taking care to not include any tough fiber from the cob.

2. Place the kernels in a medium bowl. Add the red onion, red pepper, and cilantro and mix well. Add the lime juice, vinegar, olive oil, and salt. Mix well and allow to marinate for at least 2 hours in the refrigerator.

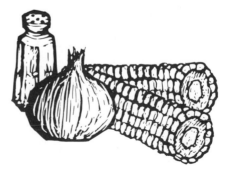

BREADS

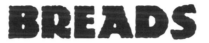

Corn Bread

Makes one 9-inch-square loaf

1 cup low-fat milk or soy milk

1 teaspoon rice vinegar or mild white wine
    vinegar

1 cup cornmeal

½ cup whole-wheat pastry flour

½ cup unbleached all-purpose flour

1 tablespoon baking powder

½ teaspoon sea salt

1 egg

3 tablespoons corn oil or melted butter

3 tablespoons maple syrup or honey

2 cups corn kernels (about 4 ears corn)

1. Preheat the oven to 375°F.

2. Place the milk or soy milk in a small bowl
with the vinegar. Allow to sit for 1 hour.

3. Mix together the dry ingredients in a large
bowl.

4. Whip together the milk mixture, egg, oil or
butter, and maple syrup or honey. Add the corn
kernels and blend. (If using fresh corn, scrape the
cob with a knife after cutting off kernels to get the
"milk" that is still in the cob. Decrease the liquid in
the recipe by ¼ cup.) Add the wet ingredients to
the dry and mix with as few strokes as possible, just
until the dry ingredients are completely coated.

5. Pour into a buttered 9-inch-square baking pan
and bake for 25 to 30 minutes, or until a toothpick
inserted into the middle comes out clean. Cool on
a rack.

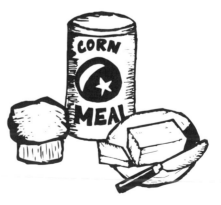

Country Corn Bread Stuffing

The sweetness of corn bread is the perfect complement to turkey. You can add oysters for an even more traditional dressing. This recipe is enough for a 10- to 12-pound turkey. For larger birds, double the recipe.

Makes enough for a 10- to 12-pound bird

1 pint fresh oysters, liquor reserved (optional)
1 cup sunflower seeds (omit if using oysters)
3 tablespoons butter or corn oil
3 celery stalks, diced
2 small onions, diced
1/2 teaspoon ground sage
1/2 teaspoon ground nutmeg
Sea salt and freshly ground white pepper to taste
1 Corn Bread (see page 216), crumbled into bite-sized pieces and left overnight to harden
1 egg
Milk, soy milk, turkey stock, or oyster liquor to moisten
1/2 cup chopped fresh parsley

1. If using oysters, drain them, reserving their liquor; set aside. If using sunflower seeds, toast them by stirring them in a dry skillet over medium heat until lightly browned; set aside.

2. Heat the butter or oil in a large skillet. Sauté the celery and onions for 5 minutes, or until tender. Add the seasonings and sauté for 2 minutes longer over medium heat.

3. In a large bowl stir together the corn bread, celery-onion mixture, and egg. Stir gently so that the corn bread does not become too crumbly. Add the milk or other liquid just to moisten the mixture, and add the parsley and sunflower seeds or oysters. Stir just enough to blend the ingredients.

4. Loosely stuff the bird *just before* it is ready to go into the oven. Remove stuffing to a serving dish as soon as the turkey has finished cooking.

Dill-Onion Quick Bread

A quick way to fill your house with the welcoming aroma of baked bread.

Makes one 9-by-5-inch loaf

1/4 cup butter or canola oil
1 cup minced onions
1 cup whole-wheat pastry flour
1 cup unbleached all-purpose flour
1 tablespoon baking powder
3 tablespoons minced fresh dill
1/4 teaspoon sea salt
1/8 teaspoon ground white pepper
1 large egg
1 cup low-fat milk or soy milk

1. Melt the butter or heat the oil in a small saucepan over medium heat. Add the onions and sauté, stirring often, for 5 minutes. Remove from heat.

2. Preheat the oven to 325°F.

3. Combine the flours, baking powder, dill, and salt and pepper in a large mixing bowl.

4. Beat the egg in a small mixing bowl and whisk in the milk. Add the onions and melted butter, mixing well. Pour the wet ingredients over the dry ones, mixing gently with a rubber spatula. Mix only enough to make sure all the dry ingredients are moistened.

5. Oil a 9-by-5-inch loaf pan. Turn the batter into the pan and bake for 50 to 60 minutes, or until the top of the bread is lightly browned and a toothpick inserted into the middle comes out clean. Allow the bread to cool in the pan for 5 minutes, remove, and place on a wire rack to cool a bit longer.

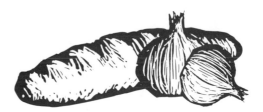

Dried Fruit and Nut Loaf

Not as rich as a fruitcake, this bread has a wonderful texture and unique flavor all its own, with fewer calories. This bread makes a great breakfast food or snack. In winter serve with warm fruit compote, in summer with berry jam.

Makes one 9-by-5-inch loaf

1/4 **cup walnut halves**
1/2 **cup pecan halves**
1/2 **cup dried apricots**
1/2 **cup dried peaches**
1 **cup low-fat milk or soy milk**
1/2 **cup maple syrup**
1/3 **cup corn or canola oil**
1 **egg**
1 **teaspoon vanilla extract**
1/4 **teaspoon sea salt**
1 1/4 **cups whole-wheat pastry flour**
1 **cup unbleached all-purpose flour**
2 **teaspoons baking powder**
1/2 **teaspoon baking soda**

1. Preheat the oven to 350°F.

2. Toast the walnuts and pecans lightly in the preheated oven for about 7 minutes. Remove, let cool, and chop; set aside.

3. Place the dried fruit in a medium bowl. Bring the milk to a boil in a saucepan and pour over the fruit. Allow the fruit to soak in the milk for at least 1/2 hour.

4. Reduce the oven heat to 325°F.

5. Drain the fruit, reserving the milk. Chop the dried fruit into bite-sized pieces. Set aside.

6. Blend together the maple syrup and corn or canola oil in a large bowl. Beat in the milk, egg, vanilla, and salt.

7. In another large bowl, sift together the flours, baking powder, and baking soda. Combine the wet and dry ingredients and stir just enough to blend; do not overmix. Fold in the nuts and chopped fruit.

8. Pour the mixture into an oiled 9-by-5-inch loaf pan. Bake for 60 minutes, or until a toothpick inserted into the center comes out clean. Cool in the pan for 15 minutes, then transfer the loaf to a wire rack and allow to cool completely before slicing.

Sweet Double-Wheat Bread

This recipe takes whole-wheat bread one step further, increasing both the nutritious germ and the fibrous bran of the wheat. It is sweetened with honey and softened with skim milk. This is a good teaching recipe: the basic steps of baking a fragrant and soul-satisfying loaf of whole-wheat bread are clearly described. Once you learn the skills of bread baking, it can become a favorite and relaxed weekend activity.

Makes two 9-by-5-inch loaves

2 **packages (4 teaspoons) active dry yeast**
1 **cup warm (100° to 105°F) water**
1/3 **cup honey**
2 **tablespoons canola or safflower oil**
1 **cup warm (100° to 105°F) skim milk**
1/2 **cup raw wheat germ**
1/2 **cup wheat bran**
2 1/2 **cups unbleached all-purpose flour**
2 **to 3 cups whole-wheat bread flour**
Extra bran to roll loaves in

1. Combine the yeast and warm water in a large bowl. Add 1 tablespoon of the honey. Within 5 minutes a foam of active yeast will appear on the surface of the water. This is called "proofing the yeast." The foam is the proof that the yeast is ready to work (sort of like a pregame warmup).

2. Stir in the rest of the liquid ingredients. The milk should be a little warmer than room temperature. Yeast will die if it is too cold.

3. Stir in the wheat germ, bran, and all-purpose flour. Add the whole-wheat flour 1 cup at a time until the dough can no longer be stirred with a spoon.

4. Turn the dough onto a large floured board. Knead more flour into the dough until it is soft but

not sticky. Continue to knead until the dough is elastic and smooth. Kneading will take between 10 and 15 minutes.

5. Put the dough into a lightly oiled large bowl and cover it loosely with a towel. Place in a warm and draft-free spot (but not too warm—not on the oven or near a heater—yeasts are creatures of comfort). Place a towel over the bowl and allow the dough to rise until doubled in bulk, about 1 hour.

6. Punch down the dough, place it on the floured board, and knead briefly until all the air pockets are burst.

7. Divide the dough in half, shape into loaves, and roll each loaf in bran. Place in greased 9-by-5-inch loaf pans. Let rise until doubled in size, 40 to 60 minutes.

8. Meanwhile, preheat the oven to 400°F. Bake the bread for about 40 minutes, or until the bread sounds hollow when tapped and the crust is a light brown.

9. Remove the loaf from the pan and allow to cool for 10 minutes before cutting (waiting will be very hard to do—this is a test of your will power).

Allergy-Free Sweet Potato Bread

This wheat-, egg-, dairy-, and corn-free recipe features flaxseed as an alternative to eggs as a binding ingredient. The natural sweetness of the sweet potato makes the maple syrup optional.

Makes one 9-by-5-inch loaf

1 medium sweet potato
2 tablespoons flaxseed, ground, or 2 eggs
$2/3$ cup water
$1/4$ cup maple syrup (optional)
$1/4$ cup safflower oil
$1/2$ cup water
1 cup rice flour
$1/2$ cup barley flour
1 teaspoon baking soda
1 teaspoon corn-free baking powder

$1^1/2$ teaspoons ground cinnamon
1 teaspoon sea salt

1. Bake the sweet potato in a preheated 400°F oven for 30 to 35 minutes, or until tender. Let cool, remove the flesh from the skin, mash the flesh, and set aside.

2. Preheat the oven to 350°F.

3. Boil the flaxseed in $2/3$ cup water for 3 to 5 minutes, or until it is the consistency of egg whites (omit this step if using eggs).

4. Cream the flaxseed mixture or eggs with the maple syrup and oil in a large bowl until smooth and creamy.

5. Add the sweet potato and $1/2$ cup water to the flaxseed or egg and maple syrup mixture. Blend well.

6. Sift together the remaining ingredients and add to the liquid mixture. Stir just enough to blend the ingredients (mixing too long will make the batter tough).

7. Pour the mixture into an oiled and floured 9-by-5-inch loaf pan and bake for 45 minutes. The bread is done when a knife inserted into the center comes out clean.

♦ **Variations:**
- Use yams, mashed potatoes, pumpkin, or puréed fruit instead of sweet potato and eliminate the $1/2$ cup added water.
- Eliminate the maple syrup and use $1/2$ cup fruit juice in place of the $1/2$ cup water.
- Substitute millet flour for rice flour.

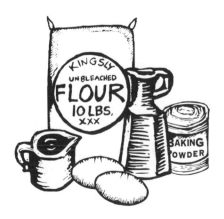

Muffins

Muffins made with whole-grain flours and unrefined oils and sweeteners are a very different sort of baked good than muffins made with refined ingredients. Whole-grain flours provide much more than fiber; they add unique flavor, freshness, and heartiness to muffins that will last you through the morning or round out a simple meal such as soup and salad.

Muffins are easy to make and add a special homemade touch to a meal. Try the techniques below while making Dill-Corn Muffins and Oat Bran Muffins. (Most of these same techniques can be used in making other quick breads, such as Dill-Onion Quick Bread.)

Tips on making perfect muffins:

- Preheat the oven for 15 minutes prior to baking. Unless otherwise stated, muffins should be baked between 375° and 400°F for 20 to 25 minutes. If the oven isn't hot enough (or is too hot) the muffins won't rise properly.
- Mix muffins very briefly; 10 to 12 seconds is enough. It's okay if the batter is lumpy. If you overmix the batter, the muffins will be tough and full of tunnels.
- Wipe the top of the muffin pan with a little oil so that batter won't stick as it rises up and over the tops of the cups.
- Fill muffin cups two-thirds full for medium-sized muffins and almost to the top for over-sized ones.
- Fill any empty cups in the muffin tin with water to prevent scorching and to keep the other muffins moist.
- Bake muffins until they are lightly browned and a toothpick inserted into the center of the muffin comes out clean. An over-baked muffin will be dry.
- Allow muffins to cool in the tin for 5 minutes. Muffins are best eaten warm, but if you prefer them cool, transfer them to a wire rack.

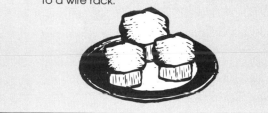

Dill-Corn Muffins

When you use whole-foods ingredients such as unrefined cornmeal, the original fresh flavor of the food is still intact. These muffins taste as if they were made from August corn still smelling of the late summer sun. This is the sort of "poetry" that is created when food retains its integrity and is not tampered with. These savory muffins make perfect companions to soups (like Cream of Cauliflower, page 164, and Moroccan Tomato, page 167) and to salads of all sorts.

Makes 12 muffins

Dry Ingredients

1 cup cornmeal
1 cup unbleached all-purpose flour
$\frac{1}{2}$ cup whole-wheat pastry flour
4 teaspoons baking powder
$\frac{1}{2}$ teaspoon sea salt
$\frac{1}{4}$ teaspoon ground allspice
3 tablespoons minced fresh dill

Wet Ingredients

1 cup buttermilk or plain low-fat yogurt
2 eggs
$\frac{1}{3}$ cup maple syrup
$\frac{1}{4}$ cup canola oil
1 cup fresh or frozen corn kernels

1. Preheat the oven to 400°F.

2. Sift together all the dry ingredients except the dill into a large bowl. Add the dill.

3. In a blender or food processor, blend all the wet ingredients except the corn kernels.

4. Add the wet ingredients and corn kernels to the dry ingredients. Mix just to blend the ingredients and scoop into oiled or paper-lined muffin cups (a soup ladle or an ice cream scoop works well for this). Fill the muffin papers about two-thirds full.

5. Bake for 20 minutes, or until a toothpick inserted into the middle of a muffin comes out clean.

6. Allow to cool for 5 minutes in the muffin pan before removing.

Oat Bran Muffins

If you are baking these muffins for cholesterol-lowering purposes, use egg whites instead of the whole egg.

Makes 12 muffins

1¼ cups oat bran
½ cup unbleached all-purpose flour
¾ cup whole-wheat pastry flour
2 teaspoons baking powder
1 teaspoon ground cinnamon
¼ teaspoon sea salt
1 cup low-fat milk or soy milk
⅓ cup honey or maple syrup
1 large egg, or 2 egg whites
¼ cup canola oil
½ cup raisins

1. Preheat the oven to 375°.

2. Thoroughly mix the oat bran, flours, baking powder, cinnamon, and salt in a large bowl.

3. Beat together the milk, honey, and egg or egg whites in a small bowl with a whisk or fork. Beat in the oil. Pour the wet ingredients over the dry ingredients and fold the two together with a rubber spatula until the dry ingredients are well moistened. Do not overmix. Fold in the raisins.

4. Spoon the batter into oiled or paper-lined muffin cups. Bake for 25 minutes, or until lightly browned and a toothpick inserted into the center of a muffin comes out clean. Let cool a few minutes before serving.

◆ **Variation:** Add ½ cup chopped walnuts or pecans to the batter.

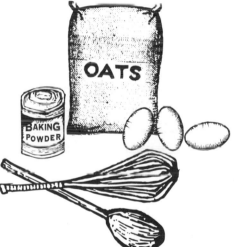

DESSERTS

Blueberry-Peach Crisp

If peaches are unavailable, this dessert can be made with just blueberries. Freeze some in the summer and you can make this dessert year-round. Serve warm with ice cream or a vanilla soy frozen dessert.

Makes 4 to 6 servings

3 cups blueberries
2 cups thinly sliced peaches
1 tablespoon arrowroot powder
3 tablespoons Sucanat or maple sugar granules
1 teaspoon grated lemon zest (organic, if available)

Topping

$\frac{1}{2}$ cup unbleached all-purpose flour
6 tablespoons Sucanat or maple sugar granules
$\frac{1}{8}$ teaspoon sea salt
$\frac{1}{8}$ teaspoon ground nutmeg
4 tablespoons butter or 3 tablespoons canola oil

1. Preheat the oven to 300°F.
2. Wash and pick over the berries. Combine the fruit and toss with the arrowroot powder, Sucanat or maple sugar, and lemon zest. Spread the mixture in an 8-inch-square or round pan.
3. To make the topping, in a small bowl, combine the flour, Sucanat or maple sugar, salt, and nutmeg. If using butter, cut it into small pieces and work it into the flour mixture until it resembles coarse meal. If using oil, drizzle it over the top of the flour mixture and work it into the flour with a fork or your fingers until the flour is coated with oil.
4. Distribute the topping evenly over the fruit. Bake until the top is lightly browned and the fruit is bubbling, about 35 to 40 minutes.

Oat-Nut Crust

This crust is a treat unto itself and is much easier to make than a pastry pie crust.

Makes one 9-inch pie crust

¹/₂ cup whole almonds
¹/₂ cup whole walnuts or pecans
1 cup rolled oats
¹/₂ cup unbleached all-purpose flour
Pinch of sea salt
3 tablespoons canola oil
3 tablespoons maple syrup
1 tablespoon vanilla extract

1. Preheat the oven to 350°F.

2. Bake the almonds and walnuts or pecans on separate baking sheets until they are fragrant and toasted: about 8 minutes for pecans or walnuts, 10 minutes for almonds. Remove from the oven and set aside to cool. Raise the oven temperature to 375°F.

3. Grind the oats in a blender or food processor until they become coarse meal. Empty into a large mixing bowl.

4. Grind the almonds and walnuts or pecans into a coarse meal and add to the oats, along with the flour and salt.

5. In a small bowl, whip together the oil, maple syrup, and vanilla. Add to the oat-nut mixture and mix well. Allow the mixture to sit for 10 minutes in the refrigerator.

6. With cold, wet hands, press the crust mixture into a well-oiled tart or pie pan. Bake for 10 to 15 minutes, or until golden brown.

Organic Citrus Zest

The rinds of lemons and oranges have a great deal of flavor in them. The outer layer of these citrus fruits contains essential oils that impart a fragrant tartness to many dishes. However, since the rind is the part of the fruit that retains the many chemicals used in the spraying of citrus fruits, it is far better to use the zest of *organic* lemons and oranges. Zest is a term used for the thin, colored layer of the rind, as opposed to the bitter-tasting white pith beneath. The easiest way to cut off the zest is to use a potato peeler or a citrus zester.

Because it is not always possible to get organic citrus, here's a way to make sure that you have organic citrus zest on hand all the time. When organic citrus is available, zest the rind and put it in small plastic bags or freezer containers. Store in the freezer and allow the zest to come to room temperature before using in recipes.

Tip: To get more juice from limes, oranges, and lemons, rub them between your palms or on a countertop before juicing.

Apple Tart

Makes one 9-inch tart

Oat-Nut Crust (see at left)
5 cooking apples, such as Cortland or
    Northern Spy
1 tablespoon fresh lemon juice
1 cup raisins or currants
1 cup apple juice
1 teaspoon vanilla extract
1 teaspoon ground cinnamon
1¹/₂ tablespoons arrowroot dissolved in
    ¹/₂ cup cold water

1. Prepare the Oat-Nut Crust and set aside to cool. Reduce the oven temperature to 350°F.

2. Wash, core, and slice the apples thinly. Place the sliced apples in a medium bowl and sprinkle the lemon juice over the slices, coating well. Place the apple slices in the precooked crust.

3. Combine the raisins or currants, apple juice, vanilla, and cinnamon in a small saucepan and simmer for 5 minutes.

4. Add the well-dissolved arrowroot to the raisin mixture and stir, over medium heat, until the mixture thickens. Pour the mixture over the apples and bake for 35 minutes.

Fresh Strawberry Tart

This tart is much lower in fat and calories than traditional fruit tarts. It is an elegant example of how whole-food ingredients can be transformed into something satisfying and sublime. The fruit is the real star of this show, so try and find some that will "sing." Agar is used to hold the filling together, and arrowroot gives the tart a delectable richness. Because no dairy products are used, this dessert is cholesterol-free.

Makes one 9-inch tart

Oat-Nut Crust (see page 223)
4 cups strawberries
1 cup plus ¼ cup apple-strawberry juice
1 tablespoon agar
Pinch of sea salt
1 tablespoon arrowroot
1½ teaspoons vanilla extract
Fresh mint leaves for garnish

1. Prepare the Oat-Nut Crust and let cool.

2. Wash, hull, and slice the strawberries. Arrange them attractively in the crust.

3. Combine 1 cup of the juice, agar, and salt in a small saucepan. Bring to a boil, reduce heat, and simmer over low heat, stirring constantly, until the agar is dissolved, about 5 minutes.

4. Dissolve the arrowroot in the remaining ¼ cup juice. Add to the agar-juice mixture, and simmer, stirring, for a few minutes over low heat until the mixture begins to thicken.

5. Remove the juice mixture from the heat and stir in the vanilla. Allow the mixture to cool for about 10 minutes.

6. Pour the juice mixture evenly over the strawberries. Chill in the refrigerator for 2 hours, or until the mixture sets. Garnish with mint leaves.

Agar

Agar is the whole-food alternative to gelatin, which is a highly refined product often made from the joints and hooves of farm animals. Agar is a sea vegetable that is dried in the form of flakes and bars and then dissolved in a liquid to create a vegetarian binding agent in recipes. Agar is very high in minerals such as calcium and magnesium and negligible in fat and calories.

Agar is usually used with fruit juice of some sort to create a jelled consistency in aspics, puddings, tarts, and other desserts. The classic agar recipe is kanten (see Kaleidoscope Kanten, next page), a refreshing fruit dessert made with agar, fruit juice, and fresh fruit. Agar flakes are the most convenient way to use agar. Use 1 tablespoon of agar per cup of liquid for a firm gelatin. If you prefer a soft gelatin, use less agar. (For another way to use agar, see Fresh Strawberry Tart, this page.)

Kaleidoscope Kanten

Kanten is a classic natural foods dessert of jelled fruit juice with fruit. It is extremely low in fat and calories, yet rich and fruity enough to satisfy the urge for something cold and sweet. Because kanten is made with agar (see sidebar), it is rich in essential minerals. You can make kanten festive by serving it in colorful glassware. Try wine, sundae, or parfait glasses.

Makes 4 servings

4 cups apple-raspberry or apple juice
5 tablespoons agar
Pinch of sea salt
1 kiwi, peeled and sliced
1 banana, peeled and sliced
1 small seedless orange, peeled, halved, and
    sliced (when peeling, cut under white pith
    with a sharp paring knife)
1 tablespoon arrowroot powder
Fresh mint leaves for garnish

1. Combine 3³/₄ cups of the juice, agar, and salt in a medium saucepan. Slowly bring to a boil, reduce the heat, and simmer for 15 minutes, stirring often to dissolve the agar.

2. Arrange the fruit in serving bowl(s).

3. Dissolve the arrowroot well in the remaining ¹/₄ cup juice. Add to the simmering juice mixture and stir until the mixture thickens slightly. Remove from the heat.

4. Pour the juice over the fruit. Let cool to room temperature, then refrigerate for 2 to 3 hours, or until set. Garnish with mint leaves.

Lemon Custard

This is a smooth alternative to dairy custards. It is much lower in fat and is cholesterol-free.

Makes 4 to 6 servings

4 cups apple juice
¹/₃ cup plus 4 tablespoons agar
Pinch of sea salt
¹/₄ cup fresh lemon juice
1 teaspoon vanilla extract
1 teaspoon grated lemon zest
2 to 4 tablespoons rice syrup or maple syrup
Sliced fresh strawberries, kiwis, bananas, or
    whole blueberries and mint leaves for
    garnish

1. Combine 3³/₄ cups of the juice and ¹/₃ cup of the agar in medium saucepan. Simmer over medium heat for 15 minutes.

2. Dissolve the remaining 4 tablespoons of the agar in the remaining ¹/₄ cup juice. Add to the juice-agar mixture and continue to cook over medium heat, stirring until thickened.

3. Stir the salt, lemon juice, vanilla, and lemon zest into the pudding.

4. Remove from the heat, add the rice syrup, and pour into an 8-by-8-inch glass baking dish. Cool to room temperature, then refrigerate for 1 hour, or until set.

5. Place the custard in a blender or food processor and blend until smooth and creamy. Pour into serving glasses.

6. Garnish with fresh fruit and fresh mint.

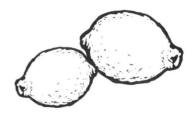

Pecan-Pumpkin Pie

This pie combines the flavor of two perennial favorites: pecans and pumpkin.

Makes one 9-inch pie

Oat-Nut Crust (see page 223)
3 cups pumpkin purée (see Note)
½ cup maple syrup
3 tablespoons molasses
1 teaspoon ground cinnamon
1 teaspoon ground ginger
½ teaspoon ground nutmeg
½ teaspoon sea salt
¼ teaspoon ground cloves
3 eggs, slightly beaten
1 cup low-fat milk
Pecan halves for garnish

1. Prepare the Oat-Nut Crust and press into a well oiled 9-inch pie pan. Bake and set aside to cool while you prepare the filling. Raise the oven temperature to 450°F.

2. Mix the remaining filling ingredients in the order given. Place in a blender or food processor (you may have to do this in batches) and blend for 1 minute (this adds air to the mixture and makes the pie light in texture).

3. Pour the filling into the prebaked crust and bake for 10 minutes. Then reduce the oven heat to 350°F and bake for another 40 minutes, or until the filling is set (a toothpick inserted into middle should come out almost clean). Garnish with pecan halves, and let pie sit for at least ½ hour before cutting.

Note: It's simple to make your own pumpkin purée, and your pie will be all the more special for it. Cut a *sugar pumpkin* in half (regular jack-o'-lantern field pumpkins will not work) and scoop out the seeds and fibrous pulp. Place cut-side down in a large baking dish or pan with a small amount of water in the bottom and bake in a preheated 350°F oven for about 45 minutes, or until the flesh is tender. Scoop the flesh from the skin and purée in a blender or food processor. Pumpkin purée can be frozen for several months for use in muffins, cookies, and pancakes. Chunks of pumpkin can also be steamed for an especially moist result.

Date Bars

The light, rather dry crust in this recipe is complemented by the natural sweetness of the moist filling. These are great for picnics and school lunches. If all you've ever eaten is packaged date bars (full of sugar, refined flour, and preservatives) you'll be amazed at how good the real thing can be.

Makes 16 bars

Filling

½ cup whole dates or figs, cut into quarters
½ cup sultana raisins
½ cup currants
Juice and rind of 1 orange
⅓ cup boiling water
¼ cup raw almonds

Crust

2 cups rolled oats
⅔ cups whole-wheat pastry flour
¼ teaspoon sea salt
¼ teaspoon ground mace or nutmeg
6 tablespoons very hard unsalted butter, cut into pieces
⅓ cup water
2 tablespoons maple syrup

1. Preheat the oven to 350°F. Grease an 8-inch-square baking pan and set aside.

2. In a 1-quart saucepan, combine the dates or figs, raisins, currants, orange juice and rind, and boiling water. Cook the mixture for 5 minutes. Let cool while you make the crust.

3. Place the oats, pastry flour, salt, and mace or nutmeg in a blender or food processor. Lightly blend ingredients, breaking up oats just a bit. Add the hard butter pieces and cut them into the oats. Add the water. Do not overmix. Press half of this mixture into the greased baking pan and reserve the remainder in a small bowl.

4. Place the warm cooked fruit mixture and the almonds in a blender or food processor and process to break up the almonds and purée the fruit. Spread all the fruit mixture on the oat crust in the baking pan.

5. Sprinkle the remaining oat mixture evenly over the filling, and press lightly to help it adhere. Drizzle the maple syrup over all.

6. Bake in the preheated oven for 20 to 25 minutes to cook and lightly brown the crust. Cool before cutting into 16 pieces.

Gingerbread Cake

Come in from the cold of fall or winter to a house filled with the smell of this heavenly dessert. Gingerbread cake is from another era and appeals to the child in everyone. Serve with warmed homemade applesauce.

Makes one 9-inch-square cake

1/2 cup maple syrup
1/2 cup corn oil or butter
1/2 cup molasses
2 eggs
1/2 cup plain low-fat yogurt
1/3 cup raisins
1 cup whole-wheat pastry flour
1 cup unbleached all-purpose flour
1 teaspoon baking soda
1 1/2 teaspoons ground ginger
1 teaspoon ground cinnamon
1/2 teaspoon ground nutmeg

1. Preheat the oven to 350°F.

2. Beat together the maple syrup, corn oil or butter, and molasses in a large bowl.

3. Separate the eggs. Set the whites aside and beat the yolks. Stir the beaten egg yolks and yogurt into the maple syrup mixture. Beat until creamy. Stir in the raisins.

4. Sift the remaining ingredients together into another large bowl. Stir in the wet ingredients just enough to blend.

5. In a large bowl, beat the egg whites until stiff. Fold into the batter. Pour into an oiled and floured 9-inch-square pan and bake for 30 to 35 minutes, or until a toothpick inserted into the center comes out clean.

Gingerbread People

Makes 2 dozen cookies

1 1/2 cups whole-wheat pastry flour
1 1/2 cups unbleached all-purpose flour
1 1/2 teaspoons ground ginger
1 teaspoon ground cinnamon
1/2 teaspoon sea salt
3/4 teaspoon baking soda
1/2 cup Sucanat
1/4 cup corn oil or butter
1/2 cup molasses
Grated zest of 1 orange
1/4 to 1/2 cup fresh orange juice
Currants, sunflower seeds, sesame seeds
    and/or almonds for decoration

1. Preheat the oven to 350°F.

2. Sift the flours, ginger, cinnamon, salt, and baking soda into a large bowl. Set aside.

3. In another large bowl cream together the Sucanat and corn oil or butter. Add the molasses and orange zest and beat until smooth with a wooden spoon or mixer.

4. Add the dry ingredients and the orange juice alternately to the wet ingredients until the dough begins to pull away from the sides of the bowl.

5. On a lightly floured surface, roll out the dough in batches to a thickness of 1/8 to 1/4 inch. Cut out gingerbread people or other shapes. (Or, the dough may be refrigerated and brought to room temperature again before rolling.)

6. Place shapes on oiled or parchment-lined baking sheets; decorate with currants, nuts, and seeds as desired; and bake for 10 to 20 minutes, depending on the size and thickness of the cookies. The bottoms should be just lightly browned.

Note: For a special touch, you may want to decorate the baked cookies with an icing made of Sucanat (see page 110 for a description of Sucanat) and water. Pulverize 1/4 cup Sucanat in a coffee or nut grinder. Place in a small cup and gradually add drops of water. Mix until a thick consistency is reached. Use a toothpick or chopstick to decorate the gingerbread people with eyes, nose, buttons, etc. The icing will be a light brown on the darker brown of the cookies.

Oatmeal-Raisin Cookies

The old-fashioned appeal of these cookies comes from the magic that occurs when whole-food ingredients, with all their rich flavors and textures, come together. These cookies taste the way oatmeal-raisin cookies were meant to taste: as if Grandma were working her spell in the kitchen

Makes 3 dozen cookies

½ cup corn oil
½ cup maple syrup
1 teaspoon vanilla extract
1 egg
1 teaspoon grated orange zest
⅛ teaspoon sea salt
½ cup whole-wheat pastry flour
½ cup unbleached all-purpose flour
2 cups rolled oats
½ teaspoon baking soda
¼ teaspoon ground nutmeg
½ cup walnuts or pecans
½ cup raisins soaked in ½ cup boiling water
   for 5 minutes and drained

1. Preheat the oven to 350°F and bake the nuts until lightly toasted; set aside. Raise the oven temperature to 375°F.

2. Beat together the corn oil, maple syrup, vanilla, egg, orange zest, and salt in a large bowl.

3. In a separate large bowl, combine the flours, oats, baking soda, and nutmeg.

4. Add the wet ingredients to the dry ingredients and stir just until the batter is well blended. Chop the nuts and fold them into the batter with the raisins. Refrigerate the batter for 15 minutes.

5. Using a cold, wet teaspoon, drop the batter onto oiled baking sheets and flatten with your fingers or palm. Bake for 10 to 12 minutes, or until lightly browned. Remove from the oven, place on a rack and allow to cool a little before eating (this will be a test of will!).

Pommes Maman

A simple but elegant way to draw a fall or winter meal to a close. This dessert from the South of France is likely to become a tradition with anyone who tries it.

Makes 4 servings

½ cup whole walnuts
½ cup currants
½ teaspoon ground cinnamon
1/4 teaspoon each ground allspice and cloves
1 tablespoon maple syrup
4 large cooking apples (Cortland or Rome)
**Fromage blanc, low-fat yogurt, or crème
   fraîche**

1. Preheat the oven to 350°F.

2. Lightly toast the walnuts in the oven for 8 to 10 minutes. Remove from the oven but do not turn the oven off. Grind the nuts in a nut grinder or blender until coarsely ground, not a powder.

3. In a small bowl, mix together the walnuts, currants, cinnamon, allspice, and maple syrup.

4. With a melon baller, core and cut a small cavity in each of the apples, being sure not to cut through the bottom. Stuff the cavities with the walnut mixture and bake for 45 minutes, or until the apples are quite soft.

5. Remove from the oven, place a dollop of fromage blanc, low-fat yogurt, or crème fraîche on each apple, and serve warm.

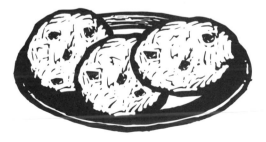

BEVERAGES

Ambrosial Punch (Nonalcoholic)

Rich apricot nectar gives this fruity punch body and a smooth taste. Be sure to chill the oranges, cider, and apricot juice before combining. Pomegranate seeds are a good alternative to cranberries.

Makes about 3½ quarts

1 cup cranberries
Mint leaves
4 large oranges, chilled
1 quart apricot nectar, chilled
2 bottles sparkling draft or crisp cider, chilled

1. Place 1 cranberry and 1 mint leaf in each compartment of an ice tray, add water, and freeze solid.

2. Halve the oranges and juice 3½ of them. Slice the remaining half into thin half-moon slices and quarter each slice. Set aside.

3. Place the orange juice in a punch bowl. Add the apricot nectar and the cider. Float the orange slices and ice cubes with cranberries in the punch.

Soothing Kuzu Drink

Strange as it may sound, this concoction can have a very settling effect on an upset digestive system.

Makes about 1 cup

1 teaspoon kuzu, ground to a fine powder
1 cup water
1 teaspoon grated ginger
1 teaspoon tamari

1. Dissolve kuzu in water in a small saucepan. Add grated ginger.

2. Bring to a boil and stir until thickened.

3. Add tamari and serve.

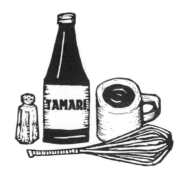

Berry-Banana Smoothie

This rich and delicious concoction is dairy- and fat-free and can be poured into Popsicle molds for tasty treats on a hot day. It is a great way to take advantage of luscious summer berries.

Makes 3 to 4 servings (about 3 cups)

1 ripe banana
7 or 8 fresh or frozen strawberries plus extra for garnish, or ½ cup blueberries or raspberries
2 cups fresh orange juice
Ice (optional)
Mint sprigs or Medjool date slivers for garnish

1. Peel the banana and slice it into ¾-inch pieces. Place in a blender.

2. Add the strawberries, blueberries, or raspberries and the orange juice and mix until a creamy consistency is reached. Add a few ice cubes for a frosty drink.

3. Serve immediately garnished with a strawberry slice, mint sprig, or Medjool date sliver.

Cool Fruit Juice Fizz

Makes 2½ quarts

1 quart fruit juice
1 tablespoon fresh lemon juice
2 cups freshly squeezed orange juice
1 quart sparkling water
Mint sprigs for garnish

Combine all the juices and chill well. Just before serving, add the sparkling water. Garnish with mint.

On-the-Porch Peach and Mint Lemonade

This drink is meant to be sipped when all cares can be released to a summer breeze.

This recipe comes from Isadora Guggenheim and Dr. Janis L. Enzenbacher.

Makes 8 to 10 servings

6 lemons
3 ripe peaches, peeled, pitted, and cut into chunks, or two cups peach juice
8 cups spring water
½ cup mild honey
Fresh mint sprigs

1. Squeeze the juice out of the lemons and set aside.

2. Purée the peaches in a blender or food processor.

3. Bring 2 cups of the water to a boil. In a heatproof pitcher, dissolve the honey in the boiling water. Add the rest of the water, lemon juice, and puréed peaches. Stir to mix well. Add a few sprigs of fresh mint. Refrigerate until very cold.

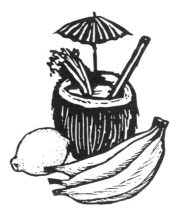

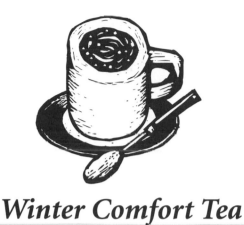

Winter Comfort Tea

This recipe comes to us from Eva Somaripa, who grows organic herbs on the Massachusetts coastline. Eva suggests adding other ingredients to taste, such as lemon balm, different types of mint, and perhaps a vanilla bean. She also suggests adding this tea to warm cider in winter and to cold fruit juices in the warmer months. Eva refuses to be more specific about measurements; making this to individual taste is part of the process of learning to cook with herbs and spices.

Makes 8 to 10 servings

2 quarts water
5 to 6 star anise
Handful of dried peppermint
1 teaspoon whole cloves
1 to 2 teaspoons orange and/or lemon zest
$\frac{1}{2}$- to 1-inch piece fresh ginger, peeled.

Bring the water to a boil. Place the rest of the ingredients in a heat-proof jar or pitcher large enough to hold the 2 quarts of water. Pour the boiling water over the herbs and spices and allow to steep for 5 to 60 minutes (depending on how strong you like your tea). Strain.

Hot Mulled Cider

This spice-and-citrus nectar is fragrant and heart-warming.

Makes 1 quart

1 quart fresh apple cider
4 whole cloves
Pinch of nutmeg
2 cinnamon sticks, broken in half
4 thin lemon slices

In a large saucepan, combine the cider, cloves, nutmeg, and cinnamon sticks. Heat without boiling for 20 minutes. Strain and serve with lemon slices.

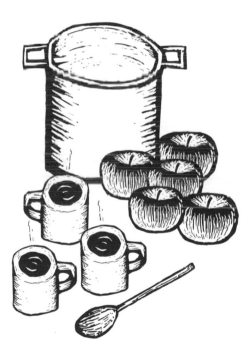

BREAKFAST & LUNCH

Sunday Morning (and Evening) Pancakes

You'll be amazed at the difference in flavor that whole-grain flours can make with a recipe such as this. We've created these pancakes to make breakfast or dinner a special meal. They're surprisingly easy to make. If you're eating them in the morning, use blueberries; for dinner or lunch, use corn and carrots and serve with broccoli or kale. If cholesterol is a concern, whip 4 egg whites instead of 2 eggs.

Makes 4 to 6 servings

³/₄ cup buckwheat flour
¹/₂ cup whole-wheat pastry flour
¹/₂ cup unbleached all-purpose flour
¹/₄ cup coarse cornmeal (not degerminated)
2 teaspoons baking powder
¹/₂ teaspoon sea salt
2 eggs or 4 egg whites
³/₄ cup buttermilk or plain low-fat yogurt
1 cup low-fat milk

2 tablespoons canola oil
1 to 1¹/₂ cups blueberries, or ¹/₂ cup corn and ¹/₂ cup coarsely grated carrot
Maple syrup (optional)
Toasted walnuts or pecans, roughly chopped (optional)

1. Mix together the flours, cornmeal, baking powder, and salt in a large bowl.

2. In a separate bowl, whip the eggs. Add the buttermilk or yogurt, milk, and oil. Blend well. Add the blueberries or corn and carrots. Add the buttermilk-blueberry or buttermilk-vegetable mixture to the dry ingredients and stir with a rubber spatula until just

The Perfect Hard-Cooked Egg

Place cold eggs in a saucepan or pot and cover them with cold water. Bring the water to a boil, then reduce the heat to simmer. Simmer for 12 minutes. Plunge eggs immediately into cold water to stop cooking. At 79 calories, an egg is a low-calorie source of protein to start off the day or to pop into your lunchbox.

blended. Do not overmix (batter will be thick). Let the batter sit, undisturbed, for 5 minutes.

3. Heat a large (preferably cast-iron) skillet and lightly coat it with oil. Give the batter a few strokes with the rubber spatula and scoop out about $1/4$ cup onto the hot skillet surface. Cook over medium heat for approximately $1^1/2$ minutes. Flip the pancake and cook another $1^1/2$ minutes on the other side.

4. Serve immediately with warm maple syrup and chopped nuts (if using blueberries). Dinner pancakes can be eaten with yogurt.

Note: It is usually helpful to scrape off any stuck batter and re-oil the skillet in between batches.

Country Torte

This recipe, which highlights the farm-fresh flavor of eggs from free-range chickens, is worth saving your cholesterol "points" for. It also uses chèvre (which is lower in cholesterol than cheese from cow's milk) and a part-skim mozzarella. A cast-iron skillet is essential to cooking this dish correctly. Serve as a late-summer meal or for brunch. Dill-Onion Quick Bread and a salad of bitter greens with Barely Tangy Vinaigrette round out a casual meal.

Makes one 10-inch torte

2 small zucchini, grated
2 small yellow summer squash, grated
2 tablespoons extra-virgin olive oil
1 bunch scallions, white and pale green parts
  only, sliced thinly
$1^1/2$ cups corn kernels (about 3 ears corn)
1 tablespoon minced fresh dill
1 teaspoon lemon zest
$1/2$ teaspoon sea salt
$1/4$ teaspoon freshly ground white pepper
$1/4$ teaspoon ground nutmeg
$3/4$ cup crumbled chèvre
$3/4$ cup grated part-skim mozzarella
4 eggs
1 teaspoon prepared mustard
Oil for cooking

Breakfasts for Children

Young children do not yet have set notions of what "should" be eaten at breakfast. You can offer them more options for healthy breakfasts if you abandon your notions and try these breakfast ideas on your children:

- Melted cheese on whole-grain English muffins. Cheese is roughly equivalent to moderately fatty cooked meat in terms of protein and fat.
- Spread cottage cheese mixed with a dash of cinnamon, a drop of vanilla, and a dab of honey on top of whole-wheat toast. Place a spoonful of unsweetened preserves on top. Broil until warm.
- Whole-grain muffin mixes with added nuts and seeds, grated carrot or zucchini or diced apple or pear.
- Warmed mochi cakes (Japanese "energy food" made from rice and found in the dairy case). Make mochi "waffles" by placing a cake in a waffle iron and cooking about 8 to 10 minutes.

1. Preheat the oven to 350°F.

2. Place the grated zucchini and squash in a dish towel or piece of cheesecloth and squeeze the excess liquid from them. Set aside.

3. In a 10-inch cast-iron skillet, heat the oil and sauté the scallions for 4 minutes, stirring often. Add the squash and zucchini, corn, dill, lemon zest, salt, pepper, and nutmeg. Stir well to blend and sauté over medium heat for 5 minutes, stirring. Do not allow the zucchini mixture to become soggy or watery. Add the cheese, mix well, and remove from the heat. Pour the mixture into a large bowl.

4. Quickly rinse out the skillet and dry. Put the skillet in the oven and heat for 5 to 10 minutes.

5. Beat the eggs with the mustard and add to the zucchini mixture. Mix well. Place a small amount of oil on a paper towel and coat the preheated skillet with oil. Pour the zucchini-egg mixture into the pan and bake for 20 to 25 minutes, or until the eggs are set. Serve immediately.

Lunchbox Ideas for School and Work

Grains

You can make a great lunch of leftover grains by mashing them with a ripe avocado. Serve with sprouts, tomato, and a little cheese on whole-wheat bread.

Sandwiches

Peanut Butter and Jelly Variations
Organic apple butter
Almond butter
Banana slices
Organic fruit spreads

Shredded Vegetable Sandwich
Mix minced onion, grated carrots, and grated cabbage and serve with a dressing of tahini, low-fat yogurt, lemon juice, and shoyu in whole-wheat pita bread. (Put the dressing in a separate container to prevent sogginess.)

Tofu Sandwich
Place firm tofu between 2 plates with a heavy object on top and let drain for at least 1/2 hour to remove excess water. Steam the tofu for a few minutes. Serve with a grainy mustard, chopped lettuce, and scallions on sourdough bread.

Autumn Sandwich
Serve sliced apple and grated Cheddar cheese on whole-grain bread with a little mustard or mayonnaise and a touch of organic apple butter.

Other Sandwich Ideas
Tahini-Miso Spread
Tofu Spread

Roasted-Eggplant Ratatouille
Tempeh with Sauerkraut, White Miso, and Mustard
Mexican Tempeh Dip in corn tortillas
Tuna Salad in Pita
Any leftover stir-fry in pita bread

Tip: Use cookie cutters to make sandwiches for young children.

Wide-Mouthed Thermos Ideas

Cooked Udon or Soba Noodles and Prepared Pasta Sauces
Add a little Parmesan cheese or leftover sautéed vegetables from dinner. (Break noodles in half before cooking to make eating easier.)

Nitrate-free chicken, turkey, or tofu dogs
Steam or bake the dogs first. Include whole-wheat buns and dabs of condiments.

Tip: Add whole-wheat alphabet noodles to kids' soups to make them more fun.

Lunchbox Snacks
Granola or fruit bars, chips, trail mixes, fruit, string cheese (a good source of protein and calcium).

Pita Pizzas
This meal can be taken cold to work or school. Spread tomato sauce, grated part-skim mozzarella, and cut vegetables (zucchini, mushrooms, peppers, etc.) on whole-wheat pita bread or whole-wheat pizza crust and place under the broiler. If you choose the toppings but let the kids make their own pizzas, you'll be surprised at the healthy ingredients they'll accept and enjoy.

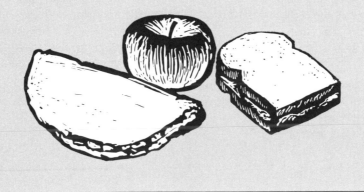

MENUS

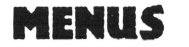

FAMILY MENUS

Baked white fish
Sweet potatoes
Steamed vegetables
Blueberry-Peach Crisp (page 222)

Whole Roasted Chicken (page 194)
Whole-grain rice, quinoa, or potatoes
Salad with Barely Tangy Vinaigrette (page 214)
Kaleidoscope Kanten (page 225)

Tostadas (page 185) or refried beans
Tortillas
Chopped tomatoes, scallions, cukes, or sprouts
Grated cheese
Whole-grain rice

Fajitas (page 192)
Guacamole
Salsa
Tortillas
Whole-grain rice
Lemon Custard (page 225)

Two-Bean Vegetarian Chili (page 182)
Corn bread, muffins, or tortillas
Green salad with Tofu Green Goddess Dressing
    (page 215)

Ground Turkey Loaf (page 196) with Creamy
    Mushroom Sauce (page 212)
Mashed potatoes
Broccoli-Carrot Amandine (page 204)

Baked Scrod with Tomato-Basil Sauce (page 189)
Greens with Garlic and Ginger (page 206)
Quinoa or Savory Grilled Polenta (page 202)
Pommes Maman (page 228)

Grilled Indian Chicken (page 194)
Carrot Salad (page 176)
Greens with Garlic and Ginger (page 206)
Cranberry Chutney (page 213)
Chapatis
Fresh fruit

Leek and Fennel Pasta e Fagioli (page 179)
French bread
Green Salad

LUNCH MENUS

Tuna in a pocket

Hummus with vegetables and blue corn chips

Pan-fried tofu or tempeh, lettuce, and tomato sandwich

Tofu Udon Salad (page 172)

Quesadillas and salad

Mushroom-Barley Soup (page 168), carrot sticks, and whole-grain bread

Leftover pasta, sauce, and vegetables

Mochi with tamari or mustard, carrot and celery sticks

Peanut butter/almond butter on celery

Fresh fruit

BREAKFAST IDEAS

Berry-Banana Smoothie (page 230)

French toast made with whole-grain raisin or Sweet Double-Wheat Bread (page 218)

Fresh fruit with Yogurt Cheese (page 161) spread

Oatmeal with tamari and tahini or raisins and apples

Sunday Morning (and Evening) Pancakes (page 232)

Quinoa with currants, cinnamon, and soy milk

Brown-rice pudding

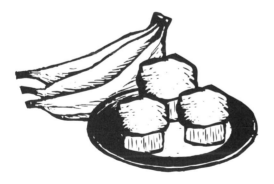

SNACKS

Fresh vegetables with peanut butter/almond butter

Mochi with mustard, tamari, or maple syrup

Tortillas or quesadillas

Popcorn with parmesan cheese

Oatmeal-Raisin Cookies (with chocolate chips) (page 228)

Tamari-roasted nuts and seeds

Toasted Sweet Double-Wheat Bread (page 218) with cinnamon or Sucanat

Date or Fig Bars (page 226)

NO CHOLESTEROL RECIPES

Appetizers

Tofu Spread (page 160)

Toasted Nut Medley (page 160)

Once Again: Hummus (page 162)

Mexican Tempeh Dip (page 163)

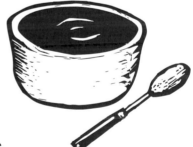

Soups

Lentil Soup (page 164)

Cream of Cauliflower Soup with Cardamom (soy milk) (page 164)

Minestrone Soup (no cheese) (page 166)

Hearty Miso Soup (page 167)

Moroccan Tomato Soup (no fromage blanc or yogurt) (page 167)

Mushroom-Barley Soup (page 168)

Ambrosial Melon Soup (page 169)

Salads

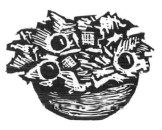

Pasta

Vegetarian Entrées

Vegetables

Sauces and Dressings

Breads

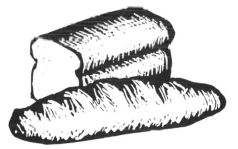

APPENDIX 1

RESOURCES

Environment

Audubon Society, 950 Third Ave., New York, NY 10022

Cousteau Society, 930 W. 21st St., Norfolk, VA 23517

Earth Island Institute, 300 Broadway, Ste. 28, San Francisco, CA 94133

Environmental Action Foundation, 1525 New Hampshire Ave. NW, Washington, D.C. 20036

Environmental Defense Fund, 257 Park Ave. South, New York, NY 10010

Environmental Policy Institute/Friends of the Earth, 218 D St. SE, Washington, D.C. 20003

Environmental Protection Agency, Public Information Center, 401 M St. SW, Washington, D.C. 20460

Global Tomorrow Coalition, 1325 G St. NW, Ste. 915, Washington, D.C. 20005

Greenpeace, 1436 U St. SW, Washington, D.C. 20009

Nature Conservancy, 1800 N. Kent St., No. 800, Arlington, VA 22209

Nationa Wildlife Federation, 1412 16th St. NW, Washington, D.C. 20036

Sierra Club, 730 Polk St., San Francisco, CA 94109

United Nations Environment Programme, DC2-0803 United Nations, New York, NY 10017

US PIRG, 25 Pennsylvania Ave. SE, Washington, D.C. 20003

World Resources Institute, 1735 New York Ave. NW, Washington, D.C. 20006

Worldwatch Institute, 1776 Massachusetts Ave. NW, Washington, D.C. 20036

World Wildlife Fund/Conservation Foundation, 1250 24th St. NW, Washington, D.C. 20037

Wilderness Society, 1400 I St. NW, Washington, D.C. 20005

Food Information

American Association of Meat Processors
P.O. Box 269, 224 E. High St., Elizabethtown, PA 17022

Food and Drug Administration, Consumer Communications, 5600 Fishers Ln., Rockville, MD 20857

Food Marketing Institute, 1750 K St. NW, Washington, D.C. 20006

Kansas Wheat Commission, 2630 Claflin Rd., Manhattan, KS 66502

The Meat and Poultry Hotline, USDA-FSIS, Rm. 1165-S, Washington, D.C. 20250

National Broiler Council, 1155 15th St. NW, Washington, D.C. 20005

National Dairy Council, Rosemont, IL 60018

National Fisheries Institute, 2000 M St. NW, Washington, D.C. 20036

Wheat Foods Council, 1620 Eye St. NW, Ste. 801, Washington, D.C. 20006

Food Safety

Americans for Safe Food, 1501 16th St. NW, Washington, D.C. 20036

Center for Science in the Public Interest (CSPI), 1501 16th St. NW, Washington, D.C. 20036

Clean Water Action Project, 317 Pennsylvania Ave. SE, Washington, D.C. 20003

Community Nutrition Institute, 2001 S St. NW, Ste. 530, Washington, D.C. 20009

Environmental Action, 1525 New Hampshire Ave. NW, Washington, D.C. 20036

Food Research and Action Center, Ste. 500, 1319 F St. NW, Washington, D.C. 20004

U.S. General Accounting Office, Washington, D.C. 20548

Institute for Food and Development Policy, 145 Ninth St., San Francisco, CA 94103

National Coalition Against the Misuse of Pesticides (NCAMP), 530 Seventh St. SE, Washington, D.C. 20003

Natural Resources Defense Council, 122 E. 42nd St., New York, NY 10168

Pesticide Action Network, 965 Mission St. #514, San Francisco, CA 94103

Public Citizen Health Research Group, 2000 P St. NW, Suite 700, Washington, D.C. 20036

Public Voice for Food and Health Policy, 1001 Connecticut Ave. NW, Ste. 522, Washington, D.C. 20036

Humane Animal Treatment

American Society for the Prevention of Cruelty to Animals (ASPCA), 411 E. 92nd St., New York, NY 10128

The Animal Protection Institute of America, 6130 Freeport Blvd., P.O. Box 22505, Sacramento, CA 95822

The Anti-Vivisection Society, Noble Plaza, Ste. 204, 801 Old York Rd., Jenkintown, PA 19046

The Earth Island Institute, 300 Broadway, Ste. 28, San Francisco, CA 94133

The Humane Society of the United States, 2100 L St. NW, Washington, D.C. 20037

The Johns Hopkins University Center for Alternatives to Animal Testing, 615 N. Wolfe St., Baltimore, MD 21205

National Anti-Vivisection Society, 53 West Jackson Blvd., Chicago, IL 60604

Organic Food Production

California Certified Organic Farmers, P.O. Box 8136, Santa Cruz, CA 95061

Demeter Association, 4214 National Blvd., Burbank, CA 91505

Farm Verified Organic Program (FVO), Mercantile Development, Inc., 274 Riverside Ave., P.O. Box 2747, Westport, CT 06880

Land Stewardship Project, 1717 University Ave., St. Paul, MN 55104

Natural Organic Farmers Association (NOFA), P.O. Box 335, Antrim, NH 03440

Northern Plains Sustainable Agriculture Society, Windsor, ND 58493

Organic Foods Production Association of North America (OFPANA), 23 Ames St., P.O. Box 1078, Greenfield, MA 01301

Organic Food Alliance (OFA), 2111 Wilson Blvd., Suite 531, Arlington, VA 22201

Organic Growers and Buyers Association, P.O. Box 9747, Minneapolis, MN 55440

Toll-Free Hotlines

Cancer Information Service, 1-800-422-6237

Meat and Poultry Hotline, 1-800-535-4555

APPENDIX 2

REFERENCES

Abdullah, Tariq H., et al. "Garlic Revisited." *Journal of the National Medical Association,* Vol. 80, No. 4, 1988.

Alliance for Food and Fiber. *Food Safety Information Kit.* Sacramento, Ca., 1989.

Americans for Safe Food. *The Safe Food Gazette.* Washington, D.C., 1988.

Anderson, Ernie and Cindy. *North America's Only Native Grain.* Cass Lake, Mn.: Northern Lakes Wild Rice Company, 1988.

Ballantine, Rudolph, *Diet and Nutrition: A Holistic Approach.* Honesdale, Pa.: Himalayan International Institute, 1978.

Belleme, John. "Miraculous Mirin," *East West,* November 1988.

Belleme, John. "Sauce," *East West,* January 1989.

Beleme, John. "The Miso-Master's Apprentice," *East West,* April 1981.

Brody, Jane. *Jane Brody's Nutrition Book.* New York: W. H. Norton & Co., 1981.

Burros, Marian. "U.S. Food Regulation: Tales from a Twilight Zone," *New York Times,* June 10, 1987.

Center for Science in the Public Interest. *Chemical Additives in Booze.* Washington, D.C., 1982.

Center for Science in the Public Interest. *Guess What's Coming to Dinner: Contaminants in Our Food.* Washington, D.C., March, 1987.

Center for Study of Responsive Law. *Eating Clean2. Overcoming Food Hazards.* Washington, D.C., 1988.

Colbin, Annemarie. *Food and Healing.* New York: Ballantine Books, 1986.

Commonwealth of Massachusetts, Division of Marine Fisheries. *Seafood: Facts Behind the Myths.* November 30, 1987.

Cross, Robert. "Atmosphere of Doubt: Private Testing Programs Pop Up in Today's Furor Over Safcty of Produce," *Chicago Tribune,* April 27, 1989.

de Langre, Jacques. *Flour from Stones and Hammers.* Berkeley, Ca.: Whole Foods Publishing Co., 1980.

DeVault, George. "The Never-Never Land of N," *The New Farm,* January, 1982.

Earth Island Institute. *The Tragedy Continues: Killing of Dolphins by the Tuna Industry.* San Francisco, Ca., Spring 1988.

Eden Foods. *Traditional Japanese Foods.* Clinton, Mi., 1986.

Eden Foods. *Ume Plum Concentrate.* Clinton, Mi., 1984.

Food and Drug Administration Pesticide Program. *Residues in Foods: 1987.* Washington, D.C., 1987.

Food Marketing Institute, Better Homes and Gardens. *A Study of Nutrition.* Washington, D.C., 1988.

Food Marketing Institute. *Antiobiotics in Livestock and Poultry Feed.* Washington, D.C., 1988.

Food Marketing Institute. *Bacterial Foodborne Illnesses.* Washington, D.C.,1987.

Food Marketing Institute, U.S. Food and Drug Adminstration, National High Blood Pressure Education Program. *Sodium Sense.* Washington, D.C.,1987.

Food Marketing Institute. *Trends: Consumer Attitutdes and the Supermarket.* Washington, D.C., 1989.

Food Marketing Institute. *EPA Announces New "Negligible Risk" Policy on Pesticides.* Washington, D.C., October 17, 1988.

Food Marketing Institute. *Pesticides in Our Food Supply.* Washington, D.C., May, 1987.

Food Marketing Institute. *Sulfites.* Washington, D.C., September 1987.

Food Marketing Institute. *U.S.-EC Food Fight.* Washington, D.C., January 1989.

Fox, Michael W., *Factory Farming.* Washington, D.C.: The Humane Society of the United States, 1980.

Fox, Michael W., *The Hidden Costs of Beef* Washington, D.C.: The Humane Society of the United States, 1989.

Fresh Produce Council and Alliance for Food and Fiber. *Issues in Food Safety.* Los Angeles, Ca., Fall 1988.

Fresh Produce Council and Alliance for Food and Fiber. *Issues in Food Safety.* Los Angeles, Ca., Winter 1989.

Frozen Food Roundtable. *Frozen Food Handling and Merchandising.* Washington, D.C., 1987.

Fulder, Stephen, and John Blackwood. *Garlic: Nature's Original Remedy.* Rochester, Vt.: Healing Arts Press, 1991.

"Gallic Hearts," *Discover,* Summer 1994.

"Going Overboard on Fish," *Health,* March/April 1994.

Goldbeck, Nicki and David. *The Goldbecks' Guide to Good Food.* New York: NAL Penguin, 1987.

Greenwald, John. "Hogging the Table." *Time,* March 18, 1996.

Hastings, John. "Is Milk from Hormone-Treated Cows Safe?" *Health,* March/April 1994.

Health, July/August 1994, p. 83.

Heritage, Ford. *Composition and Facts About Foods.* Mokelumne Hill, Ca.: Health Research, 1971.

The Humane Society of the United States. *Fact Sheet on Beef.* Washington, D.C., 1983.

The Humane Society of the United States. *Fact Sheet on Broiler Chickens.* Washington, D.C., 1983.

The Humane Society of the United States. *Fact Sheet on Dairy Cattle.* Washington, D.C., 1983.

The Humane Society of the United States. *Fact Sheet on Hogs.* Washington, D.C., 1983.

The Humane Society of the United States. *Fact Sheet on Veal.* Washington, D.C., 1983.

The Humane Society of the United States. *Livestock Cruelties State Legislative Action Packet.* Washington, D.C., 1984.

The Humane Society of the United States. "Livestock Transportation: Too Much Cruelty, Too Little Industry Concern," *The Humane Society News.* Washington, D.C., 1984.

Hunter, Beatrice Trum. *Consumer Beware!* New York: Touchstone Books, 1971.

Ingersoll, Bruce. "Meat Inspection Cuts Proposed by Reagan Are Hot Issue for Bush," *Wall Street Journal,* February 2, 1989.

Jacobson, Michael F. *Eater's Digest: The Consumer's Factbook of Food Additives.* Garden City, N.Y.: Doubleday, 1976.

Jacobson, Michael F. *The Complete Eater's Digest and Nutritional Scoreboard.* Garden City, N.Y.: Anchor Press/Doubleday, 1985.

Kleiman, Dena. "Can You Have Fat in Your Steak and Eat It Too?" *New York Times,* April 26, 1989.

Leary, Warren E. "For Dieters with a Sweet Tooth, Scientists Offer New Choices," *New York Times,* September 5, 1989.

Lecos, Cris W. "Sweetness Minus Calories = Controversy," *FDA Consumer,* Washington, D.C., February 1985.

Leibhardt, William C., and Martin Culik. "How to

Lose $42 an Acre," *New Farm,* February 1983.

Leviton, Richard. "American Miso Makes a Big Move Down South," *Soyfoods,* Summer 1982.

MacNeil, Karen. *The Book of Whole Foods: Nutrition and Cuisine.* New York: Vintage Books, 1981.

Moffat, Anne Simon. "Developing Nations Adapt Biotech for Own Needs." *Science,* July 8, 1994.

Mott, Lawrie, and Karen Snyder. "Pesticide Alert," *Organic Gardening Magazine,* June 1988.

National Coalition Against the Misuse of Pesticides. *Pesticide Safety: Myths & Facts.* Washington, D.C., 1988.

National Coalition Against the Misuse of Pesticides. *Pesticides and You.* Washington, D.C., 1987.

National Dairy Council. *Newer Knowledge of Milk.* Rosemont, Il., 1983.

National Research Council. *Regulating Pesticides in Food: The Delaney Paradox.* Washington, D.C.: National Academy Press, 1987.

National Toxics Campaign Fund. *A Consumer's Guide to Protecting Your Drinking Water.* Boston, Ma., 1989.

Nazario, Sonia L. "Big Firms Get High on Organic Farming," *Wall Street Journal,* March 21, 1989.

Nutrition Search, *Nutrition Almanac.* 2nd ed. New York: McGraw-Hill, 1975.

Pesticide Action Network. *Pesticide Action Network Newsletter.* San Francisco, Ca., Spring 1986.

Puzo, Daniel P. "FDA Discounts Peril of Pesticides," *Los Angeles Times,* December 29, 1988.

Reed, Leni. "Cheese, Milk's Leap: Everyone Loves Cheese, But Some Cheeses are More Lovable Than Others," *American Health,* September 1988.

Richards, Bill. "Sour Reception Greets Milk Hormone," *Wall Street Journal,* September 15, 1989.

Seamens, Dan, and David Wollner. *Shopper's Guide to Natural Foods.* Brookline, Ma.: East West, 1983.

Seligmann, Jean. "Guess What's Bad for You?" *Newsweek,* May 30, 1994.

Serrill, Michael S. "Mad Cows and Englishmen." *Time,* April 1, 1996.

Shabecoff, Philip. "E.P.A. Restricts Fungicide's Use on 42 Products," *New York Times,* February 17, 1989.

Schneider, Keith. "Food Industry is Testing for Toxics to Reassure Consumers on Crops," *New York Times,* March 27, 1989.

Schneider, Keith. "Pesticide Barred in 70's Is Found to Taint Poultry," *New York Times,* March 16, 1989.

Schreiber, Jim. *Milling for Quality.* Berkeley, Ca.: Whole Foods Publishing Co., 1980.

Simons, Marlise. "Concern Rising Over Harm from Pesticides in Third World," *New York Times,* May 30, 1989.

Shurtleff, William, and Akiko Aoyagi. *The Book of Miso.* Brookline, Ma.: Autumn Press, 1976.

Shurtleff, William, and Akiko Aoyagi. *The Book of Tofu.* New York: Ballantine Books, 1975.

Stevens, William K. "Officials Call Microbes Most Urgent Food Threat," *New York Times,* March 28, 1989.

Tierra, Michael. *The Way of Herbs.* New York: Washington Square Press, 1983.

Tobin, R. S., D. K. Smith, and J. A. Lindsay. "Effects of Activated Carbon and Bacteriostatic Filters on Microbiological Quality of Drinking Water," *Applied and Environmental Microbiology,* March 1981.

U.S. Department of Agriculture, U.S. Department of Health and Human Services. *Nutrition and Your Health: Dietary Guidelines for Americans,* 4th edition. Washington, D. C., 1995.

U.S. Department of Agriculture. *Meat and Poultry Labels Wrap It Up.* Washington, D.C., 1987.

U.S. Department of Agriculture. *Regulating Hormone Use in Animal Production in the United States.* Washington, D.C., November 1988.

U.S. Department of Agriculture. *Talking About Turkey.* Home and Garden Bulletin No. 243, Washington, D.C., 1987.

U.S. Department of Commerce, Bureau of the Census. *America's Agriculture: A Portrait of the Past and Present.* Washington, D.C., August 1986.

U.S. Department of Health and Human Services.

Diet, Nutrition, and Cancer Prevention: The Good News. NIH Publication No. 87-2878. December 1986.

U.S. Department of Health and Human Services. *The Surgeon General's Report on Nutrition and Health.* Washington, D.C., July 1988.

U.S. Environmental Protection Agency. *Lead and Your Drinking Water.* Washington, D.C., April 1987.

U.S. Environmental Protection Agency. *You and Your Drinking Water.* Washington, D.C., December 1986.

U.S. General Accounting Office. *Pesticides: The Need to Enhance FDA's Ability to Protect the Public from Illegal Residues.* Washington D.C., October 1986.

United States Senate, Select Committee on Nutrition and Human Needs. *Dietary Goals for the United States.* Washington, D.C., February 1977.

Wheat Foods Council. *Nature's Best: Wheat Foods.* Manhattan, KS, 1984.

Wittenberg, Margaret. *A Shopper's Guide to Whole Foods.* Austin, TX: Whole Foods Market, 1984.

Wood, Rebecca. *The Whole Foods Encyclopedia.* New York: Prentice Hall Press, 1988.

Worthington-Roberts, Bonnie. *Putting Carbohydrates into Perspective.* Washington, D.C.: The Wheat Industry Council, 1985.

INDEX